Health and Beauty Therapy

A Practical Approach for NVQ Level 3

2nd Edition

Health and Beauty Therapy

A Practical Approach for NVQ Level 3
2nd Edition

Dawn Mernagh-Ward and
Jennifer Cartwright

T

First published in 1995 by Stanley Thornes (Publishers) Ltd

Second edition published in 2001 by:
Nelson Thornes Ltd
Delta Place
27 Bath Road
CHELTENHAM
GL53 7TH
United Kingdom

01 02 03 04 05 / 10 9 8 7 6 5 4 3 2 1

A catalogue record for this book is available from the British Library

ISBN 0 7487 6078 4

Y0052775

Illustrations by Angela Lumley
Page make-up by Florence Production Ltd, Stoodleigh, Devon

Printed and bound in Italy by Canale

Contents

ACKNOWLEDGEMENTS

We wish to express our thanks to our husbands and sons, Ken and David Ward, David and Edward Cartwright and our families and friends for their patience, support and encouragement whilst researching and writing this book.

Special thanks go to Rod Fabes, Angela Barbagelata Fabes (Carlton Professional), Vanessa Puttick (The Hairdressing & Beauty Equipment Centre), Eve Taylor (Institute of Clinical Aromatherapy), John Birtwistle (Silhoutte), Simon Grogan (Cosmetronic), Jayne Lewis-Orr, Moira Paulusz (Health & Beauty Salon), Deborah Hale (Forest Mere Health Farm) Christophe Barbagelata (Endolite UK), Richard Warden (Helionova), Sharon Curtis (The International Dermal Institute) Delvis Bona, Pam Baddersley, Val Cooke, Chris Elliot, Heather Lulham-Robinson and Gaye Wensley for their technical assistance.

Acknowledgements and thanks are due to Lyn Goldberg, author of *Massage and Aromatherapy*, for work reproduced in chapter 11 of this book and Janet Simms, author of *A Practical Guide to Beauty Therapy for NVQ Level 2*, for work reproduced in chapter 12 of this book.

We are extremely grateful to our colleagues in the beauty industry, in particular the companies that have kindly allowed us to reproduce photographs and illustrations:

Front cover photograph: Image Bank
Figure 3.2 courtesy of Prestige Medical
Figures 3.7, 13.2 courtesy of Matis
Figures 3.15–13.20 courtesy of Warwickshire College
Figures 4.66, 5.8, 6.1, 6.4, 6.31, 7.7, 8.3 courtesy of Carlton Professional
Figures 4.7, 6.30, 6.34 courtesy of Cosmetronic (UK) Ltd
Figures 6.11, 6.33, 7.9 courtesy of Silhouette International
Figure 6.18, 7.13, 7.14 courtesy of The Hairdressing and Beauty Equipment Centre
Figure 6.26 courtesy of Ultratone Bodyshapers
Figure 7.1 courtesy of Totally UK Ltd
Figures 7.3, 7.8 courtesy of CACI
Figure 7.5 courtesy of BelleSante (UK) Ltd
Figure 7.6 courtesy of R. Robson Ltd
Figures 7.10, 7.11 courtesy of Endolite UK
Figure 7.12 courtesy of Bioskin las
Figure 8.2 courtesy of Vibrosaun
Figures 8.4, 8.7 courtesy of Chiva Som International Health Resort, Thailand
Figures 8.5, 8.10 courtesy of Forest Mere Health Farm
Figure 9.6 courtesy of Helionova Ltd
Figure 9.7 courtesy of Aim International School, Bangkok, Thailand
Figures 10.1, 10.3 courtesy of Rita Roberts
Figures 11.5, 11.8–11.49 courtesy of Eve Taylor Institute of Clinical Aromatherapy
Figure 13.1 courtesy of Sheila Godfrey
Figure 13.2 courtesy of Matis, Paris

INTRODUCTION

A career in beauty therapy has never been more exciting as technologies continue to advance to meet the growing demands of the public. It is, however, a very challenging profession due to the fact that by its nature it is a caring industry requiring a great deal of sympathy, empathy and understanding from the therapist. The range and breadth of the skills and knowledge covered are vast and it is essential that the therapist remembers that they will continue to learn new skills and further enhance existing ones throughout their career. Opportunities for the therapist expand every year, particularly as advancements in travel have made the world a much smaller place.

Health and Beauty Therapy: a Practical Approach for NVQ Level 3, 2nd edition, is intended as a guide for trainees studying for NVQ at level 3 in Beauty Therapy who have prior knowledge of anatomy, physiology and science. The only optional unit not covered is electrical epilation, which is considered to be a specialist area requiring a full book to study sufficiently (see *Electro-epilation: A Practical Approach, 2nd edition*, by Gill Morris, Elizabeth Cartwright and Michelle Severn). Additional reading and study is also recommended for aromatherapy, in particular *Massage and Aromatherapy* by Lyn Goldberg. Key skill areas are covered within this book and *Good Practice In Salon Management* and are linked to the beauty therapy curriculum through reception, stock control, dispensing products, costing treatments, working with others and liaising with clients and visitors. Lecturers can map the three main key skills – communication, application of number and Information Technology (IT) to these areas by setting assignments. The lecturer must ensure that the appropriate level of key skill is matched and that IT can be used to display graphs and charts of measurement and study produced by the individual student. For example, the findings from a stock control, the day's client profiles or monies taken on treatment and retail services could be displayed in a pie chart. It must be remembered that there is a requirement for uniqueness of portfolios, therefore assignment work must reflect this, perhaps by setting one research assignment in purchasing, equipping and planning the opening of a new salon. This would give a great deal of scope for individualism as well as matching the majority of key skill requirements.

This book is also a useful reference book for beauty therapy examinations offered by CIBTAC, CIDESCO, C & G, EDEXCEL, ITEC and VTCT. It will also assist in updating qualified therapists, especially those who work on their own.

Wishing you success and happiness in your future careers

Dawn Mernagh-Ward   Jennifer Cartwright

This book is dedicated to Rod Fabes for his inspirational support and guidance to the beauty therapy industry.

Sadly, Rod did not live to see publication of this book but his enthusiasm for our work and the education of future therapists remained to the end.

After working through this chapter you should:

◊ have a greater awareness of the structure and functions of the human body

◊ be able to give a brief outline of the structure and functions of the various systems of the body

◊ be able to relate this knowledge to the practical treatment situation where appropriate.

In order for the therapist to plan and perform effective treatment programmes for individual client's needs, it is essential to have an understanding of the structure and functions of the body. This chapter is designed to give an overview for therapists who have previous knowledge of anatomy and physiology and it is recommended that further study is undertaken from specialist sources.

Cells and tissues

The human body develops from a single cell called the *zygote* which results from the fusion of an *ovum* and *sperm*. Cell multiplication follows and as the foetus grows, cells with different structural and functional characteristics develop. However all cells carry the same genetic 'blue-print' as the initial zygote.

Structure of the cell

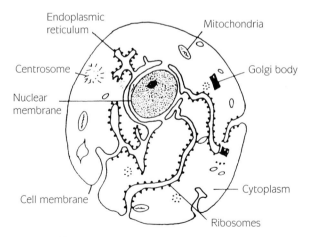

Fig. 1.1 *An animal cell*

All animal cells are composed of the following basic structures.

Cell membrane
This is really the cell wall and it keeps the cell contents intact. Substances can pass into and out of the cell across the membrane. It is a flexible structure and can change shape.

Cell fluid

Known as *cytoplasm*, cell fluid is a jelly-like substance that suspends all the cell's contents. Found within the cell fluid are folded membranes forming tubes known as *endoplasmic reticulum*, structures which function as transportation channels.

In addition to the internal system of membranes there are other structures within the cytoplasm:

Mitochondria

Food substances such as sugar are broken down chemically in the mitochondria to release energy that is needed to drive the reactions in the cell.

Ribosomes

Ribosomes play a part in building up proteins from which all cells and tissues are constructed.

Golgi bodies

Golgi bodies are specialised structures found near the nucleus. Their main function is to add carbohydrate to cell protein.

Nucleus

The nucleus is the most important part of the cell. It is a large spherical body enclosed in a special cell fluid called protoplasm but separated from it by a nuclear membrane. In the nucleus there are a number of thread-like bodies called *chromosomes*. There are 46 chromosomes in every human cell which are arranged in pairs, one member from each pair being inherited from the male parent and the other from the female. The chromosomes contain the basic hereditary information which determines the individual's characteristics and traits, such as hair and eye colour, the structure of bones and teeth, etc.

Mitosis

Mitosis is the process of cell multiplication that occurs throughout life whereby cells are formed to replace those that have died. Mitosis is divided into four phases.

1 Prophase

A structure called a *centrosome* divides into two *centrioles* which migrate to opposite sides of the cell remaining attached by thread-like *spindles*.

2 Metaphase

The nuclear membrane disappears and the chromosomes arrange themselves at the centre of the cell. They are attached to the spindles of the centrioles.

3 Anaphase

The *centromere*, a structure that connects pairs of chromosomes, divides and the identical chromosomes move apart, breaking the spindle structure.

4 Telophase

The spindles disappear completely while the nuclear membrane reappears around each of the two groups of chromosomes. A constriction occurs around the middle of the cell body until eventually the cell divides into two. The two cells are known as *daughter cells*.

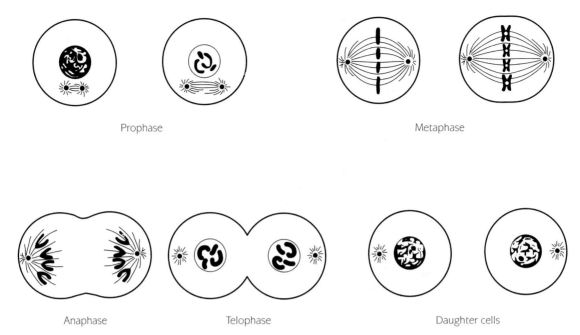

Fig. 1.2 *Cell division by mitosis*

Types of tissues

Cells unite to form tissues within the body. There are four main types:

- Epithelial.
- Connective.
- Muscular.
- Nerve.

Epithelial tissue

This is the simplest form of tissue and consists of one layer of cells in the case of simple epithelium and two or more layers in the case of stratified epithelium. This type of tissue forms the skin and is found within the linings of certain organs.

Connective tissue

There are many forms of connective tissue in the body. Adipose, bone and fibrous tissues are a few examples. Connective tissues can generally be thought of as tissue that unites other tissues together or gives support.

Muscular and nerve tissue

See pp. 13–18 for muscular tissue and pp. 26–29 for nerve tissue.

ACTIVITY

Research the different types of epithelial, connective, muscular and nerve tissue.

Progress Check

1   Describe epithelial tissue.
2   Explain briefly the process of cell division by mitosis.

The skin

The human skin is the largest organ of the body covering an area of approximately 1.2–2 square metres. Its main purpose is one of protection. It keeps the internal structures of the body covered and intact and it has to be able to withstand daily wear and tear. It also protects the body against invasion by bacteria, chemicals and other foreign substances.

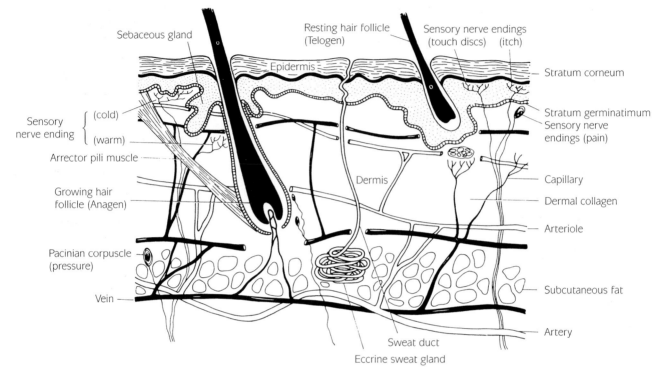

Fig. 1.3 *Vertical section of the skin*

The structure of the skin
Skin is composed of three main layers:

- Epidermis.
- Dermis.
- Subcutis.

Epidermis
This is the outer, visible layer of the skin and is itself composed of five distinctive layers. It takes approximately 30 days for this layer to renew itself and will vary in thickness on different parts of the body.

There are five distinct layers of the epidermis and these are:

1   **Stratum germinativum** (sometimes referred to as the basal layer). This is the deepest layer of the epidermis and consists of columnar cells which are mitotically active. The new cells produced by mitosis in the stratum germinativum are continually pushed up into the subsequent layers of the skin. *Melanocytes* are present within this layer and are responsible for producing the pigment *melanin*.

2   **Stratum spinosum** (sometimes referred to as the prickle cell layer). This layer is immediately above the basal layer and consists

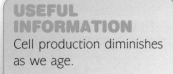

USEFUL INFORMATION
Cell production diminishes as we age.

of cells with prickle-like projections which are connected to each other. They are living cells, each containing a nucleus.

3   **Stratum granulosum**. This layer is formed from rows of flattened cells which contain a granular protoplasm. The dark granules present are *keratohyaline* which is involved in the first stage of keratinisation.

4   **Stratum lucidum**. This layer consists of light-permeable, transparent cells which contain droplets of a substance called *eleidin*. Eleidin is formed from keratohyaline and transforms into *keratin*.

5   **Stratum corneum**. This is the visible layer of the epidermis. Its cells are completely flattened, keratinised structures with no nucleus. Cells are shed from the stratum corneum and replaced on a continuous basis. The stratum corneum usually consists of many flattened cells.

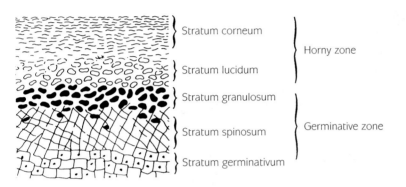

Fig. 1.4 *The layers of the epidermis*

Dermis

The dermis lies directly below the epidermis and is the thickest layer of the skin. It consists of two main layers known as the *superficial papillary layer* and the *reticular layer*. Found within the dermis are the following structures:

●   **Collagen and elastin fibres**. Collagen is a protein constituent and is responsible for giving the skin its firm contours. Elastin is formed from connective tissue. The yellow elastin fibres give the skin its suppleness. Collagen and elastin both deteriorate with the natural ageing process.

●   **Hair and hair follicles**. The hair follicle is a natural indentation within the dermis consisting of a downward extension of epidermal cells. The hair follicle is composed of an inner and outer root sheath which is surrounded by a connective tissue sheath. This sheath has a loosely-knit mesh of papillary cells overlying it, interspersed with nerves and blood capillaries. At the base of the follicle is a cluster of cells called the *dermal papilla* which provides the sole source of nourishment for the hair.

●   **Sudoriferous glands**. These are found in abundance within the dermis and are composed of epithelial cells. They produce a watery substance known as sweat which travels via a duct to the surface of the skin through a pore, or otherwise open into hair follicles. There are two main types of sudoriferous gland; *eccrine glands* and *apocrine glands*. The latter do not become active until pubescence. Both play a part in the heat regulation of the body.

- **Sebaceous glands**. These are also found in abundance within the dermis and are composed of secretory epithelial cells. They produce a fatty substance called *sebum* and normally open into a hair follicle. Sebum keeps the hair lubricated and gives some protection to the surface of the skin.
- **Arrector pilorum muscles**. These are tiny, involuntary muscles attached to the hair follicle. The muscles respond to cold and fear causing them to contract and forcing the hairs within the follicles to stand on end, giving the skin the appearance of goose flesh.
- **Sensory nerve endings**. Within the dermis are nerve endings which respond to pain, pressure, heat, cold and touch. The nerves carry impulses to the brain. Without the responses made to impulses from the sensory nerve endings serious mechanical damage could occur to the skin and the body as a whole.
- **Lymph vessels**. These are found in abundance throughout the dermis. Lymph vessels help to drain excess fluid.

Subcutis

The subcutis is the third layer of the skin and is a type of connective tissue which divides the dermis from the muscular layer. It has a rich blood supply and contains some sensory nerve endings. The majority of the cells in this layer are fat cells which act as a buffer to prevent damage to the underlying structures and also insulate the body against heat loss. The thickness of the subcutis varies on different parts of the body, for example it is thicker on the gluteal area than the forehead. It is generally thicker on women than on men.

Natural moisturising factor

The skin has a natural moisturising factor which is created within the cell regeneration and the production of the skin's acid mantle. It helps to prevent moisture loss from the epidermis. As the cells move upwards towards the surface of the skin, moisture is pushed from the inside of the cells outwards thus coating each cell with a sticky intercellular glue. This has the effect of holding the stratum corneum together.

The functions of the skin

The skin serves many important functions. The main ones are:

- **S**ecretion.
- **H**eat regulation.
- **A**bsorption.
- **P**rotection.
- **E**limination.
- **S**ensation.

Secretion

The two main substances the skin secretes are *sebum* and *sweat*.

Sebum is produced by the sebaceous glands which are situated in the dermis between the angle of the follicle and the arrector pilorum muscle. Sebum is a fatty substance which lubricates the skin's surface and the hair. Sebum is also bactericidal and so prevents bacterial infection.

Sweat is produced by the sudoriferous glands which are coiled tubules situated in the dermis. Sudoriferous glands open onto the skin's surface via a small duct (the sweat duct) and pore. There are two types of sweat gland:

- Eccrine glands are found in abundance all over the body. They secrete a clear, watery fluid.
- Apocrine glands are found under the arms (axillae) and in the groin area (inguinal). They produce a milky fluid. Apocrine glands start working from puberty onwards.

Heat regulation

Body temperature in good health is 36.9°C. For this temperature to remain constant a heat loss/production balance must be maintained. This is sometimes referred to as *homeostasis*.

Heat loss is affected by two main factors: the amount of blood circulating in the capillaries and the amount of sweat formed and its rate of evaporation.

Any increase in body temperature will have the following effects:

- *Vasodilation* occurs. The capillaries near the skin's surface dilate, allowing more blood to circulate nearer to the surface where heat will be lost by radiation and convection thus giving the skin a flushed look.
- Increased amounts of sweat are produced. This has a cooling effect as it evaporates from the surface of the skin.

A decrease in body temperature will have the opposite effects:

- *Vasoconstriction* occurs. Capillaries near the skin's surface constrict. Less blood flows near the surface and therefore less heat is lost.
- Sweat production diminishes.

Absorption

As one of the skin's main functions is to protect against the intrusion of foreign substances, the skin absorbs very little. Only tiny quantities of water and oil-soluble substances are absorbed.

However, the skin can be said to absorb radiation; in particular ultra-violet radiation. Ultra-violet rays penetrate the skin and act on a substance called *ergosterol* which is present in the subcutis of the skin, producing vitamin D.

Protection

The skin has several protection mechanisms:

- The stratum corneum (horny layer) of the epidermis contains keratinised cells which act as a buffer and are impervious to most substances.
- Sweat is acidic and has the effect of inhibiting organism growth.
- Sebum, as well as being bactericidal, acts as a lubricant preventing the surface of the skin from cracking. This also helps to prevent invasion by bacteria.
- Adipose tissue in the subcutis insulates the body and protects the underlying structures from bumps and knocks.

USEFUL INFORMATION
Together, the sweat and sebum that mix on the surface of the skin form what is known as the acid mantle, which, as the name suggests, is acidic and protects the skin from organism growth.

- Sensory nerve endings in the skin respond to painful stimuli to protect the body from mechanical and environmental damage.
- Melanin is produced in the skin in response to ultra-violet radiation. Certain types of ultra-violet radiation can cause damage to the skin, such as premature ageing and skin cancers. Melanin is produced to limit this damage.

Elimination

As has been previously mentioned the skin secretes sweat and sebum. These contain waste products that the body needs to eliminate.

Sensation

The sensory nerve endings found within the dermis protect the body from serious environmental and mechanical damage by reacting to pain, pressure, heat, cold, and touch.

pH of the skin

pH is the measurement of acidity or alkalinity. The pH scale ranges from 0–14 with 7 being neutral. The lower the number the more acidic and the higher the number the more alkaline. The skin has a pH between 4.5 and 6 making it acidic.

POINT TO NOTE

The skin is pH buffered, meaning that the pH of the skin does not change very easily (a buffer is acid and salt, the skin is lactic acid and lactate).

ACTIVITY

Describe the physiological effects of massage on the skin.

Progress Check

1 Name the layers of the epidermis and give a brief description of each.
2 List the main functions of the skin.

The skeletal system

There are two types of skeleton:

1 Exoskeleton – this is where hard material is formed mainly on the outside of the body. Crustaceans normally have an exoskeleton.
2 Endoskeleton – this is where the skeleton is formed inside the soft tissue. The skeleton is made of bone and cartilage such as in human beings.

Functions of the skeleton

The skeleton has four main functions:

- Support.
- Protection.

- Muscle attachment.
- Movement (locomotion).

Support
The skeleton supports and raises the body from the ground and allows movement. Vital organs are suspended from the skeleton thus preventing them from crushing each other.

Protection
The skeleton is uniquely designed to protect the internal organs. In particular it protects:

- the brain, which is encased in the cranium
- the spinal cord, which is encased in the vertebral column
- the heart and lungs, which are surrounded by the rib cage.

The organs are protected by the skeleton from distortion resulting from pressure and from injury resulting from impact.

Muscle attachment
The skeleton acts as a framework for the voluntary muscular system. For movement to take place a muscle must be held in place firmly at one end (this is known as the origin of the muscle) and be free to move at the other end (this is known as the insertion of the muscle). The origins and insertions of most of the body's muscles are located on the bones of the skeleton.

Movement (locomotion)
Many bones of the skeleton act as levers. When muscles pull on these levers they produce movement, such as the chewing action of the jaw, the flexing of the biceps and the inhalation/exhalation movements of the ribs. All these movements require a system of joints and muscle attachments.

Composition of the skeleton
The skeleton consists of some 204 bones in adult life.

- 22 form the cranium.
- 25 form the thorax.
- 33 form the spine.
- 120 form the upper and lower limbs.
- 4 form the pelvis.

Types of bone tissue
There are two types of bone tissue: *compact* and *cancellous*.

Compact bone
Compact bone contains large numbers of structures called *Haversian systems*. A Haversian system consists of a central longitudinal canal, called the *Haversian canal*, rich in blood, lymph and nerves, surrounded by plates of bone arranged concentrically, called *lamellae*. Spaces between lamellae contain osteocytes or bone cells called *lacunae*. The Haversian systems are covered with a tough, fibrous sheeting called *periosteum*. This tubular formation makes this type of bone strong and rigid.

> **USEFUL INFORMATION**
>
> Bone is a dry, dense tissue composed of approximately:
>
> * 25% water.
> * 30% organic fibrous material.
> * 45% minerals.

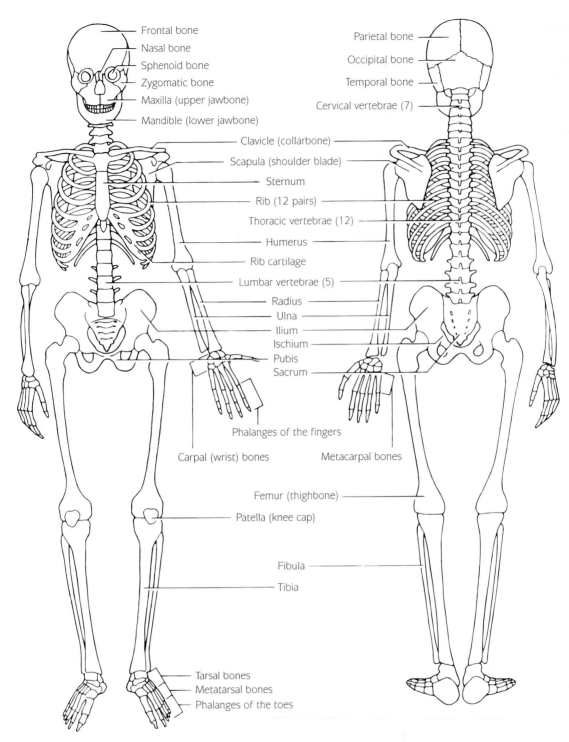

Frontal bone
Nasal bone
Sphenoid bone
Zygomatic bone
Maxilla (upper jawbone)
Mandible (lower jawbone)

Parietal bone
Occipital bone
Temporal bone
Cervical vertebrae (7)

Clavicle (collarbone)
Scapula (shoulder blade)
Sternum
Rib (12 pairs)
Thoracic vertebrae (12)
Humerus
Rib cartilage
Lumbar vertebrae (5)
Radius
Ulna
Ilium
Ischium
Pubis
Sacrum

Phalanges of the fingers

Carpal (wrist) bones   Metacarpal bones

Femur (thighbone)
Patella (knee cap)

Fibula
Tibia

Tarsal bones
Metatarsal bones
Phalanges of the toes

Fig. 1.5 *The skeleton*

Cancellous bone

Cancellous bone appears more 'spongy' than compact bone. It has larger Haversian canals with less lamellae, giving a latticework appearance. Cancellous bone contains red bone marrow.

Periosteum

Periosteum is the fibrous sheeting which covers the bone surface. It is composed of two layers. The inner layer produces new cells for bone growth. The outer, fibrous layer has a rich vascular supply.

Classification of bones
Long bones
The strongest bones of the skeleton, long bones are composed of a shaft (diaphysis) and two ends (epiphyses). The diaphysis is formed from compact bone while the epiphyses have an outer covering of compact bone with cancellous bone found within. An example of a long bone is the femur.

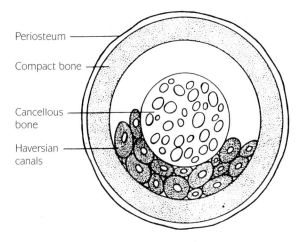

Fig. 1.6 *Cross section through a long bone*

Short bones
Short bones are the small bones found in the wrists and ankles. They consist of a relatively thin outer layer of compact bone with cancellous bone inside. Examples of short bones are the metatarsals.

Flat bones
Flat bones consist of two thin layers of compact bone joined by a layer of cancellous bone and covered by periosteum. Two sets of blood vessels pass into the bone to supply the spongy and compact tissues. Examples of flat bones include the frontal and parietal bones of the cranium.

Irregular bones
Irregular bones consist of a mass of cancellous bone covered by a thin layer of compact bone overlaid with periosteum. Examples of irregular bones are the vertebrae.

Sesamoid bones
Sesamoid bones are rounded masses of bone tissue found in certain tendons. The best example of a sesamoid bone is the patella.

Joints
Where two or more bones come together a joint is formed. There are three main classifications of joint: *cartilaginous, fibrous* and *synovial.*

Cartilaginous joints are slightly moveable joints. They are held together by strong ligaments. the bones are separated by pads of white fibro-cartilage which allow only slight movement when the fibro-cartilage pad is compressed. Examples of this type of joint include the sacro-iliac joint and the symphysis pubis.

Fibrous joints are fixed joints. They do not allow any form of movement. Fibrous tissue is found between the bones in these joints. Examples of fibrous joints are the sutures between the bones of the skull.

Synovial joints are freely moveable joints. They allow a considerable amount of movement. The joint is enclosed in a fibrous capsule supported by ligaments. The capsule is lined by a synovial membrane which secretes synovial fluid into the capsule. Synovial fluid prevents friction between articulating surfaces of the joint which are both covered in hyaline cartilage for smooth operation.

The types of synovial joint are:

- Ball and socket joints.
- Hinge joints.
- Pivot articulations.
- Gliding joints.

Synovial joints are capable of the following types of movement:

a Extension – when a limb is extended, two parts of the limb are pulled away from each other (Fig. 1.7a).

b Flexion – when a limb is flexed, two parts of the limb are pulled towards each other (Fig. 1.7b).

c Abduction – when a limb is pulled away from the midline (median line) of the body (Fig. 1.7c).

d Adduction – when a limb is pulled towards the midline of the body (Fig. 1.7d).

e Circumduction – combination of flexion, extension, abduction and adduction.

f Rotation – movement round the long axis of bone (Fig. 1.8).

g Pronation – when a limb is turned to face downwards.

h Supination – when a limb is turned to face upwards.

i Inversion – when a limb is turned to face inwards.

j Eversion – when a limb is turned to face outwards.

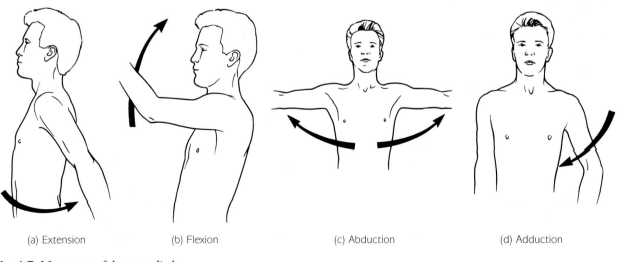

(a) Extension   (b) Flexion   (c) Abduction   (d) Adduction

Fig. 1.7 *Movements of the upper limb*

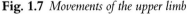

Ball and socket joints

These joints are capable of flexion, extension, abduction, adduction, rotation and circumduction. Examples of ball and socket joints include the hip and shoulder.

Hinge joints

These joints allow for flexion and extension. Examples of hinge joints include the knee, elbow, ankle and the joint between the atlas and occipital bone in the head.

Pivot articulations

These joints allow for rotation only. Examples include the joint between the radius and ulna and the axis joint of the head.

Gliding joints

In these joints the articular surfaces glide over each other. Examples of gliding joints are the tarsal joint of the ankle and the carpal joint of the wrist.

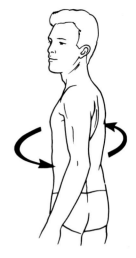

Fig. 1.8 *Rotation*

ACTIVITY

With a colleague, undertake the following activities, noting which bones and types of joints are being used:

a walking up stairs
b catching a ball
c rotating the head.

Progress Check

1　Give the functions of the skeleton.
2　Name two classifications of joints.

The muscular system

Roughly one fifth of body weight is that of muscle. It is muscle which forms the flesh of the body and moves, with the aid of the skeleton, the body. Whilst most muscles are attached to bones, there are exceptions, such as the epicranial aponeurosis. Both ends of the epicranial aponeurosis are attached to the skin. The muscle causes movements such as frowning, raising of the eyebrows, etc.

The naming of muscles is complicated. They can be named according to:

- Function, e.g. flexor or extensor, adductor or abductor, supinator or pronator.
- Attachments, e.g. sternocleidomastoid.
- Shape, e.g. trapezius.
- Formation, e.g. biceps (2 heads), triceps (3 heads), quadriceps (4 heads).
- Position, e.g. intercostal muscles (between the ribs).

USEFUL INFORMATION

The composition of muscular tissue is:

* 75% water.
* 25% solids, of which the most important is a protein called myosin.

Types of muscular tissue

There are three types of muscular tissue: *voluntary, involuntary and cardiac.*

Voluntary muscular tissue

Voluntary muscle is also called striated muscle and forms the flesh of the limbs and trunk. It consists of long fibres, made of multi-nucleate cells, which vary considerably in length according to the individual muscle. Each fibre contains numerous thread-like structures called *myofibrils*. Myofibrils are alternately striped in regular light and dark bands which is why voluntary muscle is sometimes called striated muscle. Muscle fibres are surrounded by a membrane called the *endomysium*. The fibres are bound together in bundles called *fasciculi* and surrounded by a sheath called the *perimysium*. The fasciculi in turn form a bigger bundle enclosed by a sheath called the *epimysium* which ultimately forms an individual muscle.

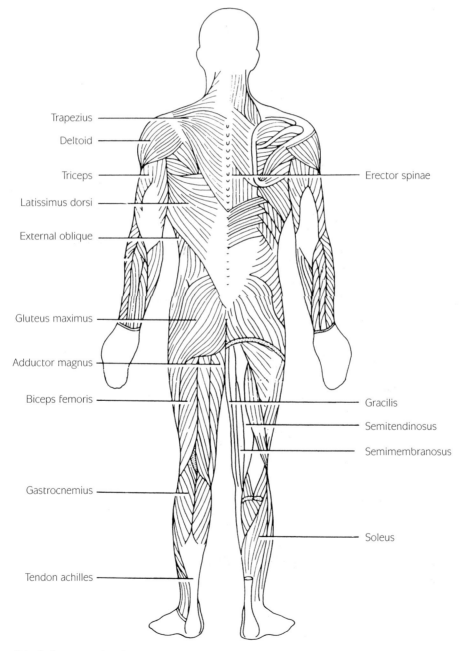

Fig. 1.9 *Muscles of the body – posterior view*

As the name suggests, voluntary muscle is under conscious control. It contracts quickly when stimulated by nerve impulses but tires rather quickly as well.

Involuntary muscular tissue

This type of muscle is found in the walls of the internal organs, e.g. stomach, bowel, uterus, etc. It consists of spindle-shaped cells, each of which contain a nucleus. These cells are unstriped and have no sheath but are bound together by connective tissue. They are not under control of will and are designed for slow contraction over a long period. Involuntary muscle, therefore, does not fatigue easily.

Cardiac muscle

This type of muscle is found only in the heart wall and is both involuntary and irregularly striped. It consists of short, cylindrical,

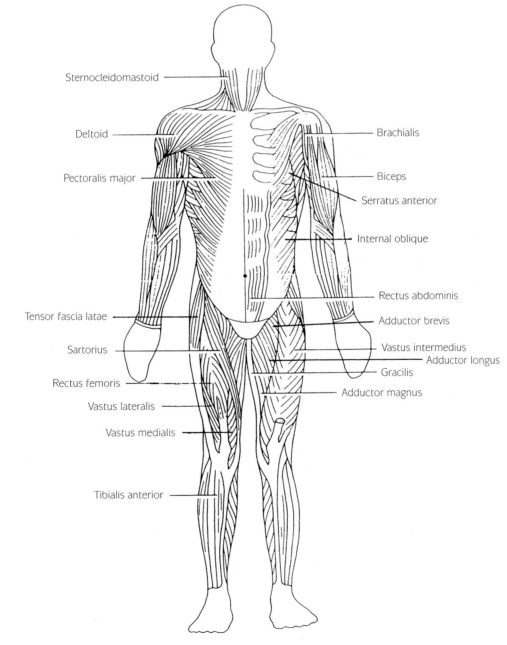

Fig. 1.10 *Muscles of the body – anterior view*

branched fibres with a centrally placed nucleus. Cardiac muscle has no sheath but is bound together by connective tissue. It is not under control of will and contracts automatically throughout life in a rhythmical pattern. The rate of these contractions is controlled by nerves which quicken or slow down the action. This is the strongest type of muscular tissue within the human body.

The properties of muscular tissue

Muscle has four main properties:

- The power of contraction.
- Elasticity.
- Fatigue.
- Muscle tone.

The power of contraction

Voluntary muscle contracts as a result of stimuli reaching it from the nervous system and many nerves have their endings in muscles. Messages passing down a nerve from the brain cause the muscle to contract when they reach it. Other stimuli such as electrical currents applied directly to the muscle or its nerve will also cause contraction.

Elasticity and fatigue

When a muscle contracts, it uses energy which is derived mainly from the respiration of glucose. Glucose is supplied to the muscle via the blood. The blood also carries oxygen which the muscle uses to 'burn up' the glucose. During normal activity, the glucose is respired *aerobically*, that is the glucose is broken down to form water and carbon dioxide. The water and carbon dioxide are removed from the muscle and it does not tire.

During heavy exercise glucose is required *anaerobically*. Anaerobic respiration produces *lactic acid* which is ultimately broken down to form carbon dioxide and water. However, lactic acid is not broken down very fast. After a certain number of contractions lactic acid begins to accumulate in the muscle. The muscle then becomes tired and is unable to contract with the same degree of efficiency. This affects the elasticity of the muscle and ultimately results in fatigue.

Muscular tone

Even when a muscle appears to be at rest it is always partially contracted and therefore ready for immediate action. This state of partial contraction is called muscular tone.

Tendons

Tendons are tough, fibrous and inelastic. They are found at the ends of muscles and their main purpose is to provide attachment to bones.

Ligaments

Like the tendons above, ligaments are strong, fibrous and do not stretch. Their function is to connect bones together.

ACTIVITY

Cut out pictures from magazines of people performing everyday activities such as cycling, walking, etc., then state which muscle or key muscle groups they are using.

Table 1.1 *The major muscles of the body*

	Position	Origin	Insertion	Action
Muscles of the neck and back				
Sternocleidomastoid	Front of the neck	Sternum and clavicle	Mastoid process	Used separately, turns the head to opposite side; used together, flexes the neck
Trapezius	Back of the neck and chest	Occiput and spines of the thoracic vertebrae	Spine of the scapula and clavicle	Draws scapula back, bracing the shoulders; pulls the occiput, extending the neck
Latissimus dorsi	Crosses the back from the lumbar region to the shoulder	Lumbar vertebrae, sacrum and back of iliac crest	Humerus	Adduction of the shoulder, drawing the arm back and downwards
Erector spinae	Between the transverse and spinal processes of the vertebrae	Sacrum	Occipital bone	Keeps the body in an upright position and produces extension of the vertebral column
Serratus anterior	Lateral chest wall	Upper nine ribs	Vertebral border of scapula	Draws shoulder forwards and rotates scapula
Muscles of the chest				
Pectoralis major	Front of the chest	Sternum and clavicle	Humerus, outer edge of the bicipital groove	Adduction of the shoulder, drawing the arm across the thorax
Muscles of the arm				
Biceps	Front of arm	By two heads from the scapula (coracoid process and above the glenoid cavity)	Radial tuberosity	Flexion of the elbow and shoulder; supinates hand
Triceps	Back of arm	By one head from the scapula and by two heads from the shaft of the humerus	Olecranon process of ulna	Extension of the elbow and shoulder
Deltoid	Over the shoulder	Spine of scapula and clavicle	Deltoid tubercle of humerus	Abducts the shoulder to a right angle
Brachialis	Crosses front of elbow	Humerus	Ulna	Flexion of the elbow
Muscles of the abdomen				
Rectus abdominis	Front of the abdominal wall	Upper border of public bone	5th, 6th and 7th costal cartilages and xiphoid process	Flexes the spine and aids respiration
External oblique	Forms the outer coat of the side abdominal wall	Lower ribs	Iliac crest	Flexes trunk together with internal oblique
Internal oblique	Forms the second coat of the side wall of the abdomen	Iliac crest	Lower ribs and fascia of the rectus abdominis	Flexes trunk together with external oblique. Produces rotation when used with the external oblique of the opposite side

Table 1.1 *The major muscles of the body (continued)*

	Position	Origin	Insertion	Action
Muscles of the buttocks				
Gluteus maximus	Large quadrilateral mass forming the prominence of the buttocks	Outer surface of ilium, also sacrum and coccyx	Upper end of femur	Extends the hip joint and rotates it laterally
Gluteus medius	Lies below the gluteus maximus	Gluteal surface of ilium	Greater trochanter of femur	Abduction of the hip joint
Muscles of the hip and upper leg				
Quadriceps	This extensive muscle mass forms the bulk of the anterior region of the thigh and is divided here into four separate muscles: the rectus femoris, vastus lateralis, vastus medialis and vastus intermedius			
Rectus femoris	Front of thigh	Ilium	Upper border of patella	Flexes the hip joint
Vastus lateralis	Lateral side of femur	Greater trochanter and linea aspera of femur	Tibial tubercle	Extends the knee joint
Vastus medialis	Medial side of femur	Lesser trochanter of femur	Tibial tubercle	Extends the knee joint
Vastus intermedius	Covers front of femur	Upper end of femur	Tibial tubercle	Extends the knee joint
Abductors of hip	Outer side of thigh	Anterior aspect of ilium	Between the two layers of a fascia lata	Abducts the hip
Adductors of hip (pectineus, adductor brevis, adductor longus, adductor magnus, gracilis)	The group lies on the medial side of the thigh	Pubic bone	Linea aspera of femur	Adducts the femur
Hamstrings (biceps femoris, semimembranosus, semitendinosus)	Back of thigh	Ischial tuberosity and femur	Tibia and fibula	Extension of hip and flexion of knee
Sartorius	Crosses over the front of the thigh	Anterior superior iliac spine	Upper part of the tibia	Weak flexor of both hip and knee joints
Tensor fascia latae	Lateral aspect of upper thigh	Outer part of iliac crest	Fascia latae	Abducts and rotates the femur and extends the knee
Muscles of the lower leg				
Tibialis anterior	Front of leg	Lateral surface of upper end of tibia	Medial cuneiform bone	Flexion and inversion of the foot
Gastrocnemius	Posterior calf area	Condyles of femur	Calcaneum	Flexes foot
Soleus	Posterior of calf area	Head and upper part of fibula and tibia	Calcaneum	Flexes foot

1   Draw and label diagrams of the main muscles of the body.
2   State the four properties of muscular tissue.

The circulatory system

The circulatory system consists of:

- Heart.
- Blood.
- Blood vessels.
- Lymph.
- Lymph vessels.

The heart

The heart is a hollow organ with walls made of cardiac muscle. It is approximately 10 cm long and weighs about 225 g in women and 240 g in men. The heart is situated in the thoracic cavity protected by the rib cage and it lies obliquely to the left hand side.

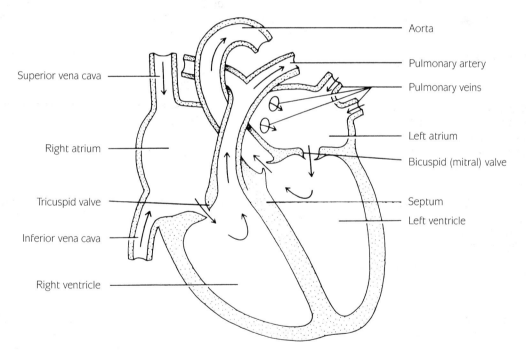

Fig. 1.11 *The heart*

The heart is composed of three distinct layers:

1   **Pericardium.** This is a smooth, membranous covering which is formed of an outer fibrous layer and an inner, serous coat. Between these layers a serous coat. Between these layers a serous fluid is secreted which allows for ease of movement between the two layers.

2   **Myocardium.** This is the muscular layer of the heart and is formed of a specialised, involuntary muscular tissue. This cardiac

muscle is exceptionally strong. The fibres are bonded together in branches and it has to be able to contact rhythmically throughout life.

3 **Endocardium.** This is the inner, lining membrane of the myocardium layer. It is very thin and consists of flattened epithelial cells.

Internal structure of the heart

The heart is divided into a right and left side with a layer of myocardium called the *septum* separating them. Each side is divided into two chambers. There are four chambers in total; the right and left *atria* and the right and left *ventricles*. Valves separate the chambers on each side of the heart from each other. The valve separating the right atrium and ventricle is called the *tricuspid valve*. The valve separating the left atrium and ventricle is called the *bicuspid* or *mitral valve*. These valves open and close when the pressure changes within the chambers.

When cardiac muscle contracts it squeezes blood out of the heart and into the arteries which carry it to all parts of the body. When cardiac muscle relaxes the heart fills with blood from the veins. This mechanism of contraction and relaxation is known as the heart beat.

Flow of blood through the heart

Deoxygenated blood returns from the body to the right atrium of the heart via the largest veins of the body, the superior and inferior vena cavae. This blood is then squeezed through the tricuspid valve into the right ventricle from where it is then forced through the pulmonary artery which carries the deoxygenated blood to the lungs. Gaseous exchange takes place between the blood and the air in the lungs; carbon dioxide is excreted and oxygen is absorbed. The now oxygenated blood returns to the heart via the pulmonary veins which empty the blood into the left atrium. It passes through the bicuspid valve and into the left ventricle, then is forced into the largest artery of the body, the aorta, which carries the oxygenated blood to the rest of the body.

POINTS TO NOTE

♦ Veins carry blood towards the heart. They normally carry deoxygenated blood. However, the one exception to this is the pulmonary vein which carries oxygenated blood from the lungs to the heart.

♦ Arteries carry blood away from the heart. They normally carry oxygenated blood. However, the one exception to this is the pulmonary artery which carries deoxygenated blood from the heart to the lungs.

♦ The left side of the heart is slightly more muscular. This is to enable it to force blood out to all parts of the body via the aorta.

Cardiac cycle

The contraction and relaxation of the heart is called the cardiac cycle and is divided into two phases:

1 **Diastole** – when blood is passing from the veins into the atria and then into the ventricles. Heart muscle is relaxed.

2 **Systole** – when the ventricles contract during systole the valves in the heart are pushed closed causing the pressure in the arteries to increase. This gives the pulse.

Blood

Blood consists of:

- Erythrocytes (red blood cells).
- Leucocytes (white blood cells).
- Platelets.
- Plasma.

Erythrocytes (red blood cells)

Erythrocytes are minute, biconcave discs made from spongy cytoplasm surrounded by an elastic membrane. Their red colour comes from haemoglobin combined with oxygen. *Haemoglobin* is a protein which contains iron and has a natural affinity with oxygen. Haemoglobin combines with oxygen to form *oxyhaemoglobin*. Red blood cells are the mechanism by which oxygen is transported around the body. Red blood cells are made in red bone marrow. Cell formation takes approximately seven days, during which time the nucleus disappears and they cease to be true cells. The life span of a red blood cell is roughly four months, after which time the cell is destroyed in the liver or the spleen.

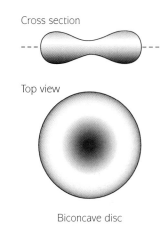

Cross section

Top view

Biconcave disc

Fig. 1.12 *Erythrocyte (red blood cell)*

Leucocytes (white blood cells)

Leucocytes are colourless cells each containing a nucleus. There are far fewer white cells than red cells; approximately one to every six hundred red cells. The main function of white cells is to fight infection and protect the body against viruses, toxins and bacteria.

There are different types of leucocytes and they have different functions within the body.

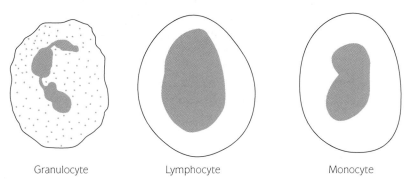

Granulocyte   Lymphocyte   Monocyte

Fig. 1.13 *Leucocytes (white blood cells)*

Granulocytes form approximately 75% of the total number of white cells. They ingest bacteria by encapsulating them and digesting them slowly – a process called phagocytosis. Granulocytes have a life span of about one week and are made in bone marrow.

Lymphocytes form roughly 23% of the total number of white cells. They are formed in lymph nodes and produce antibodies which kill foreign proteins. They can live for up to one hundred days.

Monocytes form approximately 2% of white cells. They can ingest foreign proteins in the blood.

Platelets

Platelets are formed in the red bone marrow and are fragments of red blood cells. They play an important part in the clotting process of blood.

Plasma

Plasma is a slightly alkaline, yellowish fluid in which the blood cells float. It consists of 96% water together with other important compounds such as:

- Proteins, e.g. albumem, fibrogen, globulin.
- Antibodies.
- Soluble salts, e.g. sodium chloride, potassium chloride, calcium phosphate.
- Food substances, e.g. amino acids, glucose, fatty acids, glycerol.
- Waste products, e.g. urea, carbon dioxide.
- Hormones.

Functions of blood

1 Transport of oxygen from the lungs to the body tissues.
2 Transport of carbon dioxide from the body tissues to the lungs.
3 Transport of excretory products.
4 Transport of digested food.
5 Distribution of hormones
6 Distribution of heat.
7 Clotting process of blood (this occurs to prevent loss of blood from a wound).

The blood clotting process in damaged tissue

Platelets produce a substance called *thrombokinase* which acts on *prothrombin* (which is already circulating in the blood) to change it to *thrombin*. Thrombin reacts with calcium ions in the blood producing *fibrinogen* – fibres of protein which radiate across the wound tangling red and white cells together with platelets – thus preventing blood loss.

Arteries and veins

Arteries and veins are hollow elastic tubes that transport blood which has been pumped by the heart around the body. They differ slightly in structure.

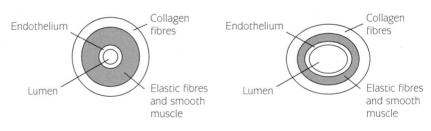

Fig. 1.14 *Cross sections of an artery and a vein*

Veins:

- have thinner walls than arteries
- contain valves to prevent the back-flow of blood
- carry deoxygenated blood (with the exception of the pulmonary vein mentioned earlier)
- have walls consisting of three layers – the tunica adventia, tunica media and tunica intima.

Arteries:

- have thicker walls than veins
- do not contain valves
- carry oxygenated blood (with the exception of the pulmonary artery mentioned earlier)
- have walls consisting of the same three layers as veins, but they are thicker than in veins.

Blood pressure

Blood pressure is the amount of pressure exerted on the arteries by blood as it flows through them. It is measured in millimetres of mercury (mmHg) using a *sphygmomanometer*.

The lymphatic system

The lymphatic system is a subsidiary or second circulatory system which drains the tissue fluid. It consists of a series of fluid-filled tubes beginning as fine, blind-ended capillaries which spread throughout most of the tissues of the body. These pass into larger lymphatic vessels which eventually drain into the great veins of the neck. The principal function of the lymphatic system is to fight infection within the body.

Lymphatic fluid

Lymph is a clear, straw-coloured liquid with a similar composition to blood plasma. Its main composition is water with some proteins, fats, hormones and salts. It contains white cells, mainly lymphocytes, together with waste products that the system is dealing with at any particular time, e.g. dead cells, micro-organisms.

Formation of lymph

Lymph is formed in the tissues of the body and is a derivative of blood plasma which passes out of the capillaries to form what is called intercellular fluid. Excess intercellular fluid drains into the lymphatic capillaries where it is known as lymph.

Lymphatic capillaries

Lymphatic capillaries are fine, hollow, blind-ended, elastic tubes, similar to blood capillaries in structure although they are wider and less regular in shape. They consist of a single layer of epithelial tissue, i.e. their walls are one cell thick, bound together with connective tissue. Because of this they are more permeable than blood capillaries, allowing for larger substances to pass through their walls. Lymph drains into them from the tissue fluids.

Lymphatic vessels

Lymphatic vessels carry lymph from the lymphatic capillaries to the great veins of the neck. They are composed of connective tissue lined with epithelial cells and they also contain valves to prevent back-flow to ensure that lymph flows away from the tissues.

Lymph nodes

Before lymph is discharged into the bloodstream it passes through at least one lymph node. Lymph nodes are situated in clusters around the body and are composed of special cells which include *macrophages* which are phagocytic, i.e. they ingest foreign particles thereby filtering the

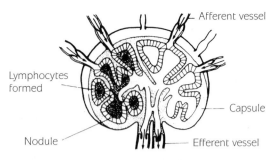

Fig. 1.15 *Cross section of a lymph node*

lymph of toxins. Major groups of lymph nodes are in the head and neck, under the arms (axillae), in the breast area, abdomen and groin (inguinal). When there is localised infection within the body the lymph nodes in that particular area will become swollen as they are engorged with toxins.

The great veins of the neck

As has been mentioned previously, lymph travels through at least one lymph node before it returns to the blood stream. The vessels which allow lymph to re-enter the blood stream are called:

- **The right lymphatic duct**. This is a dilated vessel situated at the base of the neck and feeds into the right subclavian vein. It drains lymph from the right half of the head, neck, chest area and right arm.
- **The thoracic duct**. This vessel begins at the *cisterna chyli*, a specialised lymph sac found in front of the first two lumber vertebrae. It connects into the left subclavian vein at the base of the neck. It drains lymph from the left side of the head and neck, the left arm, left side of the chest area and both legs.

The spleen

The spleen is a large nodule of lymphoid tissue which is a deep purplish-red in colour. It is situated high up at the back of the abdomen on the left side behind the stomach. The functions of the spleen are:

- Formation of lymphocytes.
- A reservoir for blood.
- Formation of antibodies and antitoxins.
- Destruction of worn-out erythrocytes.

ACTIVITY
Research the ABO system of blood grouping.

Progress Check

1   Name and describe the principle cells of the circulatory system.
2   Describe the flow of blood through the heart.
3   What is the main function of the lymphatic system?

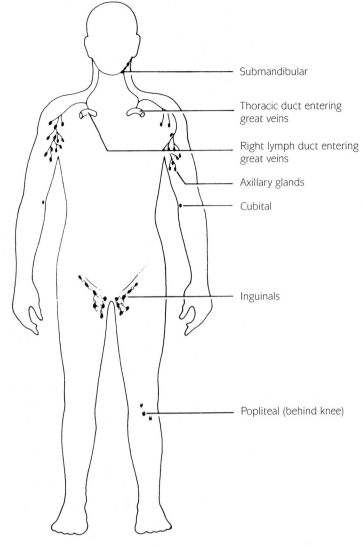

Fig. 1.16 *Lymph nodes of the body*

Submandibular

Thoracic duct entering great veins

Right lymph duct entering great veins

Axillary glands

Cubital

Inguinals

Popliteal (behind knee)

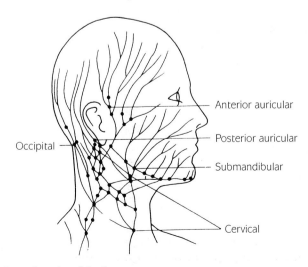

Fig. 1.17 *Lymph nodes of the face*

Occipital

Anterior auricular

Posterior auricular

Submandibular

Cervical

The neurological system

The neurological system is involved in transmitting messages from the brain to all other parts of the body. It consists of three main divisions:

1. The central nervous system.
2. The peripheral nervous system.
3. The autonomic nervous system.

The central nervous system

The central nervous system consists of the brain and spinal column and is at the centre of the neurological system.

The brain

The brain is the most important part of the entire neurological system. It receives impulses and stores them, it also transmits impulses to all parts of the body to stimulate organs to work.

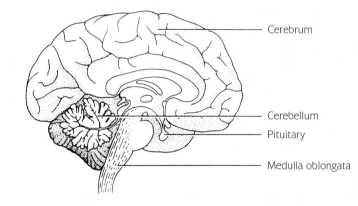

Fig. 1.18 *Cross section through the brain*

The adult brain weighs approximately 1.5 kg and contains millions of neurones. Each neurone is composed of a cell body that is similar in composition to other animal cells in that it contains a nucleus and is surrounded by cytoplasm. However it differs in that it has a long tail known as its axon. The purpose of which is to control impulses away from the cell body. Attached to the cell body are small fibres called dendrites and these carry impulses into the cell. Groups of neurones together form what are termed nerves and in order for impulses to travel along a nerve they must move from the axon of one to the dendrite of the next. Where axons and dendrites meet is called the synapse.

For neurones to remain undamaged in the brain they need to be well protected and this is accomplished firstly by the skull – a hard outer casing of bone – and secondly by a specialised layer called the *meninges*.

The meninges consist of three distinct layers. These are:

- the *dura mater* – a tough, fibrous outer membrane which cushions the brain against the inside of the cranium
- the *arachnoid mater* – the middle layer, which is much more delicate
- the *pia mater* – the inner layer which folds into the convoluted surface of the brain.

A special fluid is found between the arachnoid and pia mater which acts as a further cushion. It is called *cerebrospinal fluid*.

The brain has three main regions: the *cerebrum*, *cerebellum* and *medulla oblongata*.

1   **Cerebrum**. The largest region of the brain, it is a dome-shaped area of nervous tissue split into two halves called cerebral hemispheres. The surface of the cerebrum is made of what is termed grey matter – this is where the main functions of the cerebrum are carried out. These functions include all forms of conscious activity. Sensations such as touch, vision, taste, hearing and smell originate here. Control of voluntary muscular movements and emotion, powers of reasoning and memory are also handled in the cerebrum.

2   **Cerebellum**. This region of the brain receives impulses from the semi-circular canals in the ears and from stretch receptors in the muscles. It processes this information to maintain muscle tone and a balanced posture. It also co-ordinates muscles during activities such as walking, running, dancing, etc.

3   **Medulla oblongata**. This region is often referred to as the *brain stem* and contains a mass of grey matter known as the *vital centre*. It controls the part of the nervous system not under control of will, e.g. regulation of blood pressure, body temperature, etc. It performs these functions through connections with the autonomic nervous system. The medulla oblongata also contains nerve fibres which connect the brain with the spinal cord.

The spinal cord

As mentioned, the spinal cord is continuous with the medulla oblongata and extends downwards through the vertebral column finishing at the level of the lumbar vertebrae. It is protected by meninges and cerebrospinal fluid like the brain. Radiating from the spinal column are

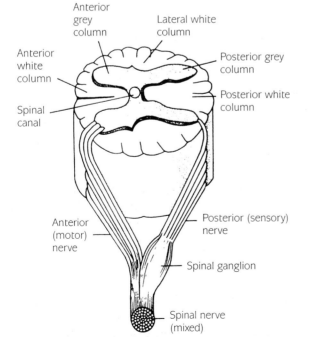

Fig. 1.19 *Cross section of the spinal cord*

12 pairs of cranial nerves and 31 pairs of spinal nerves corresponding to the segments of the vertebral column. The cranial and spinal nerves are part of the peripheral nervous system.

The peripheral nervous system

This part of the neurological system consists of all the nerves situated outside the central nervous system.

There are three types of nerve cell in the peripheral nervous system:

1　**Motor (efferent) nerves.** These nerves convey impulses from the brain through the spinal cord to the skeletal muscles, glands and smooth muscular tissue (effector organs).
2　**Sensory (afferent) nerves.** This type of nerve conveys impulses from the sensory nerves endings in organs to the brain and spinal cord.
3　**Mixed nerves.** These consist of both motor and sensory nerve fibres.

The peripheral nervous system consists of 31 pairs of spinal nerves and 12 pairs of cranial nerves.

The spinal nerves are as follows:

- 8 pairs cervical.
- 12 pairs thoracic.
- 5 pairs lumbar.
- 5 pairs sacral.
- 1 pair coccygeal.

The twelve pairs of cranial nerves are the:

- Olfactory nerves.
- Optic nerves.
- Oculomotor nerves.
- Trochlear nerves.
- Trigeminal nerves.
- Abducent nerves.
- Facial nerves.
- Auditory nerves.
- Glossopharyngeal nerves.
- Vagus nerves.
- Accessory nerves.
- Hypoglossal nerves.

The autonomic nervous system

The autonomic division of the nervous system controls areas of the body over which there is no conscious control. It is divided into two sections:

- the sympathetic system
- the parasympathetic system.

The sympathetic system

The sympathetic system is composed of a gangliated cord which is situated on either side of the anterior surface of the vertebral column. It is composed of a network of interlaced nerves termed *plexuses*. The main plexuses of the sympathetic division are:

- solar plexus – which supplies the abdominal viscera
- cardiac plexus – which supplies the thoracic viscera
- hypogastric plexus – which supplies the pelvic region.

The parasympathetic system

This division is composed mainly of the vagus nerve which has the largest distribution of all the cranial nerves. It starts from nerve cells in the medulla oblongata and passes through the neck into the thorax and abdomen.

All the internal organs have in effect a double nerve supply, one supply from the sympathetic system and one from the parasympathetic system. The two systems work antagonistically. The sympathetic system increases body activity and the parasympathetic system slows it down.

The other area that the autonomic nervous system is involved with is the *reflex action*. This is an involuntary action designed to protect the body against serious damage. A very good example of this is if you touch a hot surface, before you have had time to register the pain in the normal way the reflex action spontaneously removes the finger.

ACTIVITY
Research the nerve supply for each of the muscles listed in this chapter.

Progress Check

1   Name and describe briefly the main divisions of the neurological system.
2   List the spinal nerves.

The endocrine system

The endocrine, or hormonal, system is a series of ductless glands that secrete *hormones* (chemical messengers) which act on parts of the body other than where they were produced. Hormones are carried in the blood stream and influence many activities of the body.

The main endocrine glands of the body are:

- Pituitary hypophysis gland.
- Thyroid gland.
- Prathyroid glands.
- Adrenal glands.
- Pancreas – the islets of Langerhans.
- Ovaries (female only).
- Testes (male only).

The pituitary hypophysis gland
The pituitary gland is sometimes referred to as the master gland because all the hormones it secretes have a bearing on all the other glands in the

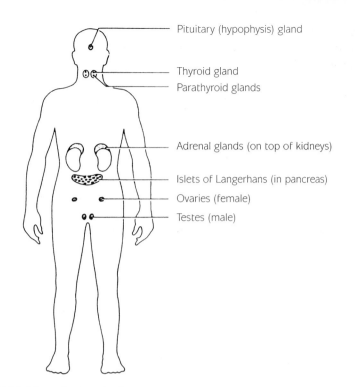

Fig. 1.20 *The endocrine glands*

system. It is situated in the head in the hypophyseal fossa of the sphenoid bone below the hypothalamus to which it is attached by an isthmus. The gland consist of a posterior and anterior lobe.

Anterior lobe

The anterior lobe of the pituitary gland secretes eight hormones in total all controlled by what is termed *the negative feedback mechanism*. This means that when the level of any particular hormone is low in the blood supplying the hypothalamus, it stimulates the anterior lobe of the pituitary to produce the appropriate releasing hormone which stimulates the target endocrine gland that produces that hormone to produce more.

The eight hormones secreted by the anterior lobe of the pituitary and their functions are:

- adrenocorticothrophic hormone (ACTH) – stimulates the adrenal cortex to secrete cortisol.
- Thyroid stimulating hormone (TSH) – stimulates activity and growth of the thyroid gland.
- Prolactin – directly affects the female breast immediately after childbirth to initiate and maintain milk secretion.
- Follicle stimulating hormone (FSH) – controls the maturation of the Graafian follicle in the ovary.
- Luteinising hormone (LH) – controls the activity of the gonads.
- Melanocyte stimulating hormone (MSH) – stimulates the production of melanin with the skin.
- Samatotrophin (HGH) – also known as human growth hormone, it promotes protein synthesis in growth and repair of all tissues.
- Interstitial cell stimulating hormone (ICSH) – controls gonad activity.

Posterior lobe

The posterior lobe of the pituitary gland secretes two hormones; *oxytocin* and *anti-diuretic hormone*.

Oxytocin promotes contraction of the uterine muscle and stimulates cells in the lactating breast to squeeze milk into the large ducts behind the nipple.

Anti-diuretic hormone (ADH) has two main functions:

- The *anti-diuretic effect* prevents water being lost from the kidneys and is influenced by osmotic pressure of the circulating blood.
- In large quantities ADH stimulates contraction of smooth muscle, especially in blood vessel walls, raising the blood pressure. This is called the *pressor effect*.

The thyroid gland

Situated in the lower part of the neck, the thyroid consists of a right and left lobe that lie either side of the trachea connected by an isthmus.

The thyroid secretes two main hormones:

- Thyroxin – necessary for controlling the metabolic rate, growth and differentiation of tissues, mental functioning and skin and hair condition.
- Calcitonin – reduces blood calcium levels by inhibiting the absorption of calcium from bones.

Parathyroid glands

The parathyroid glands are four small glands, two embedded in the posterior surface of each lobe of the thyroid gland. They secrete the hormone called *parathormone* which maintains the blood calcium concentration within its normal limits. It works in conjunction with calcitonin to control blood calcium levels.

Adrenal glands

There are two adrenal glands, one situated on the upper aspect of each kidney enclosed within the renal fascia. The glands are composed of two distinctive layers; the *adrenal cortex* and the *adrenal medulla*.

Adrenal cortex

The adrenal cortex produces three groups of hormones:

- Glucocorticoids – hormones which affect the regulation of carbohydrate metabolism, as well as helping in the formation of liver glycogen and helping *gluconeogenesis* (raising blood sugar levels). They suppress the body's inflammatory and allergic reactions and are connected with sodium and water reabsorption from the renal tubules.
- Mineral corticoids – hormones associated with the maintenance of the electrolyte balance in the body. They stimulate the reabsorption of sodium by the kidneys.
- Gonadocorticoids – sex hormones. The gonadocorticoids are *androgens* (male sex hormones) and the adrenal production is of little importance compared to the production of sex hormones by the ovaries/testes.

Adrenal medulla

The adrenal medulla is completely surrounded by the cortex, it is an extension of tissue from the same source as the nervous system and is closely linked to the sympathetic part of the autonomic nervous system.

The adrenal medulla secretes two hormones:

♦ Adrenaline (epinephrine) – associated with conditions needed for 'fight or flight'. Readies the body for immediate action. It triggers the constriction of peripheral blood vessels and the dilation of muscle fibres, enabling energy (food and oxygen) to be channelled where it is most needed. It also accelerates the conversion of glycogen to glucose.
♦ Noradrenaline (norepinephrine) – causes vasoconstriction and raises both systolic and diastolic blood pressure.

The pancreas

Hormones are produced in the pancreas by clusters of cells called *islets of Langerhans* which are distributed irregularly throughout the organ. There are three main types of cell in the islets of Langerhans. One of these cell types, the B cells, secrete the hormone *insulin* which together with glucagon, affects the level of glucose in the blood. The effect of insulin balances the effect of glucagon. Glucagon raises blood sugar levels while insulin reduces it.

The ovaries

The ovaries are the female gonads or sex glands. They are situated in shallow depressions on the lateral walls of the pelvis. The ovaries consist of a cortex and a medulla.

The ovarian cortex surrounds the medulla and contains ovarian follicles each of which contains an ovum. Throughout the reproductive years, one ovarian follicle matures, ruptures and releases its ovum during each menstrual cycle.

The ovarian medulla lies in the centre of the ovary and consists of fibrous tissue, blood vessels and nerves.

The two main hormones produced by the ovaries are:

♦ Oestrogen – influences the menstrual cycle. It stimulates the uterine lining to thicken to prepare for implantation should fertilisation occur. It is also partly responsible for breast development – the growth of milk ducts in the breast. It also influences health and growth of bones, subcutaneous fat distribution and skin condition.
♦ Progesterone – connected with the development of the placenta and the maintenance of pregnancy when it occurs. It also prepares the mammary glands for lactation.

> **USEFUL INFORMATION**
>
> Insulin plays a part in the following processes:
>
> * Conversion of glucose to glycogen in the liver and muscles.
> * Synthesis of DNA and RNA.
> * Prevention of protein and fat breakdown.
> * Storage of fat in adipose tissue.

> **ACTIVITY**
> Research the effects of pregnancy on the female body.

The testes

The testes are the male gonads. They consist of 200 to 300 lobules composed of germinal epithelial cells. Between these lobules are interstitial cells that secrete the main male hormone *testosterone*.

Testosterone is responsible for the secondary sexual characteristics that occur at puberty in males. Secondary sexual characteristics in males include:

- Increase in body hair.
- Deepening of the voice.
- Broadening of muscles.

Progress Check

1   State the importance of the endocrine system.
2   Research the main disorders of the endocrine system.

The respiratory system

The respiratory system is involved in the taking in of oxygen and the removal of carbon dioxide from the body. This process is achieved through a number of specialised organs and tissues.

The respiratory system consists of:

- Nose.
- Pharynx.
- Larynx.
- Trachea.
- Two bronchi.
- Bronchioles.
- Two lungs.
- Intercostal muscles.
- Diaphragm.

Nose

The function of the nose is to warm, filter and moisten air. This function is achieved by tiny, ciliated, columnar epithelium which trap bacteria and dust. They secrete mucous which moistens the air as well as acting as an adhesive medium to prevent bacteria and dust entering the throat. Once air has passed through the nose it moves on to the pharynx.

Pharynx

The pharynx has both a respiratory and a digestive function. The respiratory function of the pharynx is similar to that of the nose – it further warms and moistens air before it travels on to the next air passage, called the larynx.

Larynx

At the top of the larynx there is a flap of tissue called the *epiglottis* which closes to stop food entering the trachea during swallowing. Air passing over the vocal cords within the larynx produces the voice.

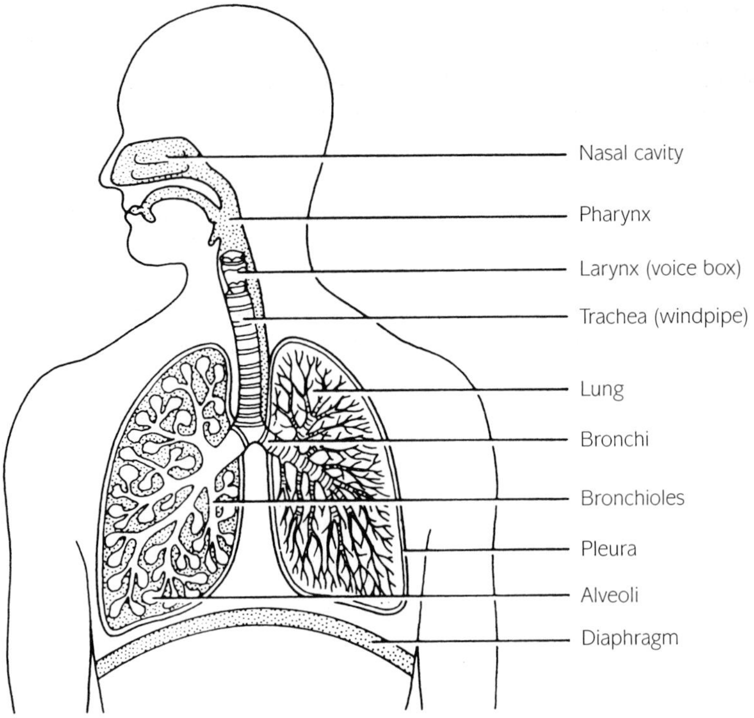
Nasal cavity
Pharynx
Larynx (voice box)
Trachea (windpipe)
Lung
Bronchi
Bronchioles
Pleura
Alveoli
Diaphragm

Fig. 1.21 *The respiratory system*

Trachea

Also referred to as the windpipe, the trachea consists of a tube surrounded by c-shaped rings of cartilage that act to keep the trachea open even when the neck is bent. It is lined with ciliated epithelium which secrete mucous – a further air-filtration system.

Bronchi

There are two bronchi; the left bronchus and the right bronchus. The bronchi are branches of the trachea that supply the left and right lungs. The right bronchus is wider and more vertical than the left. Both are further divided into a network of narrower passages called bronchioles.

Bronchioles

As mentioned above, bronchioles are narrow passageways which branch from the bronchi. They can branch many times and end in tiny air sacs called alveoli.

Alveoli

Alveoli are extremely tiny, thin-walled, elastic air sacs. They are lined by a flat epithelium and surrounded by pulmonary capillaries. The barrier between the gas in the alveoli and the blood in the vessels is so thin that oxygen and carbon dioxide can pass across it.

Lungs

The lungs are a pair of conical organs each surrounded by a specialised membrane called the *pleura*. The pleura consists of two layers moistened by a special fluid, resembling lymph, which acts as a lubricant enabling the two surfaces to glide smoothly over each other during respiration.

Intercostal muscles
There are both external and internal intercostal muscles. Both sets lie between the ribs. They are responsible for raising and lowering the chest during *inspiration* (breathing in) and *expiration* (breathing out).

Diaphragm
The diaphragm is a sheet of muscle that separates the thorax from the abdomen. It is a little unusual in that when it is contracted it becomes flattened and when relaxed it is dome-shaped. The muscle originates from the tip of the sternum, the lower ribs and the cartilages of the lumbar vertebrae and is inserted into the central aponeurosis (a flattened-out tendon). Three openings in the diaphragm allow for the passage of the oesophagus, the aorta and the vena cava. The flattening of the diaphragm increases the volume of the chest cavity, aiding inspiration. Relaxing the diaphragm decreases the volume of the chest cavity, aiding expiration.

How the respiratory system works
The processes of respiration can be summarised in four parts:

- Movement of air in and out of the lungs.
- Free passage of air down the airways.
- Gaseous exchange.
- Control of respiration.

Movement of air in and out of the lungs
During inspiration the intercostal muscles contract, moving the rib-cage upwards and outwards, and the diaphragm contracts downwards to a more flattened position. This causes the thorax to increase in volume, hence decreasing the pressure in the chest cavity. This causes a pressure difference to develop between the inside and outside of the lungs. Air moves from the region of higher pressure (outside the lungs) to the region of lower pressure (inside the lungs) until the pressure difference is removed.

During expiration the diaphragm and intercostal muscles relax and the ribcage returns to the normal position. This has the effect of reducing the volume within the thorax, increasing the air pressure in the lungs, forcing air out of the lungs.

Free passage of air down the airways
As air is breathed in through the nose it passes over hairs and mucous which filter and warm the air. The air passes through the naso-pharynx where it is further filtered and warmed, to the larynx and down the trachea. The trachea also contains mucous secreting ciliated cells which remove any debris from the inhaled air not already dealt with. The air then moves into the bronchial tree, through the bronchi and bronchioles to reach the alveoli.

The air retraces this journey through expiration.

Gaseous exchange
In the lungs, oxygen from the inspired air in the alveolus passes across the alveolar membrane and the capillary walls to combine with haemo-globin in the red blood cells. Simultaneously, carbon dioxide diffuses back from the blood into the alveolar air so that it can be exhaled.

> **USEFUL INFORMATION**
> Air is composed of approximately:
>
> * Nitrogen, 78%
> * Oxygen, 21%
> * Inert gases, 0.07%
> * Carbon dioxide, 0.03% (variable)
> * Water vapour (variable).

Control of respiration
Control of respiration is achieved through both chemical and neurological means. Respiration is controlled by nerve cells in the medulla oblongata in what is known as the *respiratory centre*. It is further controlled by chemoreceptors in the walls of the aorta and carotid arteries which are sensitive to changes in oxygen and carbon dioxide concentrations in the blood.

Progress Check

1 State the composition of air.
2 Describe briefly the mechanism of breathing.

The digestive system

The digestive system is concerned with the taking in and breakdown of food. There are two phases to digestion, mechanical and chemical.

The digestive system consists of the alimentary tract or canal and the glands secreting digestive juices which act upon the food matter.

The alimentary canal is a passage over 9 metres long leading from the mouth to the rectum. It is lined throughout with a mucous membrane which lubricates the system. Muscular walls act upon the foodstuffs eaten and help their passage along the alimentary canal. The alimentary canal consists of:

- Mouth.
- Pharynx.
- Oesophagus.
- Stomach.
- Small intestine.
- Large intestine.

The glands are:

- Salivary glands – secreting saliva in the mouth.
- Gastric glands – secreting gastric juices in the stomach.
- Pancreas – secreting pancreatic juice in the duodenum.
- Liver – secreting bile in the duodenum.
- Intestinal glands – secreting intestinal juice in the small intestine.

Mouth
Digestion commences mechanically and chemically in the mouth with the action of the teeth and salivary glands respectively.

There are 32 permanent teeth in the adult mouth of four types. Each type of tooth has a specific function in the breakdown of food; the *incisors* are adapted to break off food, the *canines* are adapted to tear at meat and the *premolars* and *molars* are adapted to grind and chew.

The tongue also plays a part in mechanical digestion. It consists of striated voluntary muscle attached mainly to the mandible and hyoid

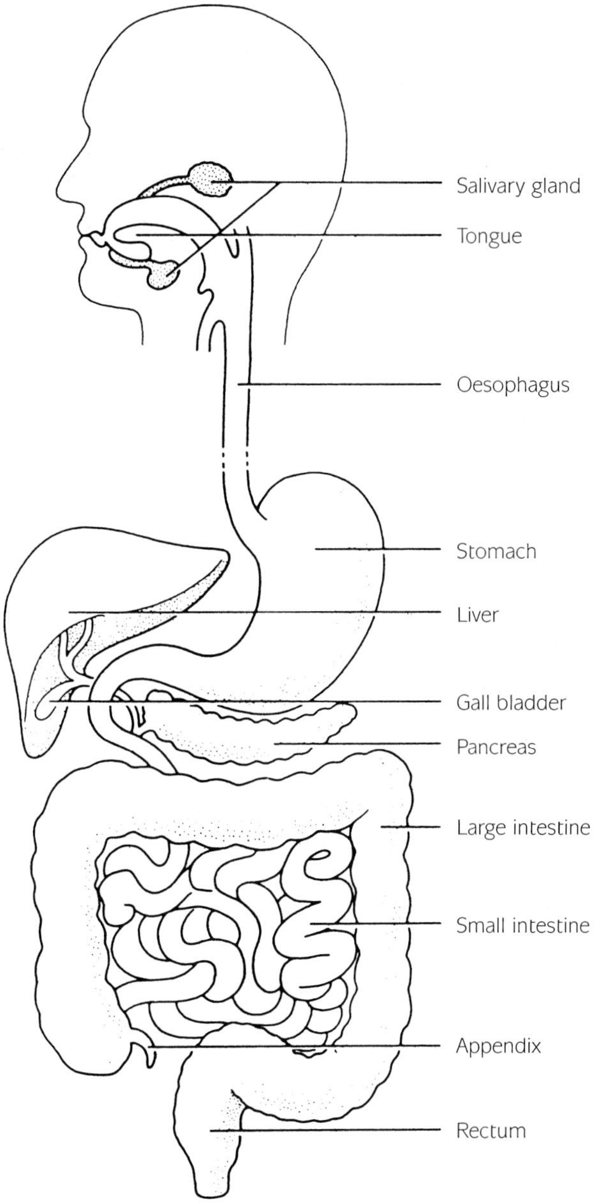

Salivary gland
Tongue
Oesophagus
Stomach
Liver
Gall bladder
Pancreas
Large intestine
Small intestine
Appendix
Rectum

Fig. 1.22 *The digestive system*

bones and helps in the swallowing action by forming the food into a suitably sized ball, or *bolus*, and moving it to the pharynx at the back of the mouth.

The salivary glands in the mouth begin chemical digestion. There are two parotid glands, two mandibular glands and two sublingual glands (the names indicate their positions in the mouth). They secrete a watery substance called *saliva* which contains the digestive enzyme *ptyalin* (amylase) which in involved in the first stage of the digestion of carbohydrates.

Pharynx

At the back of the mouth lies the pharynx which is about 13 cm long and leads backwards from the mouth. It consists of three areas – the naso pharynx, the oral pharynx and the larygeal pharynx. The oral pharynx is shared by both air and food and the larygeal pharynx merges with the oesophagus. When food is swallowed, the pharynx contracts forcing food downwards into the oesophagus.

Oesophagus

The oesophagus is a muscular tube 25–30 cm long leading from the pharynx to the stomach. It is composed of voluntary and involuntary muscle fibres which work in a wave-like motion called *peristalsis* to propel food into the stomach.

Stomach

The stomach is a muscular sac-like organ placed on the left side of the abdominal cavity beneath the diaphragm. At either end of the stomach are valves, called *sphincters*, which allow or restrict the movement of food into or out of the stomach. The *cardiac sphincter* lies between the oesophagus and the top of the stomach and the *pyloric sphincter* lies between the bottom of the stomach and the duodenum.

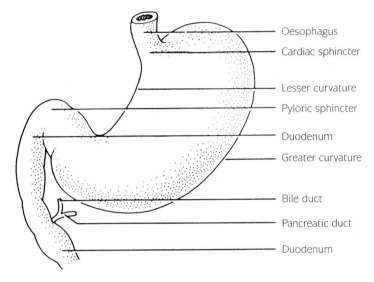

Fig. 1.23 *The stomach*

The stomach has several distinct layers. The outermost layer is called the *peritoneum* and its main function is to prevent friction with other organs in the abdominal cavity. The peritoneum is a serous membrane, that is it produces a fluid called serum which acts as a lubricant. Next there is a muscular layer, then a layer which is composed of connective tissue and is rich in blood vessels. Forming the stomach lining is a mucous layer. The layers of the stomach have the ability to expand and contract according to the amount of food consumed. The surface of the inner stomach is convoluted. This provides a greater surface area for the action of secreted acidic gastric juices on the food. Food is held in the stomach until it becomes liquefied and has been partially digested.

Chemical digestion continues in the stomach. Protein digestion commences; proteins are broken down to *peptones*. Gastric juice contains *hydrochloric acid* and the enzymes *pepsin* and *rennin*. The acid is antiseptic in action and provides the correct medium for the digestive juices to work in.

Mechanical digestion is also continued in the stomach. The food is churned with strong muscular movements and leaves the stomach in a series of gushes.

Some substances ingested are absorbed directly into the body from the stomach; these include water, alcohol and glucose.

Small intestine

This part of the digestive tract leads from the stomach to the large intestine and is 6–7.4 metres in length. It has three main sections: the *duodenum*, the *jejunum* and the *ileum*.

The duodenum is the first part of the small intestine and is attached to the back of the abdominal wall by peritoneum. It is approximately 24 cm long and curves like the letter C. Lying within the curve is the pancreas.

The jejunum and ileum form most of the total length of the small intestine and lie to the front of the abdominal cavity. The structure of the small intestine is similar to the stomach externally but internally it is puckered and covered with hair-like projections called *villi*. These have the effect of increasing the surface area of the small intestine. Digestion products are absorbed into the villi.

Within the small intestine, the digestion of protein, carbohydrate and fats takes place. Enzymes from three types of digestive juice – *pancreatic juice* from the pancreas, *bile* from the liver, *succus entericus* from the small intestine – affect this digestion. Peptones from the stomach are broken down to polypeptides and finally to amino-acids; carbohydrates are broken down to simple sugars, e.g. glucose; fats and oils are broken down to fatty acids and glycerol. Fatty acids and glycerol after absorption may be used for energy by muscles in activity, or stored.

Large intestine

The large intestine is the last stage of the alimentary tract and begins at the ileum and ends at the rectum. It is about 1.5 metres in length and is divided into three parts:

- the ascending colon
- the transverse colon
- the descending colon.

The first part of the ascending colon consists of a lined pouch called the *caecum* from which extends the *vermiform appendix*. It contains the *ileo-caecal* valve which allows on-flow, but prevents back-flow, of intestinal contents. The remainder of food undigested, plus roughage and unabsorbed digestive juice pass from the small intestine into the large intestine in a liquid form. Here the water is reabsorbed and the solid faeces are formed.

Glands of the digestive system

The liver

The liver is the largest gland in the body, weighing between 1 and 2.3 kg. It is situated in the upper part of the abdominal cavity and consists of four lobes. Blood rich in nutrients is supplied to the liver via the *hepatic portal vein* which carries blood from the stomach, spleen, pancreas and the intestines. Arterial blood is supplied to the liver via the *hepatic artery*. The right and left *hepatic ducts* carry bile from the liver to the gall bladder. The main digestive functions of the liver are:

- Production of bile, which together with lipase from the pancreas commences the first stage of fat digestion.
- Synthesis of vitamin A from carotene.
- Storage of vitamins, namely B12, A, D, E, K and iron.

The pancreas

The pancreas is a pale grey gland weighing approximately 60 g. It is situated high on the left side of the abdominal cavity behind the stomach. The pancreas consists of a large number of lobules made up of small alveoli and these secrete pancreatic juice which contains the enzymes *lipase, trypsin, chymotrypsin* and *amylase*. Lipase converts fats into monoglycerides, diglycerides and fatty acids. Trypsin and chymotrypsin convert peptones (protein) into polypeptides. Amylase converts carbohydrates (starch) into maltose.

USEFUL INFORMATION

The pancreas is both an endocrine and an exocrine gland as it secretes hormones (see p. 32) and also has a digestive function.

Progress Check

1. Explain briefly the digestive process.
2. What are the main functions of the liver?

The urinary system

The urinary system consists of:

- The kidneys.
- Ureters.
- Bladder.
- Urethra.

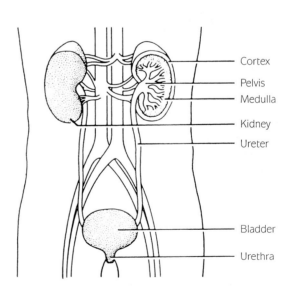

Fig. 1.24 *The urinary system*

The kidneys

There are two kidneys, each approximately 11 cm in length by 6 cm in width. They lie high on the posterior wall of the abdomen. Each kidney consists of an outer layer called a fibrous capsule, a *cortex*, an inner *medulla* which contains *renal pyramids* and the pelvis.

Each kidney receives blood at very high pressure through a renal artery. Once inside the kidney, the artery divides into smaller capillaries which carry the blood to tiny cup-shaped structures called *glomerular capsules*. The glomerular capsules are the beginning of lengths of narrow tubes, approximately 3 cm long called *nephrons*. Urine is produced in the nephrons.

Formation of urine

The capillary inside each glomerular capsule divides into a tiny bundle of inter-twined blood vessels called a *glomerulus*. Blood pressure is so high in this area that liquid is forced out through the capillary walls into the space inside the glomerular capsule. This liquid is known as *glomerular filtrate*. It contains urea to be excreted together with many useful substances (e.g. glucose, amino acids, mineral salts, vitamins and large amounts of water) which the body cannot afford to lose. These substances are reabsorbed in the nephron.

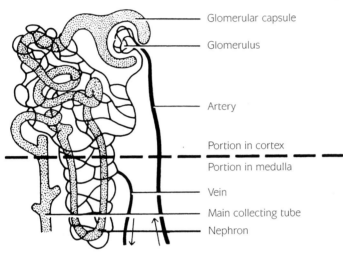

Fig. 1.25 *The internal structure of a kidney*

Reabsorption

Glomerular filtrate flows out of the glomerular capsules into the tubular part of each nephron; it is here that reabsorption occurs. The walls of the nephron extract useful substances from the filtrate and these pass into blood flowing through capillaries surrounding the nephron. What is left now is *urine*, which consists of waste products such as urea, uric acid and small amounts of mineral salts.

The ureters, bladder and urethra

A thin tube called a *ureter* which is attached to the concave side of each kidney conveys the urine to a single large bag called the *bladder*. The bladder has only one exit, a tube called the *urethra*, which leads to the body's surface. The bladder end of the urethra is closed by means of a sphincter. Urine drains continuously out of the kidneys into the ureters, where it is forced downwards into the bladder by wave-like contractions. The bladder stretches and expands as it fills with urine. When the bladder is full, the stretching stimulates sensory nerve endings in its walls which convey nerve impulses to the brain letting you know when your bladder must be emptied. The sphincter muscles around the urethra are then voluntarily relaxed allowing urine to drain from the bladder through the urethra and out of the body.

Progress Check

1   Explain briefly how urine is produced.
2   Describe the appearance of a kidney.

Anatomy of the female breast

The breasts are the accessory glands of the female reproductive system and are composed of fatty, fibrous and glandular tissues. Breasts mature in the female at puberty under the influence of the female hormones oestrogen and progesterone.

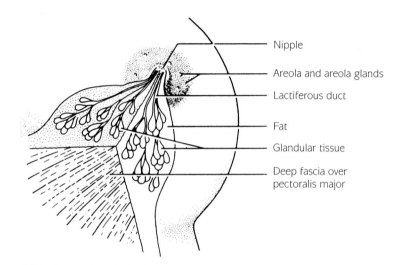

Nipple

Areola and areola glands

Lactiferous duct

Fat

Glandular tissue

Deep fascia over pectoralis major

Fig. 1.26 *Section through the breast*

The breasts are structured for breast feeding with each consisting of about 15–20 lobes of glandular tissue. These are formed from lobules and are connected by areolar tissue, blood vessels and ducts. Each lobule is made up from tiny little sacs called alveoli which collectively form lactiferous ducts. These converge towards the nipple (or *areolar*) where they form a *lactiferous sinus* whose function is to act as reservoir for milk in the event of lactation.

Fatty tissue covers the entire surface of the breast whilst fibrous tissue, in conjunction with the pectoral muscle group lying directly underneath on the chest wall, provides support for the breast.

POINT TO NOTE

Suspensory ligaments in the form of fibrous tissue give the breasts their firm contour. The firm contour decreases as we age. It is therefore extremely important to wear a good, properly fitted, supporting bra at all times.

1   What is the main function of the female breast?
2   Explain the importance of the pectoralis muscle group.

Key Terms

You need to know what these words and phrases mean. Go back through the chapter to find out.

- Blood and lymphatic circulation
- Cells and tissues
- Dermis
- Digestive system
- Endocrine glands
- Epidermis
- Female breast
- Heart
- Kidneys
- Neurological system
- Respiratory system
- Skeletal system
- Subcutis
- Types of muscular tissue

After working through this chapter you will be able to:

- list the different nutrients required for a balanced diet
- identify the different food sources for the different nutrients
- list the reasons why people may wish to gain or lose weight
- list different types of diet
- recognise the different body types
- identify a number of postural problems
- list the components of fitness
- understand the factors that should be considered when offering corrective exercise home care advice.

As many clients attend health spas and clinics to support them in a weight loss programme, it is important that the therapist has an understanding of basic nutrition. It must however be stressed that the role of the therapist is not that of a dietician who undertakes specialist training in this field. Health spas employ medical staff to carry out a client's initial consultation and will refer them to the dietician if a special diet is needed due to medical conditions such as diabetes or if the client wishes to lose weight. Many therapists in salons work in close liaison with doctors, particularly if offering specialised treatments such as alpha hydroxy acids or collagen injections, and some salons extend their range of treatments to include dietary advice under medical supervision. It is strongly recommended that the therapist should only supplement their clients' weight loss programmes with information on healthy eating. The therapist must refer the client to their doctor if they have any underlying medical problems or a serious weight condition.

Basic nutrition

In order for our body to operate efficiently it requires a well-balanced diet. In general a normal varied diet will provide all the nutrients required for health, though during illness or pregnancy the diet will require additional supplements, e.g. iron is often needed to supplement the diet of expectant mothers. During the latter half of the twentieth century there was a greater tendency for mothers to take up employment and this trend, along with the advancements in convenience foods, has been responsible for a move away from the traditional diet. However, more recently, people have become health conscious and realise that trends in lifestyle may lead to an unbalanced diet. Many people now pay more care and attention to their diet.

Nutrition, in conjunction with digestion, is the process by which the body absorbs foodstuffs and converts them to substances that it requires for life. Food is made up of differing amounts of substances and these can either be used directly by our bodies or converted into other substances our bodies need. The types of food required by a healthy

USEFUL INFORMATION

* Disaccharides consist of two monosaccharide molecules which chemically combine. Sucrose, maltose and lactose are disaccharides.
* Polysaccharides are complex molecules consisting of large numbers of monosaccharide molecules chemically combined. Starches, glycogen, cellulose and dextrin are polysaccharides. The body cannot digest all polysaccharides. For example, cellulose, present in vegetables and fruit and some cereals, passes through the alimentary canal almost unchanged.

individual are: proteins, carbohydrates, fats, water, fibre, mineral elements and vitamins.

Proteins

Proteins are used by the body for the growth and repair of body tissues. They also act as a secondary source of energy. Proteins are broken down during digestion into amino acids. Proteins are made up of varying amounts of different amino acids and can be sub-divided into two categories; first class proteins and second class proteins.

First class proteins

First class proteins are those that contain all the essential amino acids required by the body. Sources of first class proteins are meat, milk, eggs, fish and soya beans.

Second class proteins

Second class proteins are those that do not contain all the essential amino acids. Sources of second class proteins are pulses and nuts.

POINTS TO NOTE

- Proteins are made up of carbon, hydrogen, oxygen and nitrogen. Some also contain phosphorous and sulphur.
- Most sources of first class protein are of animal origin. Vegetarian diets, particularly vegan diets, can be deficient in certain essential amino acids.

USEFUL INFORMATION

Amino acids not needed by the body are broken down in the liver. The nitrogeneous part is converted into urea and excreted in urine and the rest, if needed, is used for energy or stored as fat.

Carbohydrates

Carbohydrates provide the body with energy. If an excess of carbohydrates is eaten the body converts them and stores them as fat. Sources of carbohydrates are starchy and sugary foods such as cereals, bread, potatoes, sugar, vegetables and fruits.

Carbohydrates are digested in the alimentary canal and are absorbed into the body in the form of monosaccharides, the simplest chemical form in which carbohydrates can exist. Examples of monosaccharides are glucose, fructose and galactose.

POINTS TO NOTE

- Carbohydrates are made up of carbon, hydrogen and oxygen.
- Starch forms the larger proportion of the carbohydrates we eat in our food. It must be broken down by the body into simple sugars before it can be used as an energy source.
- The body breaks down complex sugars and starch into glucose which is the form in which fuel is transported around to the different organs of the body.

Fats

The body needs a certain quantity of fat to protect organs, provide insulation, transport fat-soluble vitamins and provide energy. Excess fat in the diet is converted into fatty acids and stored until it is needed. Fats come from either animal or vegetable sources.

Examples of foods containing animal fats are meat, cheese, butter, milk and eggs. Vegetable oils and margarine contain vegetable fats.

Cholesterol is a fat-like substance which is produced naturally in the bodies of all animals. A high level of cholesterol in the blood encourages the build up of deposits of fat on the inside walls of arteries which can lead to heart problems.

Water

A large proportion of the body weight is made up of water. Water is found in the blood and tissue fluids and aids in digestion, maintaining the body temperature and health of cells. It also dilutes waste products and assists in their elimination. It is found throughout the body in varying quantities and is essential to life. The body excretes around two litres of water per day in the form of urine and perspiration. The body re-balances its fluid loss by absorbing water from drinks and food. The majority of foods we eat contain some water.

Fibre

Fibre is a nutrient that is not digestible but is required by the body to assist in the digestion process, in particular excretion. It provides the diet with bulk, helping to satisfy the appetite and provides a medium on which peristalsis can work, hence aiding the movement of food through the alimentary canal.

Mineral elements

Minerals are needed by the body to maintain health. They are not required in large quantities in the diet.

Calcium

Calcium is needed for the formation and maintenance of healthy teeth and bones and for muscular activity. It can be found in foods such as milk, cheese and eggs.

Iodine

Iodine is essential for the formation of the hormone thyroxine from the thyroid gland. It is only needed in very small quantities and can be found in foods such as watercress, seafood and iodised salt.

Iron

Iron is used by the body to manufacture haemoglobin. Women generally require more iron in their diet than men as they lose blood, and therefore iron, during menstruation. During pregnancy expectant mothers often need to supplement their diet with additional iron to maintain their own health and that of the foetus. Iron can be found in foods such as liver and green vegetables, e.g. spinach.

Magnesium

Magnesium is needed by the body for metabolism and the composition of bones, nerves and muscles. It can be found in foods such as green vegetables, wholegrain cereals and lentils.

Manganese

Manganese is necessary for metabolism and can be found in foods such as kidneys, lentils, almonds, apricots, wheatgerm and watercress.

Phosphorous

Phosphorous is needed for the formation of teeth and bones. It is a constituent of cells and plays a part in the maintenance of body fluid balance and aids in the utilisation of energy from foods. It can be found in foods such as cheese, eggs, meat, fish, yeast, wheatgerm and green vegetables.

Potassium

Potassium is needed to maintain the body's fluid balance and is also involved in the functioning of nerves and muscles. It can be found in the majority of foods, especially milk, cheese, seafood, bananas, spinach, butter and baked potatoes.

Sodium

Sodium is required to maintain the fluid balance of the body. It also plays an important role in the transmission of impulses from the nerves and in muscular contraction. It can be found in the majority of foods, in particular salt.

Sulphur

Sulphur helps with the formation of body tissues and can be found in foods such as eggs, fish, cheese, meat and beans.

Trace elements

Trace elements are found in extremely small quantities within the body and are needed for a variety of body processes such as digestion. Examples of trace elements are copper, cobalt, fluorine and zinc.

Zinc

Zinc is found in foods such as fish and nuts and is important for a healthy skin. It protects and repairs DNA and can be found in high levels in animals and fish. Oysters contain the highest dietary sources of zinc. Zinc is essential for male and female fertility and it must be noted that stress, smoking and alcohol deplete zinc.

> **USEFUL INFORMATION**
> Some vegan diets can be deficient in zinc.

> **POINTS TO NOTE**
>
> - Mineral elements are often called mineral salts.
> - Deficiency in iron leads to anaemia.
> - Calcium absorption diminishes in females over 50.
> - Anti-oxidants are nutrients that help to protect the body from damage caused by preventing and treating disease. The main anti-oxidants are considered to be Vitamins A, C, E and beta-carotene (the precursor of vitamin A found in fruit and vegetables).

Vitamins

Vitamins have no energy value but are essential organic substances required in small quantities for health and certain chemical activities of the body.

They can be categorised into two groups:

- ● Water-soluble vitamins such as B complex and C.
- ● Fat-soluble vitamins such as A, D, E and K.

> **USEFUL INFORMATION**
>
> The liver can convert carotene, which is found in foods such as carrots and spinach, into vitamin A.

Vitamin A (retinol)

Vitamin A is needed for growth of the majority of body cells and is particularly important for healthy eyesight. Deficiency in vitamin A can lead to poor night vision and dry skin. Good sources of vitamin A are milk, butter, cream, eggs, cheese, carrots, green vegetables and oily fish, e.g. sardines.

Vitamin B complex

Vitamin B includes a complex of vitamins:

- ● Vitamin B1 (thiamine) helps the nervous system to function and controls the release of energy from carbohydrates. Examples of food sources are wheatgerm, offal, yeast, eggs and nuts.
- ● Vitamin B2 (riboflavin) is needed for energy and health of the mouth and skin. It can be found in foods such as eggs, cheese, kidneys and liver. It is resistant to heat but can be destroyed by sunlight.
- ● Pantothenic acid is essential for the body's nervous system and in the burning of fat for energy. Examples of food containing pantothenic acid are liver, egg yolk and vegetables. It is present in most types of food.
- ● Vitamin B6 (pyridoxine) helps with many of the body's functions and is obtained from foods such as brewer's yeast, bread, wholegrain cereal, milk, eggs and liver.
- ● Niacin or nicotinic acid is crucial for the utilisation of energy and healthy skin. It plays parts in both the digestive and nervous systems. It can be found in food such as liver, eggs, cheese, brewer's yeast and bread.
- ● Folic acid is important for the formation of red blood cells and can be found in foods such as liver, kidneys and fresh green vegetables.
- ● Vitamin B12 is needed in the body for the production of red blood cells. Examples of food sources are meat and dairy products.
- ● Biotin is required for healthy skin and hair. It is produced naturally by the body and can be obtained from such food stuffs as liver, yeast, kidneys and egg yolk.

Vitamin C (ascorbic acid)

Vitamin C assists in the formation of connective tissue, the absorption of iron and the development and maintenance of healthy bones. It can be found in foods such as vegetables and citrus fruits, e.g. oranges.

POINT TO NOTE

Some vitamins such as B and C are sensitive to heat and can be destroyed in the cooking process.

Vitamin D (calciferol)

Vitamin D assists in depositing phosphorous and calcium in the bones and is therefore required for the formation of healthy, strong bones and teeth. Examples of foods with a rich supply of vitamin D are cheese, eggs, margarine, butter and fatty fish. The body can produce vitamin D when exposed to sunlight and is able to store it in the liver.

Vitamin E (tocopherol)

The function of vitamin E is not known, however it is thought that a deficiency prevents growth. It can be found in foods such as peanuts, milk, vegetable oils, eggs, fish, wholemeal bread and cereals. Deep-frying destroys a lot of this vitamin.

Vitamin K

Vitamin K is needed for the clotting mechanism of blood. It can be obtained from green vegetables, fruit and liver.

Vitamin P (rutin)

Vitamin P strengthens capillary walls. A rich source can be found in green buckwheat tea.

ACTIVITY

Compile lists of a child's and an adult's daily food intake and note the different nutrients that will have been absorbed by their bodies.

Progress Check

1 List the nutrients required for a balanced diet.
2 Give an example of a good food source for each of the following nutrients:
   a protein   **c** fats   **e** iron and calcium.
   b carbohydrate   **d** vitamins A and C
3 State how each of the following is used by the body:
   a protein   **d** calcium   **g** vitamin C
   b carbohydrate   **e** iron   **h** vitamin D.
   c fats   **f** vitamin A

Metabolism

Metabolism is the process by which the body makes use of the food it takes in and utilises it for energy, growth and general health. The body metabolises basic food elements in two general ways:

- Catabolism is the way in which the body releases energy by breaking down food.
- Anabolism is the way in which the body builds up or utilises cell structures from digested food materials.

Calorific requirements

The body needs a well-balanced diet to meet its individual daily requirements. The calorific requirement of an individual is the amount of energy the body needs to stay warm and do any work required of it. Fats have a higher calorific value than carbohydrates, i.e. they contain more energy per unit weight, and carbohydrates have a higher calorific value than proteins. As people vary in size, age, gender and way of life, each individual will have different nutritional needs. It is therefore impossible to state a general energy requirement to suit everybody. Women generally require less energy than men; manual workers require more energy than sedentary office workers; older people require less energy than younger people.

Basal metabolism

The basal metabolism is the minimum energy output required by the body for vital functioning, e.g. respiration, heart beat, peristalsis, etc. The basal metabolic rate varies according to gender, age, lifestyle and body size. It also tends to decrease with age. If the body absorbs more energy from foods than it needs for basal metabolism and the work it does (e.g. exercise), it will store the excess as fat around the body.

POINTS TO NOTE

- As the body ages the basal metabolic rate will fall by an average of 5% every 10 years.
- Regular exercise increases the metabolic rate as muscle cells burn up more calories than fat cells even when at rest.

Diets

Social and peer-group pressures regarding the way individuals look can create a great deal of stress in people's lives. One of the major influencing factors in how people feel about themselves often relates to how they truly feel about their body shape and size. It cannot be stated that obese people are more unhappy with their appearance than extremely thin people as feelings are individual and other factors in people's lives often alter their emotions, e.g. the excitement of a new job or home, or a loving relationship can all detract from past insecurities and can bring about weight loss or gain! There are a variety of reasons why a person may be over or under weight, e.g. a lack of, or excessive exercise, poor diet. Some people suffer with weight problems due to medical conditions such as an over or under active thyroid gland.

POINTS TO NOTE

A general indicator to assess a client's frame size is the circumference of their wrist:

- 14 cm (5 ½ inches) = Small
- 15.25 cm (6 inches) = Medium
- 16.5 cm (6 ½ inches) = Large

For figure assessment, when measuring a client:

- Remember to consider their modesty – only expose the areas you need to measure.
- Do not pull the tape measure tight.
- Always record the measurements accurately.

There are a variety of reasons why people may wish to lose or gain weight including:

- To feel healthy and fit.
- To feel happy with their appearance.
- To restore their figure after childbirth.
- To prevent coronary conditions.

It is a common misconception that it is only women who worry about weight problems. In today's society men take a lot more time and effort over their appearance and although some may not show it they often suffer in the same way as women if they are not happy with the way they look. People may wish to diet to improve their total shape whilst others may feel that they have problems with particular areas such as the abdomen, thighs and hips. For whatever reason a person wishes to lose or gain weight they must be sensible in adjusting their diet to ensure it meets the body's nutritional requirements and suits their lifestyle.

There are many books available on different types of diet and fact sheets available through doctors, hospitals and slimming organisations. The important thing to remember if wishing to lose weight is that the body stores excess energy obtained from fats, carbohydrates and proteins in the form of fat around the body. As a person continually takes in surplus energy requirements, the fat cells will increase in size and thus they will gain more and more weight. Therefore the diet will need to be balanced and they will need to increase their energy output to burn up the excess fat. For those wishing to gain weight it is often quite difficult to increase the intake of foods with a high calorific value and the process of weight gain for many people is a slow and arduous task.

POINTS TO NOTE

- Weight loss should be slow and controlled, as often people who lose weight rapidly find it returns fairly quickly.
- Individuals develop different eating habits, e.g. some people like to nibble whilst others like full meals and others need to satisfy a sweet tooth.

POINTS TO NOTE

- Body mass index (BMI) can be calculated by dividing the client's weight (in kilograms) by the square of the client's height (in metres). This can be used as a guide to five BMI groups:
- Underweight: BMI 19.9 and below
- Normal: BMI 20–24.9
- Grade 1 obesity: BMI 25–29.9
- Grade 2 obesity: BMI 30–39.9
- Grade 3 obesity: BMI 40 and above

Women

ft ins	cm	Small lbs	kg	Medium lbs	kg	Large lbs	kg
4 10	147	102–111	46–50	109–121	49–55	118–131	54–59
4 11	150	103–113	47–51	111–123	50–56	120–134	55–61
5 0	152	104–115	47–52	113–126	51–57	122–137	56–62
5 1	155	106–118	48–54	115–129	52–59	125–140	57–61
5 2	158	108–121	49–55	118–132	54–60	128–143	58–65
5 3	160	111–124	50–56	121–135	55–61	131–147	59–67
5 4	163	114–127	52–58	124–138	56–63	134–151	61–69
5 5	165	117–130	53–59	127–141	58–64	137–155	62–70
5 6	168	120–133	55–60	130–144	59–65	140–159	63–72
5 7	170	123–136	56–62	133–147	60–67	143–163	65–74
5 8	173	126–139	57–63	136–150	62–68	146–167	66–76
5 9	175	129–142	59–64	139–153	63–69	149–170	68–77
5 10	178	132–145	60–66	142–156	64–71	152–173	69–79
5 11	180	135–148	61–67	145–159	66–72	155–176	70–80
6 0	183	138–151	63–69	148–162	67–74	158–179	72–81

Men

ft ins	cm	Small lbs	Medium lbs	Large lbs
5 2	158	128–134	131–141	138–150
5 3	160	130–136	133–144	140–153
5 4	163	132–138	135–145	142–156
5 5	165	134–140	137–148	144–160
5 6	168	136–142	139–151	146–164
5 7	170	138–145	142–154	149–168
5 8	173	140–148	145–157	152–172
5 9	175	142–151	148–160	155–176
5 10	178	144–154	151–163	158–180
5 11	180	146–157	154–166	161–184
6 0	183	149–160	157–170	164–188
6 1	185	152–164	160–174	168–192
6 2	188	155–168	164–178	172–197
6 3	190	158–172	167–182	176–202
6 4	193	162–176	171–187	181–207

Fig. 2.1 *Charts to show an example of accepted weight norms of gender, height and frame size*

Types of diet

There are many types of diet available to suit individual requirements. Some of these are outlined below.

Calorie controlled diet

This type of diet limits the quantity of calories the individual takes in per day, but enables them to select the types of food they eat. It is also a useful diet for those who eat out socially as it allows them to save calories for that special meal without everyone they eat with focusing on the fact that they are on a diet. It can also assist those who have a sweet tooth by enabling them to save calories for a treat.

High protein diet

A high protein diet is suitable for people who want to build muscles. However, a diet high in protein can still produce excess energy requirements as protein is a secondary source of energy. Also, protein type foods often contain saturated fats which can increase the body's cholesterol level.

Low fat diet

A low fat diet will obviously reduce the main energy source from outside the body. Some of the fat which was laid down and stored when the body was consuming an excess to the body's requirements is utilised instead.

Low carbohydrate diet
A low carbohydrate diet means reducing the quantity of sugars and starch in the diet. Some people find this hard to do particularly if they have a sweet tooth. As the body obtains most of its daily energy requirements from carbohydrates, it works by reducing the readily available energy. The body calls on its reserve of energy, the stock-pile of fat!

High fibre diet
A high fibre diet provides a lot of bulk to the diet which generally makes the dieter feel full. High fibre diets also improve bowel conditions such as constipation.

Vegetarian diets
Over the years many people have opted to become vegetarians. There are two types of vegetarian:

- Lacto-vegetarians, who do eat some animal products such as milk, cheese and eggs.
- Vegans, who do not eat any form of animal produce.

Health diets
Health diets are prescribed by doctors or nutritionists for the benefit of their patients' health. Examples of people who require health diets are coronary sufferers and diabetics.

Commercial diet products
There is a large variety of products which can be purchased over the counter in many shops. They include solid food substances, e.g. diet bars, and powders which are mixed with water to produce liquid meals. The main problem with commercial diet products is that people tend to totally replace their diet with them and do not balance their diet nutritionally. Often these products' calorific values are way below the body's daily needs.

Slimming clubs
Over recent years the number of slimming and similar clubs has increased rapidly. Many people gain support and comfort from other dieters.

POINT TO NOTE

It is important with all diets to ensure that the body receives balanced nutrients to maintain health, repair and growth.

ACTIVITY

Analyse the dietary habits of two colleagues and research their daily calorific intake.

Alternative weight control

There is a variety of alternative ways in which weight can be controlled:

- Acupuncture. This can prove to be quite a costly method depending how quickly the dieter responds to treatment, however many people find it helps suppress their appetite.
- Hypnosis. Depending on an individual's response to hypnotherapy this method may encourage weight loss.
- Cosmetic surgery. This is a fairly drastic and expensive method to remove surplus fat.
- Tablets. There is a variety of slimming tablets that can be purchased over the counter. These are taken a number of hours before eating to suppress the appetite.
- Drugs. Doctors sometimes prescribe drugs to people whose life is threatened by their weight to help suppress their appetite.

ACTIVITY

Research the alternative weight loss methods available in your local area, noting the cost and duration of treatments.

Eating problems

There is a variety of different types of eating problems, some of which can prove to be fatal.

Stress-induced eating

Stress affects everyone differently, but it can be noted that weight is either lost or gained according to how it affects an individual's eating patterns. Some people eat more under stress as they often take comfort from eating, whilst others eat a great deal less as they find their appetite reduced. Quite often when the anxieties disappear the normal eating pattern will gradually re-emerge. It is important to note that help in some form should be sought to cope with the problem creating the stress, particularly if rapid weight loss is noted. There are many self-help groups for people suffering with stress depending on the cause, e.g. living with cancer, losing a child. However it may be just the support of family or friends that is needed to reduce anxiety and bring comfort or a relaxing massage.

Bulimia nervosa

Bulimia nervosa is a disease where sufferers will 'binge' and afterwards make themselves sick. It is sometimes very difficult to realise that a person close to you is suffering with this disease, particularly in the early stages as they mainly eat in front of people. It is important that medical help is sought as soon as possible.

Anorexia nervosa

Anorexia nervosa is a slimmer's disease where sufferers slowly starve themselves of food. This disease is often brought on by social pressure to be slim. The sufferer starts by dieting, quite often drastically, to lose weight. Once the weight is lost the suffer still perceives him/herself as 'too fat' and comes to believe that any food he/she eats will increase his/her weight. This can be a life-threatening disease and medical help should be sought as soon as possible.

Figure and postural analysis

In order to perform an effective body-treatment consultation the therapist must have an understanding of the figure and postural problems that a client may have.

Body types

Body types are generally categorised into three types; *ectomorph, mesomorph* and *endomorph*. However it should be noted that the majority of people tend to be a combination of the categorised body types.

The ectomorph

Ectomorphs tend to be recognised by:

- Narrow shoulders and hips.
- Long bones.
- Not much muscle bulk.
- Low percentage of fat.
- General lack of curves.

The mesomorph

Mesomorphs tend to be recognised by:

- Athletic build.
- Well-developed shoulders.
- Slim, 'boyish' hips.
- Well-toned muscles.
- Low percentage of fat.

The endomorph

Endomorphs tend to be recognised by:

- Rounded shoulders.
- Heavy build.
- Higher percentage of fat to muscle bulk.
- Inclination to be overweight.

USEFUL INFORMATION
Although the appearance of the body can be altered through diet and exercise the actual body type remains constant through life.

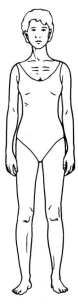 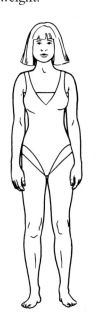

Fig. 2.2 *Ectomorph*   **Fig. 2.3** *Mesomorph*   **Fig. 2.4** *Endomorph*

Good posture

It is rare to find perfect posture. This is mainly due to the lifestyles that we lead: company representatives who spend a great deal of their day driving often suffer with tense, round shoulders; busy mothers who carry young children around on their hips or carry heavy shopping bags on one side whilst holding their child's hand for example often suffer with scoliosis.

We naturally take notice of the person who holds him/herself well. A person with good posture often creates a good first impression compared to the person who slouches. Watch men and women when they are attracted by a member of the opposite sex they automatically react by stretching their bodies upright! Besides enhancing the body's appearance good posture also maximises the lung capacity which obviously has a beneficial effect on the body.

Recent studies around the world show a relationship of blood types to diet and lifestyle and there is increased attention to the body shape according to the effects on metabolism and main areas of fat storage (and cellulite) of the endocrine glands. Body shapes/types, identified according to the predominant endocrine influence are described as four main types: gonad (G), thyroid (T), super-adrenal (S), and hypophysis/pituitary (H).

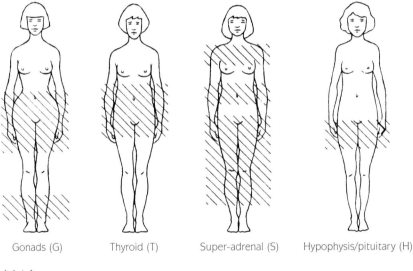

| Gonads (G) | Thyroid (T) | Super-adrenal (S) | Hypophysis/pituitary (H) |

 Main areas of body fat storage

Fig. 2.5 *Fat storage*

Points to look for in good posture

1. The head should not abnormally extend or retract beyond the mid line.
2. The arms, when relaxed, should lie evenly.
3. The spinal column should be straight.
4. The distances from the right and left scapulae to the spine should be even.
5. The abdomen should appear flat.
6. The waist curves should be level.
7. The buttocks should not protrude abnormally.
8. The legs and knees should be straight and facing forwards.

9 The feet should face forwards and should be either together or slightly apart.
10 The body weight should be evenly distributed.

If an imaginary, lateral line is drawn down the side of the body it should pass in a straight line through the ear, shoulder, elbow, waist, hip, knee and ankle. Trainee therapists often use a plumbline to assist in postural analysis.

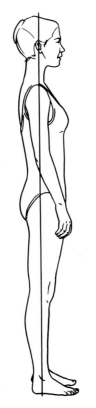

Fig. 2.6 *Correct postural stance (lateral view)*

Progress Check

1 State four reasons why clients may wish to gain or lose weight.
2 Explain briefly four different types of diet.
3 Describe three different eating problems.
4 Name the three main body types and for each give a brief description of how you would recognise them.
5 What points would you look for to establish good posture in a client?

Figure problems and postural conditions

Many clients are concerned about the distribution of their body fat which influences their shape. The most common problem in women is the rounded, heavy thighs, buttocks and hips commonly referred to as a 'pear-shape'. The therapist needs to assess the client fully and analyse whether the body fat is evenly distributed. They should also note any stretch marks and their cause, e.g. rapid weight loss or pregnancy, and the type of fat, e.g. cellulite, soft or hard. It is also important to build up a picture of the client's lifestyle, eating habits and dietary intake.

Soft fat

Soft fat is the easiest type of fat condition to mobilise. It is not firm and moves easily when touched. It is easy to manipulate and generally responds well to diet and exercise.

Hard fat

This type of fat is difficult to disperse and is firm to touch.

Cellulite

Cellulite is not a term that is recognised by the medical profession but it clearly exists and is not identifiable as any other fat type.

Cellulite affects mainly women and causes unsightly dimpling and puckering of the skin. It is normally found in the thigh and buttock areas. It gives a characteristic 'cool feel' to the skin as the blood circulation is diminished in the area. The formation of cellulite is linked to the female hormones, namely oestrogen and progesterone, which play a part in subcutaneous fat distribution. A person does not have to be overweight to be affected by cellulite. As well as being unattractive, cellulite can be painful as it can compress nerve endings. For these reasons, many women resort to the therapist for treatment. There are varying degrees of cellulite, namely hard and soft.

The stages of hard and soft cellulite development are described as Stage 1, 2, 3 or 4 according to the degree of change to the circulation pattern and aesthetic appearance.

POINT TO NOTE

Contact thermography (using special heat active material) is sometimes used to illustrate these stages prior to and during treatment.)

Stretch marks

Stretch marks, or striations as they are technically known, are caused by thinning and loss of elasticity in the dermis. On fair skins they first appear as red, raised lines becoming purple later on whereas on darker skins they initially appear as dark raised lines and eventually flatten to form shiny streaks usually between 6 and 12 mm long. They often occur on the hips and thighs during adolescent growth spurts and occur on approximately 75% of all pregnant women, especially on the abdomen and breast areas. It is for the latter reason that most women seek the advice of the therapist and provided they are caught in the early stages treatment can be effective. (See chapter 7.)

The two main reasons why stretch marks can occur are due to *endocrine cause* or *mechanical cause*.

It is known that corticosteroid hormones suppress fibre formation in the skin which in turn causes collagen found within the dermis to waste away. Consequently the organisation and texture of tissues is seriously affected and this can lead to a state of well defined marking of the skin. This is the endocrine cause of stretch marks.

It is thought that sudden and excessive weight increase does not allow the skin time to stretch gently, therefore 'ripping' of the collagen and elastin fibres occurs and leads to the appearance of stretch marks. This is a mechanical cause.

Figure and postural conditions

Deviation in body alignment can lead to a variety of figure and postural conditions, the main ones being outlined below.

Dowager's hump

This is a condition associated with old age. Fatty deposits build up at the back of the neck over a period of time as the client holds his/her head forward of the normal postural alignment.

Protruding abdomen

This often relates to the postural condition of lordosis. However it may also be the result of fatty deposits around the area or as a result of weak abdominal muscles, a condition often found in postnatal mothers.

Midriff bulge

This is a fairly common condition, often associated with the over 35 age group, where as a result of the ageing process, fatty deposits accumulate in this area. It tends to be more apparent in women than men.

Flat feet

Flat feet is a condition due to the absence or sinking of the medial longitudinal arch of the foot, caused by weakness of the ligaments and tendons.

Hallux valgus

Hallux valgus is a condition recognised by a deviation of the big toe from the mid-line. It is commonly referred to as a bunion.

Tibial torsion

Commonly referred to as 'knock knees', tibial torsion is generally due to a slack tendon supporting the knee. This results in the knees rotating inwards towards the mid-line.

Winged scapulae

The shoulder blades protrude as they are adducted towards the mid-line. This is a fairly common condition in backpackers who carry heavy weights on their backs.

Round shoulders

Round shoulders are generally a result of the postural condition kyphosis. The pectoral muscles shorten creating a 'barrel chest'. Round shoulders are often associated with tall people who round their shoulders to appear smaller, ladies with large chests who try to conceal the size of their breasts and people suffering with severe asthma.

Kyphosis

Kyphosis may be recognised by the client's rounded shoulders. This shortens the pectoral muscles and curves the thoracic area of the vertebral column outwards. In women it can lead to sagging breasts as the suspensory ligaments and pectoral muscles normally hold the breasts upright. This condition is quite common in young girls with large breasts who through embarrassment curve their shoulders round to conceal themselves. It is also common in office workers, drivers and therapists whose everyday bodily posture involves rounding their shoulders.

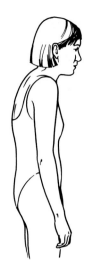
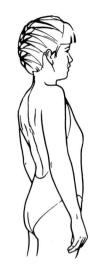
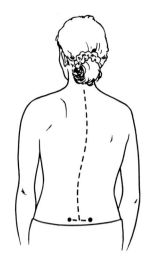

Fig. 2.7 *Kyphosis*   **Fig. 2.8** *Lordosis*   **Fig. 2.9** *Scoliosis*

Lordosis

Lordosis is recognised by the hollow back created by the inward curvature of the lumbar area of the spinal column. The muscles of the back tighten and this often leads to back ache. In severe cases the pelvis tends to tilt forward, the abdomen and gluteals appear to protrude the knees will hyper-extend, shortening the hamstrings in order to counter-balance the body weight. This condition is common in small people who often, through trying to appear taller, hollow out their backs. Gymnasts and ballet dancers can also suffer with this condition.

Scoliosis

Scoliosis is recognised by a lateral deviation of the vertebral column. The shortening of muscles on one side of the body can lead to dropped shoulders, uneven waist and scapulae and a tilting pelvis. Busy mothers who tend to hold their children on one side of their waist can suffer with scoliosis. Carrying heavy bags or standing with the body weight to one side can also lead to this condition.

POINT TO NOTE

Some spinal curvatures are structural and cannot be altered by the therapist.

Postural assessment of the client

1   The therapist first assesses the client by observing their postural stance from a side view and notes any deviations to the points listed on pp. 56–57.
    Note. Whilst training it is common practice to use a weighted string (plumb line) as a guide to check that the body is in alignment or whether the client's head, shoulders, abdomen, pelvis, buttocks or knees are protruding forwards or behind the plumb line.
2   The therapist assesses the anterior then posterior view of the client.
    Note. It is common practice whilst training for the trainee to:
    ◆ mark the individual vertebrae to see if there is any curvature of the spine

- mark the scapulae and measure the distance between them and the spine
- place their hands on either side of the waist to see if they are even
- place their hands on both shoulders to see if they are even.

3   The therapist observes the client's normal seating position noting the position of the head, shoulders, arms, waist, pelvis, legs, knees and feet.

4   The therapist notes the client's normal walking pattern, observing the gait of movement, the positioning of the skeleton and the distribution of body weight.

ACTIVITY

Perform a postural analysis on three different colleagues. Note your findings and research suitable corrective exercises for postural improvement.

POINT TO NOTE

The majority of postural conditions can be assisted by gentle corrective exercise undertaken by the client at home.

Corrective exercise as home care advice

In order for the therapist to assist the client in gaining the maximum benefit from some salon treatments, e.g. neuro-muscular electrical stimulation, they need to have a basic understanding of the use of corrective exercise. A number of therapists develop an interest in exercise and take up specialist exercise courses which enable them to teach and fully advise on exercise programmes. There are also a great many books on types of exercises, mobility, muscle strength and fitness testing that would be useful further study.

Before advising any corrective exercises it is important to consider the:

- Age and mobility of the client.
- Muscle strength of the client.
- General health of the client.
- Past history of exercise of the client.
- Environment in which the exercises will be carried out.

POINTS TO NOTE

- Youth does not always indicate that the fitness and mobility of a client are good.
- Muscle strength can be determined by testing through resistance-type exercises the strength of the client's muscles in different areas of the body.
- Exercise should not be performed for at least two hours after eating.
- Advise clients that they must not continue if they feel dizzy or if they feel any discomfort.

Isotonic exercise

Isotonic exercise is a form of exercise that produces lengthening and shortening of the muscle fibres by movement of the joints, e.g. active exercise (exercise with movement).

Concentric and *eccentric* muscle work relates to isotonic exercise. Concentric is where the fibres, through shortening, become thicker, e.g. the biceps when the arm is bent. Eccentric is where the muscle fibres, through movement, lengthen, e.g. the triceps when the arm is bent.

Isometric exercise

Isometric exercise causes the muscle fibres to contract without an overall change of length in the muscle, e.g. passive exercise (exercise without movement).

Corrective exercise

Corrective exercises may be recommended to supplement salon treatments providing the therapist is happy that there are no underlying medical conditions.

The normal pattern of exercise sequences would include warm-up exercises, aerobic exercises, strengthening and stretching exercises and a cool-down/relaxation period.

Warm-up exercises

Warm-up exercises prepare the body's physiology for action and so reduce the risk of injury. They should include:

- ◆ Mobility exercises (within the normal range of movement).
- ◆ General activity to gradually increase the heart and respiration rates and to stimulate circulation.
- ◆ Static stretches of the muscles to be exercised, held for 6–8 seconds.

Aerobic exercises

Aerobic exercises provide a sustained period of exercise at the correct level of intensity to increase the heart rate into the training zone. They should include:

- ◆ Build-up aerobics.
- ◆ Peak aerobics.
- ◆ Cool-down aerobics.

Strengthening and stretching exercises

Strengthening and stretching exercises are used to build up muscle strength and improve mobility. They can be used to correct postural conditions. Examples of exercises follow.

1 Arm lift – a strength exercise for kyphosis

Purpose – To strengthen scapular adductors and help prevent or correct round shoulders and kyphosis.

Position – **a** Least difficult: lie prone with arms in reverse 'T'; forehead resting on floor.

    – **b** More advanced: same as before except arms are extended overhead and held against the ears.

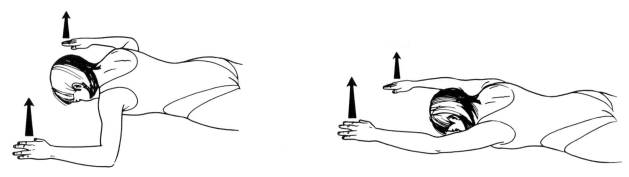

Fig. 2.10 *Arm lift*

Movement – Maintain the arm position and contract the muscles between the shoulder blades, lifting the arms as high as possible without raising head and trunk. Hold, relax and repeat.

2 Wand exercise – a stretch exercise for kyphosis

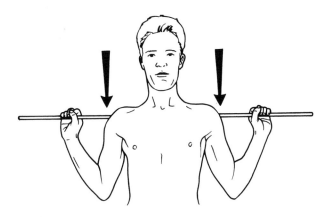

Fig. 2.11 *Wand exercise*

Purpose – To help prevent and correct round shoulders and kyphosis by stretching the muscles on the anterior side of the shoulder joint.

Position – Sit with wand grasped at ends. Raise wand overhead. Be certain that the head does not slide forward into a 'poke neck' position. Keep the chin tucked and neck straight.

Movement – Bring the wand down behind the shoulder blades. Keep spine erect. Hold.

Hands may be moved closer together to increase stretch on chest muscles.

3 Pelvic tilt – a strength exercise for lordosis

Purpose – To strengthen the abdominals and help prevent or correct lumbar lordosis and backache.

Position – Supine with knees bent.

Movement – Tighten the abdominal muscles and tilt the pelvis backward; try to flatten the lower back against the floor. At the same time, tighten the hip and thigh muscles. Hold then relax. Breathe normally during the contraction, do not hold the breath.

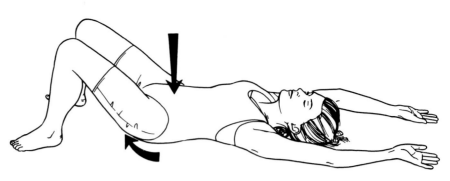

Fig. 2.12 *Pelvic tilt*

4 Low back stretcher – a stretch exercise for lordosis

Purpose – To stretch hip flexors and lumbar muscles, and help prevent or correct lumbar lordosis and backache.

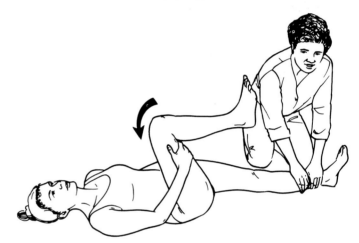

Fig. 2.13 *Low back stretcher*

Position – Supine position.

Movement – Draw one knee up to the chest and pull it down tightly with the hands, then slowly return it to the original position. Repeat with other knee. Do not grasp knee, but the thigh. If a partner or a weight stabilises the extended leg, the hip flexor muscles of that leg will also be stretched.

The therapist needs to advise on suitable exercises to stretch the shortened muscles and strengthened the lengthened muscles ensuring the starting position is appropriate to the client's mobility, muscle strength, balance and age range, e.g. an older client with unsteady balance would be more suited to exercises performed in a sitting position on a steady chair.

Isotonic and isometric exercises can be used and gradually, as muscle strength improves, resistance exercises using available home weights, e.g. jars of coffee, can be used to strengthen the arm muscles.

Cool-down/relaxation period
Cool down/relaxation exercises allow the body to cool down gradually and control breathing.

◆ The types of exercise selected and the number of repetitions would vary according to the area being exercised and the mobility, strength and balance of the client.

◆ It is important to remind the client to continue breathing smoothly throughout exercise to maintain the intake of oxygen and exhalation of carbon dioxide.

◆ If the client's needs are greater than the therapist can offer, the therapist should recommend appropriate, qualified exercise specialists.

Progress Check

1 Describe how you would recognise the following conditions:
   a soft fat   **c** cellulite   **e** dowager's hump
   b hard fat   **d** stretch marks   **f** midriff bulge.

2 Explain what is meant by the following terms:
   a kyphosis   **b** lordosis   **c** scoliosis.

3 Before recommending corrective exercise home care advice what factors would you take into consideration?

4 Define the following terms:
   a isotonic exercise   **c** concentric muscle work
   b isometric exercise   **d** eccentric muscle work.

Physical fitness

Every physical activity undertaken needs the body to produce energy from food digested and absorbed by the body. There are two systems which release energy from food; the *aerobic* system and the *anaerobic* system.

The aerobic system provides energy for prolonged activity, i.e. for most activity. The anaerobic system provides energy for short periods of activity (up to ten seconds) and can be thought of as an 'emergency' system. The aerobic system utilises carbohydrates and fats to obtain energy whereas the anaerobic system utilises only carbohydrates. The body switches to the anaerobic system when the aerobic system cannot produce enough energy for the body's needs. Once the anaerobic system cannot produce enough energy, the body tires and needs to rest until waste products produced by the anaerobic system are removed. How well the aerobic and anaerobic systems work is one measure of physical fitness and is important for health.

Components of physical fitness may be classified as either health related components or skill related components.

Health related components of physical fitness are:

◆ Cardiovascular fitness.
◆ Muscular endurance.
◆ Muscular strength.
◆ Flexibility.
◆ Body composition.

Skill related components of physical fitness are:

- Agility.
- Balance.
- Co-ordination.
- Speed.
- Power.
- Reaction time.

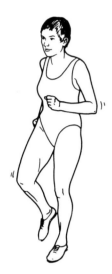

Fig. 2.14 *Running in place*

Cardiovascular fitness

Cardiovascular fitness is a measure of the efficiency of the respiratory and circulatory systems. It is a term used to how effectively oxygen is taken into the body and transported to the working muscles for energy and how effectively the waste produced is removed by the body.

A person who is considered to have a high cardio-respiratory endurance, i.e. they can exercise for a fair period of time at increased heart rate and recover reasonably fast, can be assumed to be 'aerobically fit'.

Exercise to test for cardiovascular fitness – running in place

Run in place for one and a half minutes (at a rate of 120 steps per minute). Rest for one minute and count the heart rate for thirty seconds. A heart rate of 60 or lower passes.

Examples of aerobic activity, i.e. activity that improves cardiovascular fitness, are jogging, swimming, brisk walking and aerobics.

Muscular endurance

This refers to the individual's ability to repeatedly use the same muscle or muscles without getting tired. Many athletes display high muscular endurance, e.g. swimmers and long distance runners.

Exercise to test for muscular endurance – side leg raise

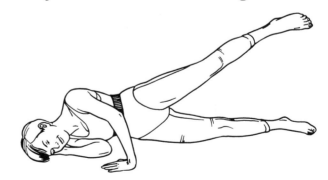

Fig. 2.15 *Side leg raise*

Lie on the floor on your side. Lift your leg up and to the side of the body until your feet are 24–36 inches apart. Hold for as long as possible. Perform 10 repetitions with each leg.

Isometric examples of muscular endurance exercises are; gluteal squeeze, pelvic tilt, arm press.

Isotonic examples of muscular endurance exercises are; squats, curl ups, back extensions.

Muscular strength

Muscular strength describes the amount of force an individual muscle or group of muscles can produce in overcoming a resistance in one maximum voluntary contraction, e.g. lifting a heavy weight.

Muscular strength can be tested by using dynamometers or manual tests for different parts of the body, e.g. press ups for the arms and chest.

Exercise to test muscular strength – press ups

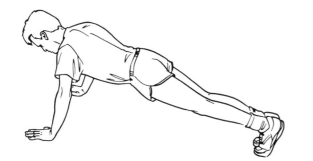

Fig. 2.16 *Press ups*

Lie face down on the floor. Place the hands under the shoulders. Keeping the legs and body straight, press off the floor until the arms are fully extended. Women repeat once, men three times.

Examples of muscular strength exercises are press ups and exercises done with variable resistance machines and free weights.

Flexibility

Flexibility can be measured by a person's range of movement. Flexibility will actually determine how an athlete can perform, as if muscles are tight and joints are inflexible, agility, range of movement, balance and speed are all restricted.

Exercise for testing flexibility of the hamstrings and lower back – toe touch

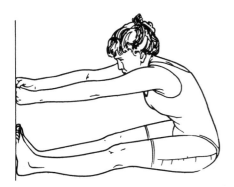

Fig. 2.17 *Toe touch*

Sit on the floor with your feet against a wall. Keep the feet together and the knees straight. Bend forward at the hips. Reach forward and touch your closed fists to the wall. Bend forward slowly, do not bounce.

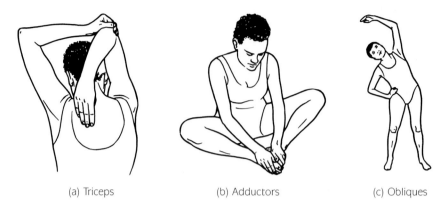

(a) Triceps   (b) Adductors   (c) Obliques

Fig. 2.18 *Examples of flexibility exercises*

Body composition

The composition of a person's body refers to the relative percentages of muscle, fat, bone and other tissues that make up the body. It can be thought of as a measure of whether a person is under or over weight, i.e. has a low or high percentage of body fat.

Body composition can be measured by using calibrated skin callipers. Four measurements are taken from different parts of the body. These measurements are then compared with a chart of accepted norms and an estimate of the percentage of body fat read off. This test can also be performed manually.

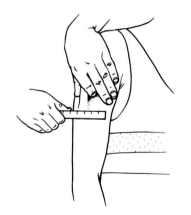

Fig. 2.19 *Measuring body composition*

Manual measurement of body composition – the pinch

Have a partner pinch a fold of skin on the back of your upper arm halfway between the tip of the elbow and the tip of the shoulder. Measurements of 1 inch for men and 1½ inches for women are acceptable.

Agility

Agility is the ability to rapidly and accurately change the direction of the entire body in space. Examples of sports that require agility are skiing and wrestling.

Balance

Balance is the maintenance of equilibrium whilst stationary or moving. Balance is very important in gymnastic beam exercises and water skiing.

Co-ordination

Co-ordination is a person's ability to use the senses, e.g. sight and hearing, in conjunction with the body parts to perform motor tasks smoothly and accurately. Good co-ordination is needed for golf.

Speed

Speed is the ability to perform a movement in a short period of time, e.g. running.

Power

Power is a person's ability to transfer energy into force at a fast rate. Discus throwing requires power.

Reaction time

A person's reaction time is the time elapsed between stimulation and the beginning of reaction to that stimulation, e.g. from starting block to sprint take-off.

Fitness testing

Before anyone undertakes an exercise regime in a professionally supervised leisure club or gym it is usual, after their initial consultation, that they be given a test to establish their level of fitness. A fitness test is used to assess where an individual's strengths and weaknesses lie, to meet the perceived needs of the client and to prevent injury.

Tests vary in their degree of sophistication depending upon the requirement of the client. Such tests should include measurements of:

- Height and weight.
- Peak flow.
- Cardiovascular fitness.
- Body composition, i.e. percentage body fat.

Conclusions are reached on an individual's fitness by comparing test results against accepted norms related to age, sex and body type.

ACTIVITY
Perform tests to identify a client's level of cardiovascular fitness, muscular strength and endurance and flexibility.

POINTS TO NOTE
- Every exercise if not performed correctly is potentially dangerous.
- Muscular strength and endurance exercises are usually combined.
- Breathing should be natural throughout the exercise.

Considerations for safe exercise

All the following should be taken into consideration when assessing whether exercise at a particular level is safe for a client:

- Heart conditions; high blood pressure; dizziness.
- Severe respiratory conditions; asthma.
- Fever.
- Recent operations.
- Broken bones.
- Other medical conditions such as diabetes, epilepsy and pregnancy.
- Whether the client has eaten a heavy meal or consumed alcohol.

Always remember that every exercise if not performed correctly is potentially dangerous!

ACTIVITY

Devise a suitable exercise plan for:

a a 50 year old female client with lordosis
b a 30 year old female office worker with kyphosis
c a 40 year old postman with scoliosis.

Name   Date

Address

Tel. no.

Date of birth

Medical history

High blood pressre   Medication

Asthma   Number of pregnancies

Dizziness/fainting   Ages of children

Anaemia

Weight   Frame size

Height   % Body fat

Reason for exercise:

Lose fat ( )   Change appearance ( )   Gain strength ( )   Feel fitter ( )

Sports performance ( )   Doctor's advice ( )   Social ( )   Other

---

Fig. 2.20 *Example of an exercise consultation card*

1   Explain the difference between the aerobic and anaerobic systems.
2   Describe the following components of health-related fitness:
     a cardiovascular fitness
     b muscular strength
     c muscular endurance
     d flexibility
     e body composition.
3   Explain the different components of skill-related fitness.
4   State the considerations for safe exercise.
5   List the points that should be noted on an exercise consultation card.

Key Terms

You need to know what these words and phrases mean. Go back through the chapter to find out.

- Basal metabolism
- Body types
- Carbohydrates
- Components of fitness
- Eating problems
- Fats
- Good posture
- Isotonic and isometric exercise
- Metabolism
- Mineral elements
- Nutrition
- Proteins
- Fibre
- Types of diets
- Vitamins

After working through this chapter you will be able to:
- list different types of infections and infestations
- carry out emergency procedures
- describe the activities undertaken in the reception area
- deal with telephone messages
- make a number of appointments for clients
- understand the purpose of stock control
- explain the purpose of a consultation
- carry out an effective facial and body consultation.

Hygiene

It is paramount that the therapist ensures the highest standards of hygiene within the salon. Because of the close proximity of therapist and client good hygiene is essential to prevent infection, cross-infection and infestation.

Protecting against disease

We spend a great deal of our lives surrounded by what are commonly known as 'germs'. Some germs are harmless, some are even beneficial, but others present a danger to us because they cause disease.

The germs which cause disease are usually spread by:

- Unclean hands.
- Contaminated tools.
- Sores and pus.
- Discharges from the nose and mouth.
- Shared use of items such as towels and cups.
- Close contact with infected skin cells.
- Contaminated blood or tissue fluid.

Viruses

Viruses are the tiniest germs, yet they are responsible for an enormous range of human diseases. Viruses can only survive in living cells. The following are examples of viral infections:

- **Common cold**: the virus is spread by coughing and sneezing and is carried through the air as a droplet infection.
- **Herpes simplex** (cold sores): the virus remains dormant in the mucous membranes of the skin. It can be activated by sunlight or general debility. Cold sores are most likely to spread when they are weeping.
- **Warts**: there are several types of wart. Verruca plantaris is a wart which occurs commonly on the soles of the feet and is spread by close contact.

Bacteria

Bacteria are single-celled organisms. They grow from spores which are very resistant to attack and multiply very quickly. Bacteria are capable of breeding outside the body and can therefore be caught easily through personal contact or by touching a contaminated article.

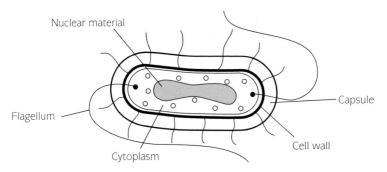

Fig. 3.1 *A typical bacterial cell*

Some bacteria causes diseases and infect wounds. The following are examples of bacterial infections:

- **Impetigo**: bacteria enter the body through broken skin and cause blisters which weep and crust over. The condition is highly infectious and can be spread easily by dirty tools.
- **Boils**: these can occur when bacteria invade the hair follicle through a surface scratch or by close contact with an infected person.
- **Whitlow**: this can be caused by the bacteria invading the pad of the finger through a break in the skin which has often been caused by a splinter.

Fungi

Fungi are yeasts and moulds. Moulds break down all sorts of materials but rarely cause disease. Yeasts are single-celled fungi which can cause disease. Fungal infections are very easily transmitted by personal contact or by touching contaminated articles. The following are examples of fungal infections:

- **Tinea pedis** (athlete's foot): the fungus thrives in the warm, moist environment between the toes and sometimes on the soles of the feet. The condition is picked up easily by direct contact with recently shed, infected skin cells.
- **Tinea unguium** (ringworm of the nail): may result from contact with the fungus present on other parts of the body, e.g. toenails may become infected during an outbreak of athlete's foot, which if touched could then be spread by contact to the nails.

Animal parasites

Animal parasites are small insects which cause disease by invading the skin and using human blood or protein as a source of nourishment. Diseases caused by animal parasites usually occur as the result of prolonged contact with an infected person. The following are examples of diseases caused by animal parasites:

- **Scabies**: tiny mites burrow through the outside layer of the epidermis and lay their eggs underneath the skin surface. The condition is very itchy and causes a rash and swelling. Characteristic line formations show where the burrows have been formed.
- **Head lice**: small parasites which puncture the skin and suck blood. They lay eggs on the hair close to the scalp. The unhatched eggs are called *nits* and can be seen as shiny, pearl-coloured, oval bodies which cling to the hair shaft.

To protect against the spread of disease you must:

- Provide each client with clean towels and gown.
- Carry out a consultation before each treatment to ensure contra-indications are spotted in time.
- Use only tools which have been cleaned and sterilised.
- Use correct treatment techniques to avoid injuring the client.
- Dispose of waste properly after each treatment.
- Wash your own hands before each treatment and as necessary throughout the treatment.
- Maintain high standards of personal hygiene.

GOOD PRACTICE

- Dirt and bacteria accumulate in cracks. You must not use tools with a damaged edge as they cannot be sterilised effectively.
- You have a responsibility to yourself, your clients and your colleagues to always work hygienically and to do everything you can to avoid the spread of infection.
- All work surfaces should be cleaned regularly with hot water and detergent. The treatment couch, trolley, sink and stools should be wiped down at the end of each working day with a solution of disinfectant.
- Waste should not be handled or exposed. Make sure that the waste resulting from your treatments is placed in a lined container, tied up and disposed of in a large sealed refuse sack with other salon waste.

ACTIVITY
Research the different skin conditions caused by bacterial, viral and fungal infections. Note their names and characteristics.

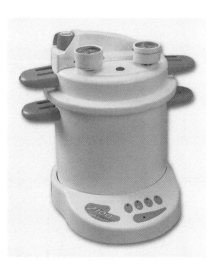

Fig. 3.2 *Small bench top autoclave*

Sterilisation and disinfection
Sterilisation is the destruction of all living organisms. It is very difficult to maintain sterile conditions. Once sterilised items have been exposed to the air they are no longer sterile. Articles which have been sterilised and stored hygienically for a short period are safe to use on the client.

Autoclave
The most effective method of sterilisation is steaming at high pressure in an autoclave. This works on exactly the same principle as a pressure cooker. Steam is produced from a reservoir of water and is contained under pressure at a minimum of 121°C for 15 minutes. Modern autoclaves use thermochromic indicators which change colour when the

required temperature has been reached. Stainless steel and glass items are suitable for sterilisation by this method. A stacking facility is usually providing so that the articles can be placed at different levels in the autoclave. The temperatures used in autoclaves vary from 121°C to 134°C and with correct time and heat exposure kill all spores. However the range of temperature can affect certain materials, e.g. soft plastics. Most hardened plastics are suitable for autoclave exposure but always check first with the manufacturer of the item to be sterilised.

Sanitisers

Sanitisers operate by irradiating implements with ultra-violet light. This would normally inactivate any bacteria, but as all implements cannot be fully exposed directly to the ultra-violet light, these units are now only recommended for storage of sterilised implements.

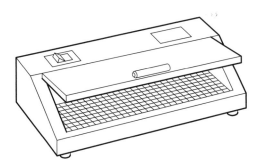

Fig. 3.3 *Sanitiser*

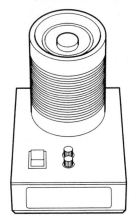

Glass bead sterilisers

Glass bead sterilisers reach temperatures between 190°C and 300°C (374–572°F) depending on the model. This temperature has to be maintained for 30–60 minutes prior to use. If extra items are put into the steriliser during this period, the temperature of the beads drops and the effects are lost. Timing has to begin again. Glass bead sterilisers can hold only very small items, e.g. tweezers, and the very high temperatures are suitable only for implements made of high-grade stainless steel or discolouration occurs. They therefore have limited use in the salon.

Fig. 3.4 *Glass bead steriliser*

Chemical methods of sterilisation

Concentrated liquid chemical agents are available which have to be diluted for use. Some chemical agents act as a sterilant, depending on the strength of the solution and the time for which items are kept in contact with them. Some liquid chemical sterilisers are very harmful to the skin and great care is needed when handling them.

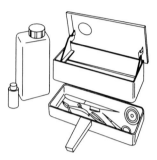

Fig. 3.5 *Chemical sterilisation equipment*

Disinfection

Disinfectants work against bacteria and fungi, but they just remove contamination; they do not necessarily kill spores. Disinfectants only reduce the number of organisms. Examples of good chemical disinfectants are:

- **Gluteraldehyde**: a 2% solution is used which remains active for 14–18 days, after which time it must be discarded. Gluteraldehyde is particularly useful for soaking metal instruments and applicators, but must be handled with great care. (See COSHH, Chapter 13.)
- **Alcohol**: alcohol disinfectants have a very effective bactericidal effect. They must be used once only and then discarded.
- **Quartery ammonium compounds**: these are bacteriostatic cleansing agents. They prevent bacteria from spreading but are not effective against very resistant organisms.
- **Hypochlorites**: these products contain sodium or calcium hypochlorite and are often used for general cleaning purposes as they are relatively cheap. Some are corrosive and should not be used for soaking metal instruments.

Antiseptics

Antiseptics are disinfectants used specifically on the skin and for treating wounds. Ready-for-use swabs impregnated with 70% isopropyl alcohol are often used for convenience.

ACTIVITY

Research the different cleaning and sterilising methods used in two salons. Make a note of any special instructions on diluting, using and disposing of the chemical disinfectants and sterilising agents used.

Emergency first aid

You need a basic knowledge of first aid so that you can assist with minor accidental injuries or unexpected situations which happen from time to time in the salon. More serious injuries, for example those involving acute pain or loss of consciousness or serious bleeding, should be dealt with by a qualified first aider, doctor or nurse.

First aid kit

The Health and Safety regulations require the salon to have a first aid kit readily available. The contents are specified and are intended to cover most emergency situations.

The first aid kit must include:

- A first aid guidance card
- Assorted plasters (preferably waterproof)
- Different sizes of sterile dressings
- Bandages
- Sterile eye pads
- Scissors
- Tweezers
- Safety pins.

Useful additions to this list are:

- Surgical adhesive tape
- Antiseptic cleansing products, i.e. liquid and cream
- An eye bath
- Gauze
- Crepe bandages
- An antihistamine cream
- Medical wipes
- Cotton wool.

If the salon has a fridge with a freezer compartment it is a good idea to keep an ice pack for injuries which produce swelling.

It is advisable to keep a stock of disposable gloves to wear when dealing with open wounds. These give some protection from hepatitis B and AIDS if an infection is present.

All staff should know what the first aid box looks like and where it is kept. It is recommended that the box is green with a white cross marked on it and that it is dustproof and free from damp.

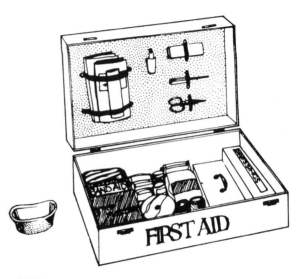

Fig. 3.6 *First aid kit*

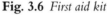

AIDS (Acquired Immune Deficiency Syndrome)

AIDS is caused by the human immuno-deficiency virus (HIV). The virus attacks the body's natural immune system and makes it very vulnerable to other infections which eventually cause death. Some people are known to be HIV positive, which means that they are carrying the virus without the symptoms of AIDS. HIV carriers are able to pass on the virus to someone else through infected blood or tissue fluid, for example through cuts or broken skin. The virus does not live for long outside the body.

Table 3.1 *First aid situations the therapist may have to deal with*

Problem	Priority	Action
Minor cuts	To stop the bleeding	Apply pressure over cotton wool taking care to avoid contact with the blood.
Severe cuts	To stop the bleeding	Keep applying pressure over a clean towel until qualified help arrives. Put on disposable gloves as soon as possible.
Electric shock	To remove from source of electricity	Do not touch the person until they are disconnected from the electricity supply. If breathing has stopped, artificial respiration will need to be given by a qualified person. Ring for an ambulance.
Dizziness	To restore the flow of blood to the head	Position the person with their head down between their knees and loosen their clothing.
Fainting	To restore the flow of blood to the head	Lie the person down with their feet raised on a cushion.
Nose bleed	To constrict the flow of blood	Sit the client up with the head bent forward. Loosen the clothing around the neck. Pinch the soft part of the nose firmly until bleeding has stopped. Make sure breathing continues through the mouth during this period. If bleeding has not stopped after half an hour, medical attention must be sought.
Burns	To cool the skin and prevent it from breaking	Hold the affected area under cool, running water until the pain is relieved. Serious burns should be covered loosely with a sterile dressing and medical attention sought.
Epilepsy	To prevent self-injury and relieve embarrassment	Do not interfere forcibly with a person during an attack. Gently prevent them from injuring themselves. Ensure the person's airways are clear and wipe away any froth which forms at the mouth. After the attack, cover with a blanket, comfort and give reassurance until recovery is complete.
Objects in the eye	To remove the object without damaging the eye	Expose the invaded area and try stroking the object towards the inside corner of the eye with a dampened twist of cotton wool. If this is not successful, help the person to use an eye bath containing clean warm water.
Falls	To determine if there is spine damage. To treat minor injuries if the fall is not serious	If the person complains of pain in the back or neck, then do not move them: cover with a warm blanket and get medical aid immediately. For less serious falls, treat the bruises, cuts, sprains or grazes as appropriate.
Bruises	To reduce pain and swelling	Apply cold compresses for 30 minutes using a towel wrapped round an ice-pack or very cold tap water. Keep the compress in place with a bandage. Replace it if it dries out.
Grazes	To clean wound and prevent infection	Soak a pad of cotton wool with an antiseptic and gently clean the graze, working outwards from the centre. Replace the cotton wool regularly throughout the cleaning. Apply a sterile gauze dressing, preferably a non-adherent type, to protect the wound as it heals. If dirt or foreign matter has become embedded in the graze, the person should be referred to a doctor who may want to give a tetanus injection.
Sprains	To reduce swelling	Apply cold compresses to the area (see treatment for bruises) and support the affected joint with a bandage firmly applied. Refer the person to a doctor.

Hepatitis B

This is a disease of the liver is caused by a virus (HBV) which is transmitted by infected blood and tissue fluids. The virus is very resistant and can survive outside the body. People can be very ill for a long time with a hepatitis B infection. It is a very weakening disease which can be fatal.

Strict hygiene practices are essential to prevent hepatitis B from spreading in the salon.

POINT TO NOTE

It is important to protect against all diseases which are carried by blood and tissue fluids. Many people feel most threatened by AIDS: this is mainly because of intense media pressure, during 1993–4, which emphasised the high mortality rate. In fact there is a much higher risk of cross-infection with hepatitis B, because the HBV virus is so resistant and can survive outside the body.

ACTIVITY

With a colleague role play emergency first aid procedures for each of the following:

a nose bleed
b dizziness
c object in the eye
d fainting.

Progress Check

1   Give an example of each of the following types of infection:
    a viral   **b** bacterial   **c** fungal   **d** animal parasite.
2   Define the following:
    a sterilisation   **b** disinfection   **c** antiseptic.
3   Explain why it is advisable to wear protective gloves when treating an open wound.
4   State the first aid treatment for a client suffering with:
    a a burn   **b** a nose bleed   **c** an epileptic fit.

Reception

The reception is the central pivot for the staff and clients of the salon. It is an area that everyone has to walk through either as a member of staff entering work and greeting clients or as a client when making and waiting for appointments. Everybody's day revolves around the salon's appointment schedule, and therefore the reception area.

First impressions do count so it is paramount that the reception area is inviting to the client. Therapeutic music rather than a loud, thudding pop record will aid relaxation for the majority of clients, and the use of essential oils either through burners or fans can saturate the air with a

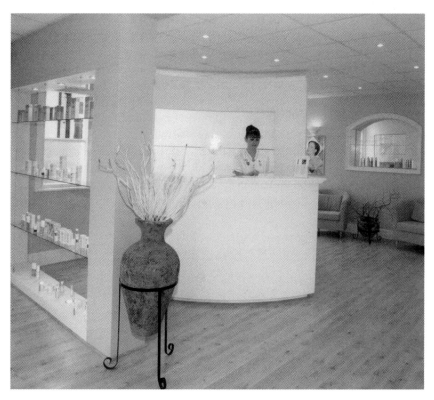

Fig. 3.7 *Reception area*

pleasant aroma. The seating should be comfortable in order to allow the client to begin to relax prior to treatment. The décor should reflect the type of premises and clientele the salon is marketing itself to, it should be continually refreshed to keep it in pristine condition and should be kept clean and tidy:

- All surfaces should be dusted and cleaned and waste bins should be emptied on a regular basis.
- Cups and glasses should be removed as soon as possible after use.
- Salon leaflets should be replaced before they become torn or out of date.

The receptionist

Some establishments employ a receptionist, in others the therapists share the responsibility. The receptionist is the first point of contact clients and visitors have with the salon. It is therefore essential that the receptionist has a thorough understanding of the workings of the establishment and is extremely professional in their approach and appearance. It is also beneficial if the receptionist has an understanding of the benefits of the treatments and retail products on offer in the salon.

Many employers are fully aware of the benefits of offering retail products to their staff at cost price together with ensuring that they have experienced all of the salon treatments on offer to the clients as well as having treatments to benefit their individual needs. The image of the salon is reflected by the appearance of the staff. Just think: when was the last time you saw a sales assistant in a top fashion retail outlet dressed in scruffy clothes?

POINT TO NOTE

It is useful for therapists to have treatments in the salon and role play the treatment as a realistic client, noting the way the reception area looked and how the receptionist and therapist interacted with them and each other.

The reception area is the life-line of the salon. It is here that:

- The appointment book is kept. This is the central control of the salon, everybody plans their activities for the day around this.
- Appointments are made either by telephone or in person.
- Clients are greeted and made welcome by the receptionist.
- Clients and visitors to the salon, e.g. cosmetic company representatives, are taken care of whilst waiting. (It is extremely important, however, that staff do not discuss any business matters in an area where clients may overhear financial purchasing arrangements, etc.)
- Enquiries are dealt with, e.g. information on salon treatments, products, planned salon events, directions to another shop in the area.
- Products are ordered, received, recorded, priced, displayed and sold.
- Salon services are advertised.
- Payment is taken for treatments and retail products.

All of the tasks outlined above are generally undertaken by the receptionist, whose job role mainly involves taking, receiving and recording information either by telephone or in person.

Dealing with clients, visitors and reception enquiries

In order for a receptionist to deal either with clients or visitors to the salon they need to fully understand the workings of the salon including the:

- Roles and responsibilities of each member of staff.
- Recording mechanisms of the salon.
- Treatments offered by the salon and their benefits.
- Retail products sold by the salon.

The receptionist must remain courteous to all clients and visitors and treat them all as equals. Generally clients are polite and friendly, however some people can demand a great deal of attention and at times be aggressive and rude. The receptionist must stay cool, calm and collected; she represents the salon and as the first point of contact will create an impression of the salon to the client or visitor. A friendly smile and voice can often help to calm an aggressive visitor. We all have bad days, but when working in a service industry our moods have to be left at home. Clients and visitors may not always manage to do this so remember that you are probably just an outlet for their emotions, it is likely that it isn't personal and shouldn't be taken as such.

Telephone enquiries

For many clients the telephone is their contact with the business. A good receptionist never forgets that all calls are from individuals and that each one of them is a prospective client.

You should always:

- Answer promptly – on the second or third ring. This gives both sides time to prepare themselves without the caller becoming impatient.
- Be friendly – give the name of the salon and say who you are. Note the client's name so that you can use it in the conversation.
- Smile when you pick up the receiver. Smiles definitely do travel down the telephone!
- Be enthusiastic – ask how you may help the caller. Enthusiasm is infectious and shows you enjoy being helpful.
- Listen attentively – it is very off-putting for a caller if they sense you are being distracted by someone else.
- Leave a good impression. Remember that you are the salon to the caller. Repeat back to them any important points discussed and thank them for calling. Don't forget to use their name!

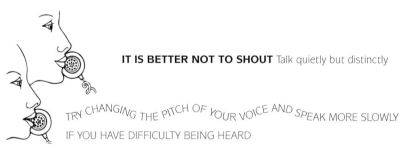

IT IS BETTER NOT TO SHOUT Talk quietly but distinctly

TRY CHANGING THE PITCH OF YOUR VOICE AND SPEAK MORE SLOWLY IF YOU HAVE DIFFICULTY BEING HEARD

Fig. 3.8 *Tips for using the telephone*

Taking messages

It is essential that all messages are accurately recorded and promptly dealt with. The receptionist or therapist must ensure they record who the message is for, who it is from, the telephone number where the caller can be contacted, the date and time of the message and the actual message and state whether the caller wants their call returned, will call again or was returning a call. The person taking the message should also record their own name in case there are any queries. An example of a message recording sheet is shown in Fig. 3.9.

To: Date:

From: Time:

Tel. no.:   Taken by:

Message

Please return their call

Will call again

Returning your call

MAKE SURE ALL INFORMATION IS CLEARLY RECORDED AND PASSED ON
PROMPTLY.

Fig. 3.9 *Message recording sheet*

Recording appointments

Recording appointments is an extremely important part of the receptionist's job and it is essential that all staff understand the appointment system that the salon operates. Appointment sheets are always made up in advance thus enabling clients to book courses of treatments.

The receptionist has to:

- Ensure that the reception desk is supplied with appointment cards, pens, pencils, ruler and rubber.
- Prepare pages in the appointment book at least six weeks in advance, to show the availability of each therapist on a particular day.
- As appointments are arranged, transfer the details to the appointment book in pencil, stating the client's name, their telephone number and the treatment required.
- Make out an appointment card for the client, recording details in pen and stating the date, day, time, therapist's name and treatment booked.
- Check the accuracy of both sets of records before handing over the appointment card to the client.
- Record the client's arrival at the salon by drawing a diagonal line in pencil across their details in the appointment book.

- When the client has gone through for treatment, draw a diagonal line across the first one to record that they are being attended to.

Clients who arrive unexpectedly may be treated provided that there is a therapist available. The receptionist should always check first and then record the client's details on the day in the appointment book.

DATE Monday October 17th   **COMPLEXION**

	LOREEN	SAIDA	LIZ	JEAN	PAUL	SUNBED
8.30						
8.45						
9.00	Ms. Warner	Mrs Cogin	Miss Williams	Mrs Lacey		Mrs Turvey
9.15	Hydra Plus		AHA	705 7997		646 2216
9.30			424 5780	Mrs Farmer		Miss Bates
9.45		BODY WRAP		Cellulite treat		777 3434
10.00	221 4477		Mrs Rees Ultratone	292 398?	Morning off	Ms. Faulkner 273 2727 DNA
10.15			252 3790	Mrs Peet		
10.30				Massage		Miss Laidlaw
10.45	Mrs Perry Dynatone	707 2700	Mrs Christopher Back massage 551 9829			827 1343
11.00				499 2000		Mr Cartwright
11.15	417 9173	Mrs Loy Massage	Mrs Cooke Massage	Mrs Dowding Dynatone		266 0479
11.30	Ms. Harris Massage					
11.45						
12.00		303 2768	448 4790	550 4171		Mr Burke
12.15	335 3939	Mrs Fabes				324 1567
12.30		Indian head	LUNCH	Miss Lulham	Mr Ashford	Mrs Wensley
12.45	LUNCH	923 5625		Hydra Plus	Massage	417 9894
13.00		Ms. Puttick				Ms Sullivan
13.15		Ultratone	Mrs Walker	217 9239	842 9111	344 3916
13.30		292 7652	AHA		Mr Lakin Back Massage 978 3493	Mrs Godfrey
13.45	Mrs Turner Massage					237 8999
14.00		LUNCH	506 4455	LUNCH	Mr Ward Massage	Mrs Bona
14.15						462 3911
14.30					320 3493	Ms. C Bailey 121 3790

☐ Available Time	⊠ Client has been taken for treatment
◹ Client arrived and is awaiting treatment	DNA Did Not Attend – Client did not inform: make a note on record card
	C Last minute cancellation

Fig. 3.10 *Example of a completed page of an appointment book*

In some salons the receptionist prepares a list for each therapist which shows their schedule for the day. This is kept by the therapist and provides a useful quick reference.

GOOD PRACTICE

- It is important that the appointment pages are kept neat and tidy. The correct codes and abbreviations must be used and the start and finish times of treatments made clear.
- Sometimes clients have to cancel or change their appointment. When details are recorded in pencil, they can be rubbed out neatly and the space used for another client.

Maintaining stock and the retail area

In many salons stock taking and ordering are undertaken by the receptionist. However it may be a task given to a therapist or the salon manager. It is extremely important that retail products are accessible and a good stock level is maintained or sales could be lost.

If the receptionist is responsible for the salon's stock they must:

- Keep the retail area clean and tidy: the counter, shelves and stock should be dusted every day and where possible have regular changes of display. Stock which is grubby and dusty will lose its value.
- Inform clients of current promotions: the receptionist should draw special offers to the attention of the clients and make sure the promotional material is displayed where it will catch the client's eye.
- Carry out stock checks: stock checks should be carried out weekly to monitor how well different products are selling and to make sure that popular lines are re-ordered before being sold out.
- Price the retail products: identical products must not be priced differently. Price tickets should be checked as part of regular stock checks. Old price tickets should be removed before putting on new ones so that a lower price is not disguised.
- Store stock correctly so that it does not deteriorate or become damaged. Keep fast-moving lines at the front of the shelves and slower moving ones nearer the back. Do not block aisles or passageways with containers of stock; keep it in a locked cupboard or secure room.
- Display stock attractively: displays should be set up with the minimum disruption to business. If all retail stock is to be displayed, extra space is needed for the fastest selling lines. Shelving should be clean, safe and undamaged and strong enough to take the weight of the products on display. Packaging should be displayed with the product. Take care with flimsy packaging and stack heavier goods lower down than more fragile items.
- Keep accurate stock records. The quality of a product cannot be guaranteed once its expiry date has passed. Stock which has been stored beyond its 'shelf-life' has either to be sold off cheaply or, ideally, disposed of.
- Store stock in a cool, dark place.

- Do not pile boxes too high.
- When an order arrives, bring old stock to the front and store new stock behind. This method of stock control is called FIFO, i.e. first in, first out.

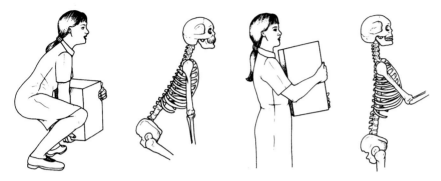

Fig. 3.11 *Correct lifting and carrying technique; avoid straining your back when moving heavy items*

The stock sheet lists the number of items in stock per product line. The details of a stock check are recorded on a stock sheet before being transferred to the stock book.

The stock book identifies reorder levels, and the receipt and sales of stock.

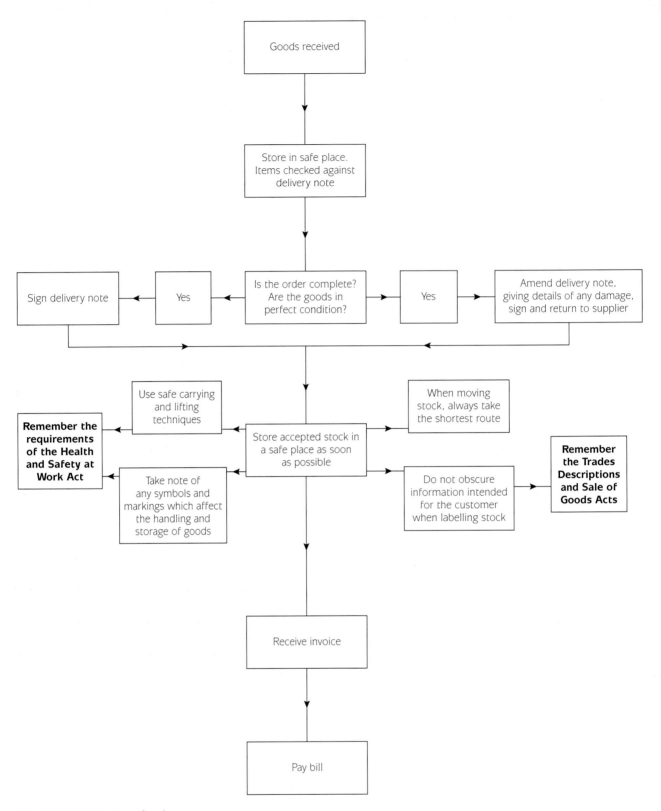

Fig. 3.12 *Distribution of stock*

	Stock List	
1	Aromatic oil for vapouriser or steam cabinet	30ml
2	Aromatic oil for body massage	30ml
3	Desincrustation gel	250g
4	Ionto gel DS	250g
5	Ionto gel GS	250g
6	Ionto gel SS	250g
7	Ionto gel DC	250g
8		
9		
10		

Fig. 3.13 *Example of a stock sheet*

No.	PRODUCT CODE	PRODUCT	STOCK LEVEL Min	STOCK LEVEL Max	Date 5/8/01 COUNTER STOCK	STOCK ROOM STOCK	TOTAL STOCK (I)	ORDER	RECEIVED	TOTAL STOCK (II)	SOLD	Date 5/8/01 COUNTER STOCK	STOCK ROOM STOCK	TOTAL STOCK (I)	ORDER	RECEIVED	TOTAL STOCK (II)	SOLD	
1	00070	Aromatic oil for vap/sc 30ml	10	14	6	2	8	2	–	8	–	6	2	8	–	2	10	–	
2	00071	Cellulite cream 150g	6	8	3	3	6	2	–	6	2	3	1	4	2	2	6	1	
3	000072	Stretch mark cream 250g	6	8	4	4	8	–	–	8	1	3	4	7	–	1	8	–	
4	000073																		
5	00074																		
6	00075																		

Fig. 3.14 *Example of a stock book*

ACTIVITY

With a colleague, discuss the following and compare your answers with other members of your group:

a What could be the possible reasons for discrepancies at a stock check?

b How do you think that seasonal variations might affect the allocation of space given to stock?

c When are the best times for changing displays and attending to stock?

d Why should the salon aim for a fast turnover of stock?

e What sort of things should be considered when fitting out a stock room?

1 List the roles of a receptionist.
2 Describe how the reception can be used for marketing.
3 List the important points that should be noted when taking a telephone message.
4 State why pencils are often used to record information in the appointment book.
5 Give the reasons for carrying out regular stock checks.
6 What is the main purpose of:
   a a stock sheet   **b** a stock book?

Computers

Businesses are becoming increasingly aware of the benefits of computerised record keeping. All sorts of information, such as clients' details, appointments, stock records and sales figures can be stored on a disc. The information can be retrieved easily by a trained person. Some manufacturers produce software (programmes) specially for use in a salon.

If you use a computer you should copy recorded information on to a second disc to provide backup in case of loss or damage to the main disc.

Many salons are now developing their own websites or joining those set up by professional bodies.

Risk assessment

In 1999, The Management of Health and Safety at Work Regulations were amended and require all business owners or managers to carry out risk assessments for the health, safety and welfare of both employees and clients. If the salon has more than five employees then formal risk assessment records must be kept, however it is recommended that all employers keep formal records. These regulations also take special notice of employees under the age of eighteen requiring employers to carry out risk assessments of their work activities identifying any particular hazard they could be exposed to and then indicating the controls the employer will put in place to ensure the employees' safety. The potential hazards can be considered under three headings: physical, biological and mechanical.

There are five steps involved in carrying out risk assessments.

- Firstly, identify all the potential hazards in all areas of the salon.
- Secondly, determine who could be at risk and how they may be at risk.
- Thirdly, evaluate these risks and decide whether the control mechanisms in place are adequate or whether more needs to be done to prevent possible accidents.
- Fourthly, formally record all your findings (see pp. 91–97).
- Fifthly, monitor and review the risk assessments on a regular basis and ensure all staff are aware of them.

RISK ASSESSMENT

Warwickshire COLLEGE
ROYAL LEAMINGTON SPA & MORETON MORRELL

Programme area/Unit/Department: Beauty Therapy and Hairdressing

Logical assessment unit: Reception

Completed by: Dawn Edwards

Date: 1 May 2001

Review date: Oct. 2001

Authorised by: Dawn Ward

Principal: Ioan Morgan

PERSONNEL AFFECTED – KEY

Staff	ST	Public	P	Young Persons	YP
Students	S	Contractors	C		

RISK RATING

SEVERITY		LIKELIHOOD	
Fatality	3	Probable	3
Major injury	2	Possible	2
Minor injury	1	Unlikely	1

Activity	Personnel affected	Hazards	Risk (Severity × Likelihood)	Existing control measures	Residual risk (Severity × Likelihood)	Existing control measures
Meeting clients in seated area	P	Large amount of people at any one time	$1 \times 2 = 2$	Signing in procedures	$1 \times 2 = 2$	
				Wearing protective gown	$1 \times 2 = 2$	
Retail product area	P, ST, S	Chemical	$1 \times 2 = 2$	Metal cabinet for storage	$1 \times 2 = 2$	
				Dummies on display		

Fig. 3.15 *Example of a risk assessment record: Reception area*

RISK ASSESSMENT

Programme area/Unit/Department:	Beauty Therapy and Hairdressing
Logical assessment unit:	Hairdressing M406/M408/M407
Completed by:	D Edwards
Date:	10 April 2001
Review date:	Sept. 2001
Authorised by:	Dawn Ward
Principal:	Ioan Morgan

PERSONNEL AFFECTED – KEY

Staff	ST	Public	P	Young Persons	YP
Students	S	Contractors	C		

RISK RATING

SEVERITY		LIKELIHOOD	
Fatality	3	Probable	3
Major injury	2	Possible	2
Minor injury	1	Unlikely	1

Activity	Personnel affected	Hazards	Risk (Severity × Likelihood)	Existing control measures	Residual risk (Severity × Likelihood)	Existing control measures
Use of hairdryer	S ST	Electricity	2×2=4	PAT tested/maintenance Supervision of students Inspection of cables and connections by users	2×1=2	
Use of scissors/ razors	S ST P	Cutting	2×2=4	Supervision of students Safe working practices	1×1=1	
Chemicals: bleach/tint perms	S ST P		2×3=6	Supervision of students Instruction on mixing peroxide Metal cabinet/fridge for storage Skin test for skins prior to all applications	1×1=1	
Hair cutting on floor	S ST P	Slipping up	2×2=4	Supervision/instruction Safe systems of work	1×1=1	
Washing hair	S ST P	Hot/cold water (spillage)	1×2=2	Instruction to students Safe systems of work	1×1=1	
Styling products: gels hairsprays etc	S ST P	Flammable products	2×2=4	Metal cabinet for safe storage Safe systems at work	1×1=1	

Fig. 3.16 *Example of a risk assessment record: Hairdressing department*

Warwickshire COLLEGE
ROYAL LEAMINGTON SPA & MORETON MORRELL

RISK ASSESSMENT

Programme area/Unit/Department: Beauty Therapy and Hairdressing

Logical assessment unit:	Laundry room	
Completed by:	Dawn Edwards	
Date:	1 May 2001	
Review date:	Oct. 2001	
Authorised by:	Dawn Ward	
Principal:	Ioan Morgan	

PERSONNEL AFFECTED – KEY

Staff	ST	Public	P	Young Persons	YP
Students	S	Contractors	C		

RISK RATING

SEVERITY		LIKELIHOOD	
Fatality	3	Probable	3
Major injury	2	Possible	2
Minor injury	1	Unlikely	1

Activity	Personnel affected	Hazards	Risk (Severity × Likelihood)	Existing control measures	Residual risk (Severity × Likelihood)	Existing control measures
Washing towels etc	S ST	Electricity	2×2=4	PAT tested, maintenance Service contract Instruction for users	1×2=2	
Tumble dryer	S ST	Electricity	2×2=4	PAT tested. Maintenance Instruction for users	2×1=2	
		Disposal of excess fluff	2×2=4	Extraction for fluff	1×1=1	
Ironing	ST	Electricity	2×1=2	PAT tested Safe practices of work	1×1=1	
Washing towels	ST	Chemical bleach	2×2=4	Safe practices at work Chemical in the metal cabinet Diluted as per instruction	1×1=1	

Fig. 3.17 *Example of a risk assessment record: Laundry room*

RISK ASSESSMENT

Programme area/Unit/Department: Beauty Therapy and Hairdressing

Logical assessment unit: Beauty M401/M403/M409/M502

Completed by: Dawn Edwards

Date: 10 April 2001

Review date: Sept. 2001

Authorised by: Dawn Ward

Principal: Ioan Morgan

PERSONNEL AFFECTED – KEY

Staff	ST	Public	P	Young Persons	YP
Students		Contractors	C		

Staff S (note: Staff = S, Students = ST)

RISK RATING

SEVERITY		LIKELIHOOD	
Fatality	3	Probable	3
Major injury	2	Possible	2
Minor injury	1	Unlikely	1

Activity	Personnel affected	Hazards	Risk (Severity × Likelihood)	Existing control measures	Residual risk (Severity × Likelihood)	Existing control measures
Use of hairdryer for mendhi	S ST	Electricity	2×2 = 4	Pat tested/maintenance Supervision of students Inspection of cables and connections by users	1×1 = 1	
Use of autoclave for sterilisation	S ST	Scald with steam Handling hot implements	2×2 = 4	Supervision of students Safe working practices	1×1 = 1	
Electrolysis	S ST P	Needle insertion Needle disposal	2×2 = 4	Supervision of students Safe systems of work Safe disposal in sealed bins collection by council	1×1 = 1	
Electrolysis blend machine	ST P S	Galvanic burn	2×2 = 4	Student supervision Safe systems at work	1×1 = 1	
Galvanic body machine	S ST P	Galvanic burn	2×2 = 4	Safe practices of work Student supervision	1×1 = 1	
Nail extension machine	S ST P	Hygiene/ infection	1×2 = 2	Student supervision induction	1×1 = 1	

Fig. 3.18 *Example of a risk assessment record: Beauty department (continued on opposite page)*

Activity	Personnel affected	Hazards	Risk (Severity × Likelihood)	Existing control measures	Residual risk (Severity × Likelihood)	Existing control measures
Nail varnish remover Surgical spirit	S ST P	Flammable	2×2=4	Storage in metal cabinet. Used in safe areas i.e. open area; well ventilated	1×1=1	
Electrical magnifying lamps	S ST P	Electrical	1×2=2	PAT tested Maintenance	1×1=1	
Chemical products	ST S P	Flammable	2×2=4	Storage in metal cupboard Skin test prior to tint applications	1×1=1	
Waxing	ST S P	Electricity and spillage of the wax	2×2=4	PAT tested appliance Safe systems at work	1×1=1	
Hand washing	ST S P	Spillage	2×2=4	Safe working practices	1×1=1	

Fig. 3.18 *Example of a risk assessment record: Beauty department (continued)*

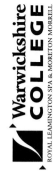

RISK ASSESSMENT

PERSONNEL AFFECTED – KEY

Staff	ST	Public	P	Young Persons	YP
Students	S	Contractors	C		

Programme area/Unit/Department: Beauty Therapy and Hairdressing

Logical assessment unit: Stock rooms

Completed by: Dawn Edwards

Date: 1 May 2001

Review date: Oct. 2001

Authorised by: Dawn Ward

Principal: Ioan Morgan

RISK RATING

SEVERITY		LIKELIHOOD	
Fatality	3	Probable	3
Major injury	2	Possible	2
Minor injury	1	Unlikely	1

Activity	Personnel affected	Hazards	Risk (Severity × Likelihood)	Existing control measures	Residual risk (Severity × Likelihood)	Existing control measures
Storage of chemicals and aerosols	ST	Flammable	2×2=4	Locked storage room with metal cabinet for flammable chemicals and aerosols	1×1=1	
			2×2=4		1×1=1	
Storage of equipment	ST		2×1=2	Unused equipment stored on shelves, safety ladder available to reach	1×1=1	

Fig. 3.19 *Example of a risk assessment record: Stock rooms*

RISK ASSESSMENT – ACTION PLAN

Logical assessment unit:

ACTION	ACTION BY	TARGET DATE	DATE COMPLETED

Fig. 3.20 *Example of a risk assessment action plan*

POINTS TO NOTE

- Risk assessment is an essential management tool, which defines what is or could be hazardous and the controls that the employer will put in place to protect its workforce and clients.
- A hazard is the potential of something to cause harm e.g. chemicals that may be used in the salon.
- A risk is the likelihood that harm will be caused by exposure to the hazard e.g. not wearing protective clothing when handling chemicals.

GOOD PRACTICE

- Risk assessment will form part of an employee's induction programme but it should not stop there, as it is essential to continually monitor and review risk assessments and update and remind all staff.
- Display your risk assessments record alongside the COSSH regulations within the salon.

Consultation

In order to achieve a beneficial treatment plan for an individual client it is essential that the therapist carries out a thorough consultation to establish a clear picture of the client's needs and constraints. This can prove to be a lengthy process for the trainee therapist but with time and practice the process will become easier and quicker.

There are many reasons why a client books an appointment for a particular treatment:

- They have heard about its benefits from friends.
- They have read about it or seen advertisements in magazines or local/national papers.
- It has been arranged by a relative or friend as a gift.
- They have, in their eyes, a problem, e.g. excess weight, poor skin condition, cellulite, stretch marks, tension in the muscles.

♦ They have a problem but don't have the confidence to book the type of treatment needed for this and so they have booked another type of treatment hoping the therapist will boost their confidence and recommended a suitable treatment plan for them.

When carrying out a consultation there are a number of things that the therapist needs to establish: medical details, personal details, body condition, skin analysis.

Medical details

Information regarding the client's past and present medical history should give the therapist clear indicators as to the possible underlying causes of the client's problems such as: the contraceptive pill causing an increase in appetite leading to weight gain; steroid medication for asthma causing weight gain; restricted mobility due to recent scar tissue causing poor muscle tone; previous acne causing skin-pitting-type scarring; childbirth causing poor abdominal muscle tone. Taking medical details also enables the therapist to identify possible contraindications to treatments.

Note. Specific contraindications to individual treatments are dealt with in each chapter.

Personal details

The therapist will take note of personal client details such as name, address and telephone numbers for their client data base. A data base can be used for a variety of things such as for marketing purposes, e.g. notifying customers of special offers and new product/equipment launches. They are also useful in case of emergencies, such as therapist illness, where an appointment needs to be altered or confirmed.

Taking personal and medical details during the consultation procedure enables the therapist to establish a professional rapport with the client, to put apprehensive clients at ease and to build up a clear picture of the individual client. Information on the client's lifestyle and occupation assist in analysing the client's constraints (time and finances) which have to be taken into consideration when organising a treatment plan for the client. This can also help the therapist in analysing the cause of the client's problem, e.g. a sales representative's job would generally involve a great deal of driving which could led to tension in the trapezius muscle and kyphosis.

A therapist would automatically consider the general health of their client as this can affect many different aspects such as skin condition, posture, etc. It is also useful to consider the client's intake of such things as alcohol, coffee and tea, particularly if the client suffers with cellulite or fluid retention. Tobacco smoking can cause dehydration of the skin as well as generally being an unhealthy habit. Diet plays a large part in our health so this should be taken into consideration as well. A poor diet can affect many of the body functions and systems, e.g. insufficient water could lead to constipation which in turn can bring about poor skin condition.

Female clients may suffer with skin related problems such as 'breakouts' due to their menstrual cycle, or they may suffer with pre-menstrual syndrome which may affect their general well being and cause many problems such as dehydration of the skin due to stress. The menstrual cycle brings about many changes in the client's body due to the hormonal balance and it is very useful to establish the time of the month prior to treatment, e.g. pre-menstrual, post-menstrual or mid-cycle.

Exposure to ultra-violet radiation is also noted in the consultation process as this can effect the client's skin condition and the sensitivity of the skin.

POINTS TO NOTE

⬧ A client who suffers with lower back ache in pre-menstrual cycle may benefit from a back massage for relaxation.
⬧ Sunburn in the area of treatment is a contraindication.
⬧ Exposure to ultra-violet radiation can cause dehydration and aging of the skin.
⬧ A professional therapist will always consider the client as an individual and where needed recommend an alternative therapist for treatments that they are not qualified to offer. For example, if a client has superfluous hair due to hormonal change such as pregnancy, the therapist would recommend electrical epilation or intense pulse light (IPL) or laser treatment.

Body condition

At the initial consultation for body treatments the therapists would establish the client's weight, height, frame size and body type, e.g. ectomorph, endomorph, mesomorph or combination. If the client was extremely sensitive about their weight at the initial consultation the therapist could offer a questionnaire with a number of weight variables to ascertain an approximate guide for organising a treatment plan.

Testing of the client's muscle tone is undertaken to establish any weak areas. The therapist would also note types of adipose tissue, e.g. cellulite, soft tissue and the area of the deposits along with any varicose veins or broken capillaries which may contraindicate treatment and the condition of the client's circulation, e.g. good, poor, fluid retention.

A thorough figure and posture analysis is carried out to highlight any problem areas and the client's reasons for treatment are recorded. All of these points will have assisted the therapist in establishing a total picture of the client's needs in order for them to develop a realistic treatment plan for the individual client.

Figure 3.22 shows an example of a trainee's consultation card for body treatments.

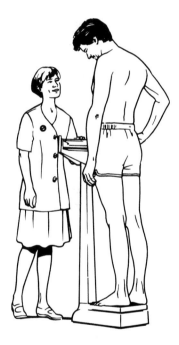

Fig. 3.21 *Body condition*

POINTS TO NOTE

Before stress can be dealt with effectively the therapist must be able to recognise its symptoms.

⬧ Physical symptoms of stress: tension headaches; indigestion; muscle tension; dry mouth and throat; tiredness; menstrual problems; diarrhoea/frequent urination; constipation; clumsiness.
⬧ Emotional symptoms of stress: rapid mood swings; lack of concentration; indecision; feeling tearful.
⬧ Behavioural symptoms of stress: sleep problems; overeating or loss of appetite; withdrawal from friends and work colleagues; increase in smoking/alcohol intake.

Medical details	Personal details
Name of doctor:	Name of client:
Present medication:	Address:
Past medication:	
Number of pregnancies:	Home tel.: Work tel.:
Ages of children:	Date of birth:
Operations: Hysterectomy ( ) Caesarean section ( ) Others	Lifestyle:
	Occupation:
	Smoker (Y/N) Number per week:
Contraindications: Diabetes ( ) Epilepsy ( ) Pacemaker ( ) Heart condition ( ) Asthma ( ) Thrombosis/phlebitis ( ) Metal pins/plates ( ) Skin diseases/disorders ( ) Oedema ( ) Blood pressure (high/low) Recent scars (up to 12 months) ( ) Hepatitis/blood infections (up to 24 months) ( ) Cuts/bruises ( )	

Body condition		
Height: Weight:	Frame size (small/medium/large)	
Body type (ectomorph/endomorph/mesomorph/combination)		
Muscle tone (please use the following symbols: +good, =medium, −poor):		
Biceps/triceps ( ) Abdominals ( ) Abductors ( ) Adductors ( ) Gluteals ( ) Other		
Types of adipose deposit (hard/medium/soft/cellulite)		
Areas of adipose deposit:		
Areas of cellulite:		
Varicose veins/broken capillaries:	Circulation (good/poor/fluid retention)	
Figure/posture analysis: Scoliosis ( ) Kyphosis ( ) Lordosis ( ) Other		
Reason for treatment		

Treatment plan	
Recommended retail/home care advice:	Recommended salon treatments:
Eyes	
Face	
Neck	
Décolleté	Recommended salon products:
Bust	Dietary/exercise advice:
Body	

Note. The reverse of this card can be used for recording a client's measurements when undertaking figure improvement programmes.

Indemnity: I confirm that to the best of my knowledge the answers that I have given are correct and that I have not withheld any information.

Signatures of: Client: Date:

                              Therapist: Date:

Fig. 3.22 *Example of a trainee's consultation card for body treatments*

Skin analysis

Analysis of the client's skin condition and turgor (tone) will enable the therapist to evaluate their needs. On a consultation card used for training a list of the main muscles or areas affecting expression lines could be listed to assist the trainee in recalling the key areas to consider along with possible problems the client might experience, e.g. comedones, areas of flakiness, poor elasticity, acne rosacea. An area for the therapist to note additional comments such as if the client has used products like Retinoic A which could contraindicate them to treatments such as waxing, or to note previous treatments and products used. The reason for treatment needs to be established during the consultation procedure to ensure that the therapist can organise an effective treatment plan. Skin analysis can be studied in depth in *A Practical Guide to Beauty Therapy* by Janet Simms published by Nelson Thornes.

Figure 3.23 shows an example of a trainee's consultation card for facial treatments.

POINT TO NOTE

After six treatments it is recommended that a new consultation card is completed.

POINT TO NOTE

Retinoic A is a topical skin care product developed in the 1960s to treat acne. It speeds up exfoliation by reducing the stratum corneum from 14 cells thick to 4. Following the interest in Retinoic A other types of acids have been examined and used to speed up skin exfoliation. (See Chapter 7).

Treatment plan

The therapist is now able to recommend salon treatments, identify a suitable salon range of products and the appropriate retail products for the client and where applicable on complementary diet and exercise. (See Figs. 3.22 and 3.23.)

Figure 3.24 shows an example of a body treatment record card.

POINTS TO NOTE

- A client is a potential client for all treatments and retail products that would benefit their skin and body condition, not just for the treatment they have booked.
- A client is paying for your professional advice and experience not just a treatment. It is their choice as to whether they adopt your recommendations, but they should always be offered.

Medical details	Personal details
Name of doctor:	Name of client:
Present medication:	Address:
Past medication:	
Number of pregnancies:	Home tel.: Work tel.:
Ages of children:	Date of birth:
Operations: Hysterectomy ( ) Caesarean section ( ) Others	Lifestyle:
	Occupation:
	Smoker (Y/N) Number per week:
Contraindications: Diabetes ( ) Epilepsy ( ) Pacemaker ( ) Heart condition ( ) Asthma ( ) Thrombosis/phlebitis ( ) Metal pins/plates ( ) Skin diseases/disorders ( ) Oedema ( ) Blood pressure (high/low) Recent scars (up to 12 months) ( ) Hepatitis/blood infections (up to 24 months) ( ) Cuts/bruises ( ) General health (good/poor)	Drink (units per week): Alcohol ( ) Coffee ( ) Tea ( ) Diet: Digestion: General health (good/poor) Exposure to ultra-violet/skin condition:

Skin analysis	
Muscle tone (please use the following symbols: +good, =medium, −poor):	
Decollete ( ) Neck ( ) Mandible ( ) Zygomaticus ( ) Orbicularis occuli ( )	
Skin turgor (tone):	Areas of pigmentation:
Areas of broken capillaries:	Type of pigmentation/vein
Skin texture:	
Oedema:	Collagen/elasticity:
Open pores:	Comedones (open/closed/micro)
Papules:	Pustules:
Moles:	Superfluous hair:
Area of flakiness:	Area of shininess:
Seborrhea:	Acne rosacea:
Acne vulgaris:	Dermatitis/eczema:
Psoriasis:	Skin tags:
Dehydration:	Scarring
Skin type:	
Comments:	
Reason for treatment	

Treatment plan	
Recommended retail/home care advice:	Recommended salon treatments:
Eyes	
Face	
Neck	
Décolleté	Recommended salon products:
Bust	Dietary/exercise advice:
Body	

Indemnity: I confirm that to the best of my knowledge the answers that I have given are correct and that I have not withheld any information.

Signatures of: Client: Date:

                         Therapist: Date:

Fig. 3.23 *Example of a trainee's card for facial treatments*

Body treatment record card			
Name of client: Address:		Home tel.: Work tel.:	
	Date	Treatment, products and equipment	Therapist
Client's views on previous treatment			

Fig. 3.24 *Example of a body treatment record card*

1   Explain why you should consider the following when carrying out a client consultation:
    a personal details   **c** body condition
    b medical details   **d** skin analysis.
2   What two key areas form a treatment plan?
3   List three examples of:
    a physical symptoms of stress
    b emotional symptoms of stress
    c behavioural symptoms of stress.
4   State the information that should be recorded on a client record card.

Key Terms

You need to know what these words and phrases mean. Go back through the chapter to find out.

- AIDS
- Animal parasites
- Antiseptics
- Autoclave
- Bacteria
- Chemical methods of sterilisation
- Consultation
- Dealing with clients, visitors and reception enquiries
- Disinfection
- Emergency first aid
- Fungi
- Glass bead steriliser
- Hepatitis B
- Maintaining stock in the retail area
- Reception
- Receptionist
- Sanitiser
- Sterilisation
- Viruses

After working through this chapter you will be able to:

- explain the equipment required for massage
- describe how a welcoming environment can be created for a client having a body massage
- list the contraindications to massage
- name the main massage movements and their effects on the body
- describe the effects of massage
- perform an effective massage treatment for a range of clients including: male, female, apprehensive, for stress and relaxation, muscular aches and pains, weight loss, poor muscle tone and for a variety of times, e.g. one hour, half an hour
- identify different types of massage.

Introduction

Massage is much more than just manipulation of soft body tissue; it has deep psychological implications. Records show that ancient civilisations practised massage in varying forms before medicine was developed. Our earliest childhood memories of when we were injured are of adults insisting on 'rubbing' it better. Hippocrates, who is regarded as the father of modern medicine, made reference to the benefit of physicians being able to rub and knead.

So it can be seen that massage has firmly established itself as a therapeutic treatment and one which enjoys re-discovered popularity in our stress-laden times.

Over the last decade, massage therapy has expanded greatly. It is widely practised as a specialist field but is also offered by beauty therapists in salons, health farms, leisure centres, etc. One of the main benefits the therapist can offer the client is relaxation to release stress which can lead to aches and pains, postural problems, and physical and emotional illness.

Every client from the high-powered executive to the busy houseperson will suffer at some time, if not for a large part of their life, with stress, whether through day-to-day problems encountered at work or in their social life or through a particular crisis. Stress can cause physical and emotional illness and therefore it is paramount that the therapist truly considers each client as an individual and views information gathered in the consultation to establish a full picture of that individual client.

A professional massage can be extremely exhausting both physically and emotionally for the therapist as they are not just laying on hands but giving of themselves. The majority of massage therapists ensure that they have booked sufficient time between each client to gather themselves and re-focus on the next person.

The consultation period spent with each client is highly important, it gives the therapist and client an opportunity to establish a professional bond and it enables the therapist to assess the individual clients' needs. On average the therapist would allow approximately thirty minutes at the first appointment and thereafter a minimum of five minutes should be taken prior to the massage to assess the client's reaction to the previous treatment and to establish their individual needs for this treatment.

Throughout the world, trainee therapists may learn different European massage routines depending on their individual tutor. When a trainee commences a massage programme the instructor will design an introductory massage routine which will encompass the classical massage movements and is generally designed to cover the whole of a female body and to last for one hour. This form of massage predominantly affects the muscular and circulatory systems and is seen as a starting point to introduce the trainee to massage and develop their:

- manual dexterity and postural stance
- understanding of rate, rhythm, pressure and contact
- understanding of the classical massage movements and their benefits
- communication, organisation and management skills
- ability to analyse the individual's needs.

From the commencement of their training until the day they decide to stop practising and learning, the therapist will broaden their knowledge and technical skills by:

- observing various techniques by different instructors
- observing technical representatives from product companies
- observing fellow therapists in the industry
- watching demonstrations at beauty exhibitions
- receiving treatment from other therapists
- reading text books on massage.

Once a trainee has learnt an introductory massage routine, mastering the correct posture, stance, rhythm, rate, pressure and client care, they will be encouraged to adapt their massage by drawing on their instructors' and other trainees' knowledge to suit the individual client's needs, e.g. male client massage is generally much firmer; clients suffering from stress in the upper back may prefer the time they have booked to be spent concentrating on this area.

Classification of massage movements and their effects on the body

Massage movements are generally divided into five main categories; effleurage, petrissage, tapotement, frictions and vibrations.

Effleurage
Effleurage can be defined as a stroking movement in the direction of venous return involving the passage of the hand or part of the hand over the skin. The hand should be moulded to the area being treated and the fingers and thumbs should be kept together. It is important that the

pressure is constant and even throughout the movement. The pressure will vary depending on the area being treated; therefore effleurage movements can be subdivided into two forms.

Superficial stroking
As the name suggests, superficial stroking is performed using a very light pressure. The hand should be flexible and under perfect control so that the entire palmar surface is in contact with the area being massaged.

Deep stroking
Deep stroking refers to the depth of pressure on the tissues rather than the use of force. Again the movement is performed using the entire palmar surface of the hand, but a greater depth of pressure is applied. The return stroke should be of a superficial nature, otherwise it may reverse some of the effects achieved, i.e. return of venous circulation and lymph.

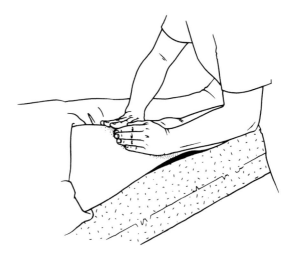

Fig. 4.1 *Deep effleurage*

The beneficial effects of effleurage
- Aids venous circulation and return to the heart by the mechanical effect on the tissues.
- Aids lymphatic circulation by the mechanical effects on the tissues.
- Speeds the absorption of waste materials.
- Promotes relaxation by the reflex effect on the tissues.
- Enables the client to become accustomed to the therapist's hands.

Petrissage
Petrissage can be defined as pressure and/or relaxing of pressure. The movements consist of repeatedly grasping and releasing the tissues with one or both hands in a lifting, rolling or pressing fashion. Petrissage movements are often named according to the part of the hand used and include palmar kneading, palmar lifting, wringing, thumb kneading, finger kneading, skin rolling and picking up.

Although the pressure is intermittent, care must be taken to avoid pinching the skin. This is prevented by gently relaxing the pressure as the bulk of the tissues diminishes.

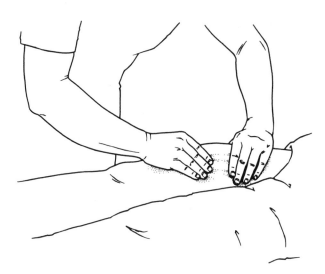

Fig. 4.2 *Petrissage*

The beneficial effects of petrissage
- Aids venous circulation.
- Increases lymphatic flow.
- Improves absorption of substances within the tissues.
- Loosens adherent tissues.
- Moves the tissues over bone.

Tapotement
Tapotement movements are sometimes defined as percussion-type movements which can be light tapping to beating movements applied in a brisk fashion. The whole hand of part of the hand can be used depending on the type of tapotement movement being given.

Tapotement movements include:

- Tapping – using the fingertips only.
- Hacking – using the ulnar border of the hands.
- Cupping – using the fingers and palms of the hands in a concave position.
- Pounding – using the ulnar border of a lightly clenched fist.
- Beating – using lightly clenched fists palms down.

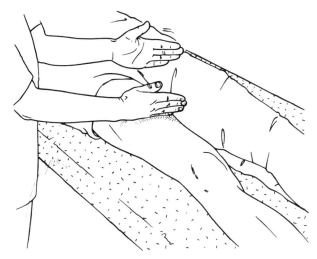

Fig. 4.3 *Hacking*

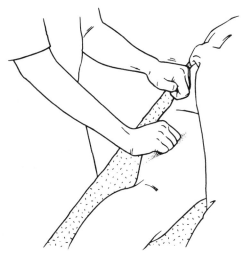

Fig. 4.4 *Beating*

The beneficial effects of tapotement

- ◊ Very stimulating – causes erythema.
- ◊ Produces localised heat.
- ◊ Stimulates muscle fibres.
- ◊ Increases cellular activity.

Frictions

Frictions are normally performed with either the palms or the fingers or the thumbs. The superficial tissues are moved over the underlying structures keeping the hand in firm contact whilst performing small circular movements in a restricted area before gliding on to the next part. The movement is applied in a direction which produces tension on the tissues and has a loosening effect. Pressure should not be too firm otherwise bruising may occur.

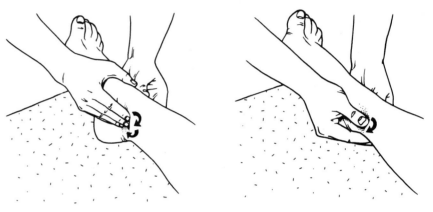

Fig. 4.5 *Frictions*

The beneficial effects of frictions

- ◊ Loosens adherent tissues.
- ◊ Greatly increases localised circulation.
- ◊ Speeds cellular activity.

Vibrations

Vibrations are defined as rapid muscular contractions of the therapist's arms being transmitted through the fingers or palms to produce a highly stimulating, shaking-type movement. Vibrations are normally applied on areas overlying muscular motor points.

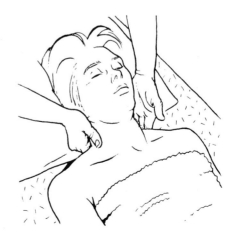

Fig. 4.6 *Light vibrations*

The beneficial effects of vibrations

- Increases blood circulation.
- Stimulates localised nerve endings.

Preparation for massage

Treatment area

Massage treatment areas vary in appearance depending on the environment in which they are found. Some salons have individual rooms for therapists to work in, designed to allow complete privacy for the client. Others screen the salon into the number of cubicles by using rails and curtains, like those you see in hospitals.

Equipment required for massage
Beauty couches

In order for the massage to be performed, a sturdy, comfortable treatment couch of the correct height for the individual therapist is needed. There are a wide variety of couches available for the therapist or salon owner to choose from.

A general purpose massage or treatment couch with an adjustable back support is available in standard heights. They can be purchased with a 'breathe hole' which can be removed when performing back and neck massage to allow the client to breathe easily. A face cushion can also be purchased and used where the couch does not have a breathe hole or when the therapist or client feels the need to use one to aid comfort during the treatment.

A multi-purpose couch/chair is available in standard heights. It enables the therapist to convert the couch from a massage plinth to a couch suitable for facial treatments by lifting and lowering the client's legs for comfort and raising the back support.

Adjustable-height couches have been developed over recent years to enhance the working life of the therapist as they can be adjusted to suit the height of the individual and/or the particular treatment they are performing.

There is a wide selection of adjustable-height couches/chairs and they are very useful. Their versatility is an important factor when different height therapists work from the same room, as for example in massaging or waxing, and where a treatment room is multifunctional and used for body and face treatments. The height-adjustable chair/couch is especially recommended for body wrapping treatments when client mobility is restricted and lower bed height is advantageous.

The heavy-duty hydraulic height-adjustable bed or chair/couch will have a central hydraulic pump, operated by the foot to adjust plinth height – the usual range being about 18 to 20 centimetres. On some models the head and leg sections are raised and lowered with either a gas strut-assisted mechanism or a foot-operated hydraulic system.

The heavy-duty electrically operated hydraulic bed or chair/couch is considered to be the present top-of-the range choice. It has all the advantages of the standard hydraulic operation but can also have the additional advantages of a greater height range (up to 50cm); often leg and head sections that are operated electronically; and for a chair/couch model it is also possible to have an electronic tilt to the mid-section for greater client comfort. Wheels and brakes to the base frame are often standard and are advantageous as they afford easy positioning around a room and cleaning of the floor area.

It is important to note that hydraulic couches:

◆ Protect therapists and employees from possible postural problems due to the use of couches of incorrect height and thus enables the therapist to perform a treatment more accurately.
◆ Enable a variety of therapists of differing heights to perform different treatments in the same treatment area.

Prior to the client's arrival the therapist or their assistant should ensure the couch is covered with clean linen, towels and/or blankets depending upon the salon policy or the client's preference. The couch may be covered with paper towels to maintain hygienic conditions, protect the linen and reduce laundry bills. Pillows or rolled towels should be available for client comfort throughout the treatment.

Couch steps

Couch steps are available to assist clients who are particularly small or who for medical reasons have difficulty getting onto the general purpose non-hydraulic couch. They should be used with care and always with the therapist in attendance.

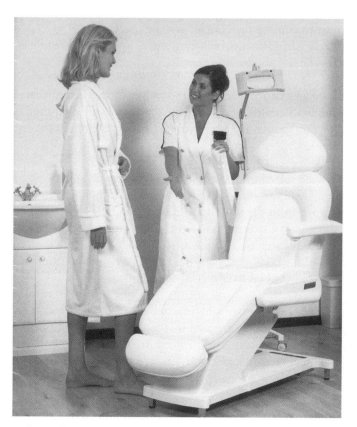

Fig. 4.7 *Electrically operated beauty couch*

Beauty chairs (stools)

As part of some massage treatments, the therapist may need to sit to ensure they are able to apply the appropriate pressure and at the same time protect their own posture. Therefore there will be a need to ensure an operator's chair or stool is in the treatment area. Two important things to note with this piece of furniture are that it has well oiled castors to allow the therapist to manoeuvre into different positions smoothly and prevent any unnecessary noise and that it should be adjusted correctly to suit the height of the therapist.

It is important to observe general safety in the treatment area by ensuring the chair or stool is safely stored to prevent any accidents.

Beauty trolleys

Most therapists use a sturdy trolley with easy-moving castors to hold the products and materials needed to perform a massage. Some holistic therapists may use a convenient surface such as a table rather than a traditional trolley to lessen the clinical aspect of massage.

Whatever surface is being used it is essential that it is cleaned and prepared with the necessary items before the client arrives and is suited for the purpose.

First impressions count, so it is essential that the therapist and treatment area are well prepared for each client.

> **ACTIVITY**
> Research the variety of massage equipment available. Draw up a chart detailing cost, durability and features of each piece of equipment.

The therapist

To establish a professional ethos, the therapist should take great care of his or her appearance and personal hygiene, particularly for massage treatments where they will be working in close contact with their clients.

They should always note the following:

- A high standard of personal hygiene should be observed at all times.
- Professional dress should be worn in the salon environment. It should be non-restrictive, clean and pressed.
- Items required to ensure personal hygiene can be maintained throughout the day should be kept in the therapist's locker, e.g. soap, towel, deodorant, a change of clothes, toothbrush and toothpaste.
- Hair should be clean and well groomed. Long hair should be styled to prevent it from falling into the client's or therapist's face.
- Comfortable, supportive, low-heeled, closed-in shoes should be worn to prevent poor posture and subsequent back problems.
- Nails should be short so that they do not disturb the flow of the massage or cause discomfort to the client and should be unvarnished for hygienic practice and in case of client allergy.

- Jewellery should be removed from the wrists and hands, along with dangling earrings or chains, again to ensure the flow of the massage and so as not to disturb the client's relaxation.
- A calm, relaxed, reassuring therapist is essential for a massage treatment.

Items required for massage
Essential items:

- Massage medium (lubricant).
- Tissues.
- Cotton wool.
- Protection for the client's hair.
- Waste receptacle.

Optional items:

- Eau de cologne (for refreshing client's feet and/or removing oil/cream).
- Hot, damp towels (for removing excess oil/cream).
- Hot, dry towels (for therapeutic purposes).
- Footspray (for refreshing client's feet).

Massage mediums
Traditionally a variety of massage mediums have been used.

Oils
Oil still tends to be the most popular lubricant for body massage as it gives the therapist more slip. The oils selected by today's therapists generally have a base of vegetable or plant oils and may have other active ingredients added to create a particular effect on the body, e.g. lemon (stimulating). Aromatherapy is a specialised massage treatment using essential oils for therapeutic purposes. This can be studied in depth by attending specialised training courses.

Modern therapists tend not to use mixtures high in mineral oil as these are generally considered to be comedogenic.

Creams
Cream is not a particularly popular medium for a full body massage, though it has been used in the past for spot areas of massage or because of a client's preference. Today you are far more likely to find creams being used as part of a particular manual body treatment for skin improvement, i.e. cellulite or stretch mark treatments.

Talcum powder
Talcum powder tends to be used as a lubricant when an electrotherapy treatment is carried out in conjunction with massage and the client or therapist does not want to use an oil or cream, e.g. during high frequency treatments. Talcum powder is popular with reflexologists as it gives 'slip' to the therapist's hands. It is often believed that greater depth can be achieved by using talcum powder as the massage medium.

In recent years product manufacturers have greatly developed products available for salon massage treatments as well as for complementary home care use. It is more popular to find a salon using one or two product companies' ranges rather than the old fashioned bulk products of the late twentieth century. One of the main reasons for this has been the huge technological advances of the new millennium, and a great increase in the general public's awareness of product knowledge combined with their thirst for improved appearance and health. Therapists have also realised the professional and financial rewards which can be gained from retailing products such as body scrubs and lotions.

ACTIVITY

Research the different professional massage mediums available. Compare their ingredients and costs.

Creating a welcoming environment

As one of the main benefits of massage is relaxation, it is extremely important to create the right environment to enhance the massage treatment. This can be done in a number of ways.

Heating
As the client will be undressed during the massage, it is important to ensure they are kept comfortable.

- The room or treatment area may be heated to a higher than normal working temperature prior to the client's arrival and the temperature reduced as necessary throughout the treatment.
- Blankets can be used to wrap the client up snugly.
- Towels can be warmed over a radiator or in a tumble drier and placed on the couch for the client or over the area that has just been worked on, particularly on cold, damp, winter days.

Electronically heated under- and over-blankets are now available which offer safe, professional and controllable heating ranges. These add great client comfort-value and gentle sedation is very beneficial for many of the new spa-type salon treatments involving envelopment/cocoon protocols.

GOOD PRACTICE

- Consideration should be given to the climate, e.g. in hot, humid countries the majority of clients like therapists to work in cool, air-conditioned rooms and to use cold (iced) towels on the areas that have been treated.
- Consideration should be given to the client's needs. Some people feel the cold more than others, e.g. in warm weather one client may not want to be wrapped up snugly in blankets and warm towels whereas another may prefer it.

Ventilation
A well-ventilated treatment area is essential to prevent cross-infection of communicable diseases. It also ensures stagnant air, saturated with carbon dioxide due to exhalation from clients and therapists, is removed. A build

up of stale air, containing heat, odours and carbon dioxide, can make the treatment room uninviting and the therapist lethargic which can affect the therapist's work.

Aroma

The treatment area needs to be inviting to the client and one of the ways the therapist can enhance this is by introducing aroma essence into the area. Qualified aromatherapists use essential oils for treatment and this obviously can create a pleasant smell in the treatment area. As no two clients are alike, the therapist must ensure that they know their client's likes and dislikes in smells. The introduction of a smell the client dislikes will automatically prevent the client from relaxing and returning for further treatment.

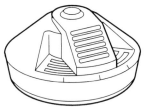

Fig. 4.8 *Aroma diffuser*

Recently, a number of manufacturers have developed a small piece of equipment, a diffuser, which is used to introduce aromas into the atmosphere. Aromatherapy burners may also be used to further enhance the environment.

Colour

When planning a treatment area of a salon, the therapist should spend a great deal of time considering the decor (wall and floor coverings, towels, etc.) to ensure they create the right sort of environment for their clients. Generally therapists select warm colours, e.g. pinks, or relaxing colours, e.g. greens. The type of client plays a large role in selection of colour schemes, e.g. sports therapists may select white as a clinical colour and a beauty salon with mixed gender clients would generally avoid what are considered by some people to be feminine colours, e.g. pinks.

Colour used in a superficial form, such as in decor, towels and lighting can contribute to a client's relaxation and should therefore be considered by the therapist when preparing the treatment area.

In recent years colour therapists have undertaken a great deal of research not only into the therapeutic effects of colour but into the use of light to heal (chromatherapy).

Lighting

Ideally the lighting of the treatment area for massage should be soft to induce relaxation. The use of strong bright lights can be very distracting to clients.

POINT TO NOTE

Chromatic light therapy (using the pure colours of the visible light spectrum, see page 254) is used to help improve problem skin conditions and promote good body equilibrium.

Sound

The therapist can perform the massage in a tranquil area and/or they may wish to compliment the treatment (with the client's agreement) with therapeutic music to aid relaxation. Some therapists retail taped music to clients who need to unwind and relax between treatments.

Health, safety, legislation and local bye-laws

Health and safety is of paramount importance and should be foremost in the therapist's mind. Therefore the therapist must be aware of certain legislative requirements in order to practise massage therapy. These are:

- The Health and Safety at Work Act 1974.
- The Office, Shops and Railway Premises Act 1963.
- Local government bye-laws relating to massage, e.g. Birmingham City Council Act 1990.
- Public Liability Insurance.
- Employers Liability Insurance.

(For further information of these legislative requirements and principles of good practice see Chapter 13.)

ACTIVITY

Through work experience, discuss with your colleagues how different salons have created a welcoming environment.

Massage consultation and assessment

The introduction to massage given in the earlier part of this chapter along with the chapter on consultation highlight the importance of performing a thorough consultation prior to the massage treatment to establish the individual client's needs, their views, preconceived ideas and to develop a professional relationship.

When training in massage therapy it is important to use a detailed consultation card which acts as a reminder to the trainee therapist to ensure they use all sources of information in order to establish a clear picture of each client. Once qualified, the therapist can purchase professional record cards or design their own for recording consultations and treatment depending upon their environment, e.g. salons offering a variety of treatments may use a multi-purpose record card whereas health centres specialising in alternative therapies may use a specialised record card.

In order to perform an effective consultation the therapist must know what the general effects of massage are along with the conditions which may prevent the client from having treatment.

The general effects of massage
- Improves blood circulation, therefore hastening the interchange of oxygen, nutrients, carbon dioxide and waste.
- Relieves muscular tension due to removal of waste.
- Increases lymphatic circulation, again hastening the removal of toxins.
- Causes hyperaemia which temporarily increases heat in the area of treatment.
- Helps to soften fatty tissue deposits depending on the movements used.
- Softens and nourishes the skin, depending on the medium chosen.

- Causes slight desquamation, thus improving the skin's texture.
- Skin tone and elasticity are improved.
- Stimulates or soothes the sensory nerve endings, depending on the massage movements used.
- Deeply relaxing – it gives the client a feeling of well-being.
- Helps to prevent stress-related disorders.

Contraindications
to massage

- Skin diseases.
- Infectious skin disorders.
- Vascular conditions – history of thrombosis, severe varicose veins.
- Heart disorders, high/low blood pressure (medical approval should be obtained before giving treatment in these cases).
- Unidentified swellings or lumps.
- Oedema.
- Raised body temperature.
- Burns/sunburn.
- Later stages of pregnancy (avoid abdominal massage once pregnancy is known).

POINTS TO NOTE

- If in doubt about the client's medical condition, refer the client tactfully to their medical practitioner without causing the client concern.
- Do not attempt to diagnose a medical condition.
- Some conditions do not prevent entire treatment, only treatment to specific areas or the omission of certain movements.

Points to note in performing a consultation
On greeting the client, the therapist takes them through to the treatment area to carry out the consultation.

Details taken in the consultation should include:

- General details, e.g. the client's name, address and contact telephone number.
- Medical history details.
- General physical health details.
- Lifestyle details.
- Posture/figure analysis.
- Further salon treatments.
- Retail and home care advice.

(For further information on the reception of clients and client consultation see Chapter 3.)

Principles of good massage practice

1   Perform a detailed consultation so as to be able to devise the most appropriate form of massage to be given. The consultation is the basis to establish how best to treat the client's needs, i.e. type, duration and frequency of massage. The consultation is also needed to rule out contraindications.

2   Maintain good posture throughout massage. The therapist needs to ensure that throughout the massage routine he/she maintains correct postural stance for the movements and area of the body being treated to provide a beneficial treatment for the client and to prevent fatigue of the therapist. When working on the body in a longitudinal direction use walk-standing and when working in a transverse direction use stride-standing (see Figs. 4.9 and 4.10).

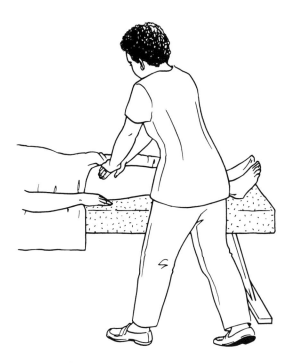

Fig. 4.9 *Walk-standing – keeping the back straight, commence effleurage on client's foot, then glide up the leg rocking the body weight forward from heel to toe*

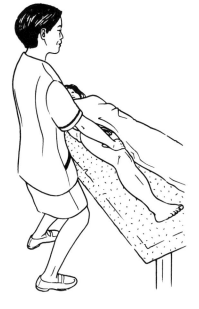

Fig. 4.10 *Stride-standing – knees bent, back straight*

3   Maintain an even rate and rhythm. Massage movements should be gentle, slow and rhythmical – with the exception of tapotement. The acceptable rate of coverage is 18 cm (7 inches) per second and this should remain consistent throughout the massage to give the most beneficial effects.

4   Ensure hand flexibility. Manual massage treatment involves the use of the hands for manipulation of body tissues. It is therefore essential that the therapist has complete control of his/her hands in order to mould them to the area being treated and provide the optimum treatment. When commencing training you should practise simple hand and wrist exercise to increase mobility and flexibility and use these exercises prior to a massage if the hands and arms are not suitably relaxed.

5   Adapt pressure according to the area being treated and the individual client's needs. The secret of a successful massage is to vary the pressure so as to be of maximum benefit to the client, but

without being too heavy as to be uncomfortable or cause pain or bruising. Pressure should be increased or decreased gradually.

6 Always maintain contact with the client during the massage. When changing movements always keep a reassuring hand on the area to avoid breaking continuity of the sequence.

Preparation for treatment

- Ensure the treatment room creates a welcoming environment.
- Ensure the couch is protected appropriately.
- The therapist should present him/herself professionally.

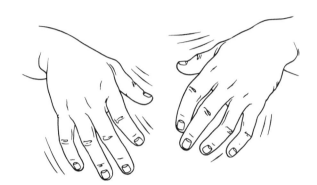

Fig. 4.11 *Hand and wrist exercise – loosely shaking hands and wrists*

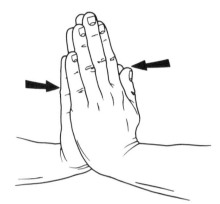

Fig. 4.12 *Hand and wrist exercise – hands in prayer position, using alternate resistance push from side to side*

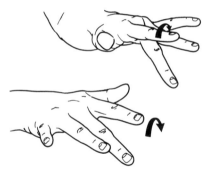

Fig. 4.13 *Hand and wrist exercise – rotate each finger and thumb individually in a circular fashion clockwise and anticlockwise*

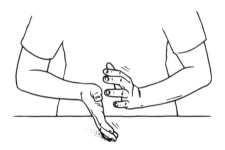

Fig. 4.14 *Hand and wrist exercise – using the ulnar borders of both hands, with relaxed fingers and wrists alternately flick the hands lightly onto a hard surface*

Massage treatment

- The client is greeted at reception and taken to the changing area.
- Consultation is carried out to check for contraindications, to establish the client's needs and to explain the benefits of the treatment.
- The client may have a selected heat treatment to relax the muscles ready for massage and this treatment is carried out first.
- The client relaxes on the couch, and using the selected massage medium the therapist performs a massage routine to benefit the individual client.

The client is allowed time to relax and then offered a drink of mineral water. If the client wishes, the oil can be removed, either by the therapist or by showering. (Aromatherapy oil is generally left on the skin.)

Progress Check

1 State the equipment needed to perform a body massage.
2 List six factors that will contribute towards a welcoming environment.
3 Give six contraindications to massage treatment and explain why each is a contraindication.
4 List the five classical types of massage movement and describe two benefits of each type.
5 State five specific effects of massage.

Introductory massage routine (for a female client)

The client should first be prepared by being asked to undress and put on a clean towelling robe. If possible, it is better to offer a heat treatment before commencing massage to relax the client and warm the body tissues. The heat treatment could be a steam bath, sauna, jacuzzi or even just a warm shower.

In the prepared treatment area, ask the client to remove their gown and get on to the couch lying face upwards (supine), assisting the client and providing couch steps where needed. Then cover the client in clean, warm towels.

POINT TO NOTE

The movements in the introductory massage routine (for a female client) are repeated a number of times to suit an individual client's needs.

Front of leg massage

Preparation

a Remove the towel from the front of the leg area, keeping other parts of the body well covered for warmth.
b Apply the selected massage medium to the area by first warming it on your own hands and then applying it to the client's leg from foot to thigh following the effleurage pattern.
c Ensure your posture is good with a straight back.

Massage sequence

1 **Effleurage to the whole leg**

Place the entire palmar surface of both hands on the dorsal surface of the foot. With one hand leading, keep fingers and thumbs together and glide hands along the entire leg to the top of the thigh. Glide hands apart laterally, lightly returning to ankle. (Main muscles affected: tibialis anterior, soleus, quadriceps, abductors, adductors.)

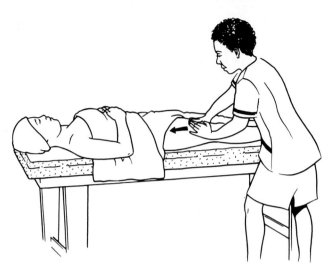

Fig. 4.15 *Effleurage to the whole leg*

2 **Deep wringing of the quadriceps**
a Slide hands to the interior aspect of the thigh and then with hands parallel, pick and lift the tissues and squeeze gently in a wringing action. Work the entire quadriceps area.
(Main muscles affected: quadriceps, abductors, adductors.)
b Effleurage to the quadriceps area.

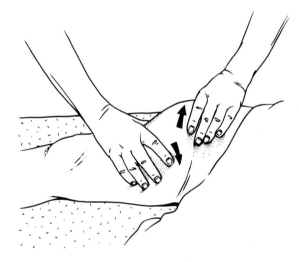

Fig. 4.16 *Wringing to the quadriceps*

Fig. 4.17 *Effleurage to the quadriceps area*

3 **Alternate palmar lifting of the quadriceps**
a Starting with hands on either side at the top of the thigh, use the entire palmar surface of both hands to gently compress the tissues against each other and lift from side to side. Keep repeating until the knee is reached and then slide the hands back up the leg.
(Main muscles affected: quadriceps, abductors, adductors.)
b Effleurage to the quadriceps area.

4 **Hacking to the quadriceps**
a Using the ulnar border of both hands, briskly but lightly hack the quadriceps area in a rhythmical pattern.
(Main muscles affected: quadriceps, abductors, adductors.)
b Effleurage to the quadriceps area.

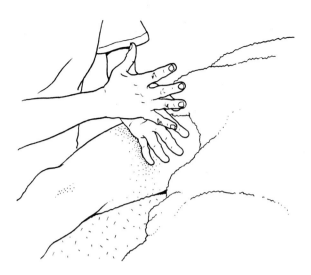

Fig. 4.18 *Hacking to the quadriceps*

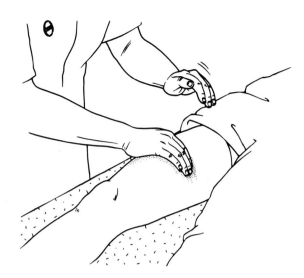

Fig. 4.19 *Cupping to the quadriceps*

5 **Cupping to the quadriceps**
   a Holding the fingers and palms of the hands in a concave position, briskly but lightly cup the quadriceps area.
   (Main muscles affected: quadriceps, abductors, adductors.)
   b Effleurage to the quadriceps area.
6 **Beating to the quadriceps area**
   a Using lightly clenched fists, palms down, lightly beat the quadriceps area.
   (Main muscles affected: quadriceps, abductors, adductors.)
   b Effleurage to the quadriceps.
7 **Thumb friction circles around the patella**
   a Using the thumb digits, gently perform friction circles around the patella.
   (Main muscles affected: tibialis anterior, coleus, quadriceps, abductors, adductors.)
   b Effleurage the whole leg.

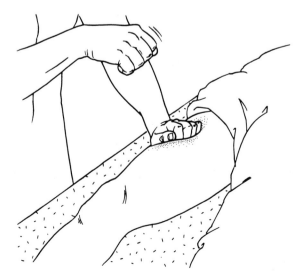

Fig. 4.20 *Beating to the quadriceps*

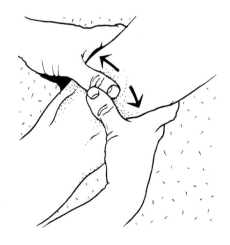

Fig. 4.21 *Thumb friction circles around the patella*

8 **Palmar kneading to the soleus**
Using the thenar eminence of the hand push upwards along the soleus muscle towards the knee. Continue using the thenar eminence of the hand to apply friction circles in a clockwise movement, slowly working down towards the ankle.
(Main muscle affected: soleus.)

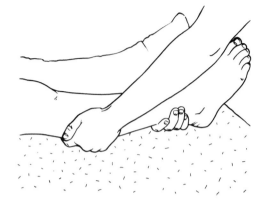

Fig. 4.22 *Palmar kneading to the soleus*

9 **Deep stroking around the ankle malleolus**
Using the digits of both hands gently stroke around the ankle malleolus.

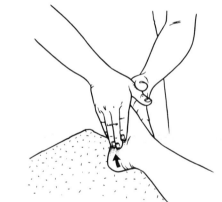

Fig. 4.23 *Deep stroking around the ankle malleolus*

10 **Friction circles between the metatarsal bones**
Using the thumbs of both hands apply friction circles between the metatarsal bones.

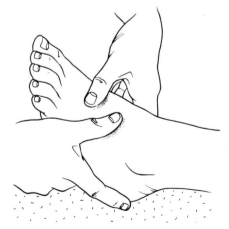

Fig. 4.24 *Friction circles between the metatarsals*

11 Toe circles

Support the toe joints with one hand underneath the foot and the other on top. Circle hands in a clockwise then anticlockwise direction a number of times.

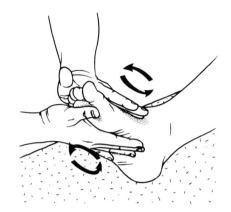

Fig. 4.25 *Toe circling*

12 Scissor friction on the sole of the foot

a Using the thumbs of both hands, friction in a scissor pattern down the sole of the foot returning with a deep push back.

b Effleurage to the whole leg to finish.

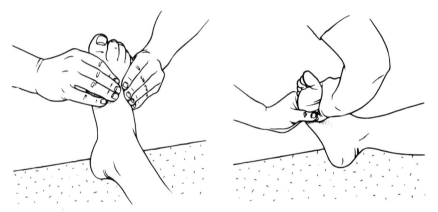

Fig. 4.26 *Scissor friction on the sole of the foot*

Arm massage

Preparation

a Ask the client to gently lift her arm out of the towel covering.

b Apply the selected massage medium to the area using effleurage movements.

Massage sequence

1   **Effleurage to the whole arm**

Place the entire palmar surface of one hand on the client's wrist and support with the other hand. Glide up the arm, around the deltoid, then lightly return.

(Main muscles affected: biceps, triceps, brachialis, deltoid.)

2   **Deep stroking to the deltoids**

Using the palmar surface of both hands, alternately effleurage around the deltoid area.

(Main muscle affected: deltoid.)

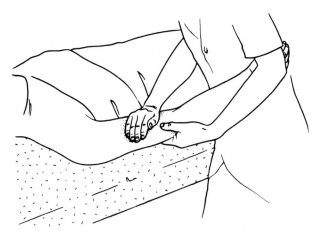

Fig. 4.27 *Effleurage to the whole arm*

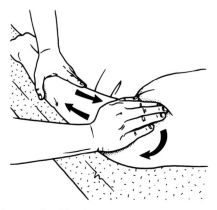

Fig. 4.28 *Deep stroking to the deltoids*

3 **Wringing and hacking to the biceps and triceps**
   a Slide hands to the biceps area and with both parallel, pick and lift the tissues and gently squeeze in a wringing action.
   b Effleurage the area.
   c Using the ulnar border of both hands, briskly but lightly hack the area in a rhythmical pattern.
   d Effleurage the area.
   e Gently rest the client's arm in a crooked position at the side of her head (a towel support may be used under the wrist) and repeat wringing, effleurage and hacking movements to the triceps area.

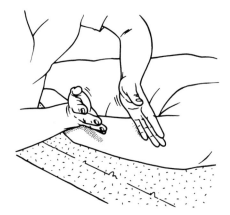

Fig. 4.29 *Hacking to the biceps*

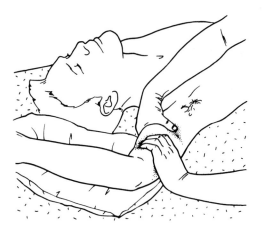

Fig. 4.30 *Wringing to the triceps*

f Return the client's arm to its previous position and effleurage the top of the arm.
(Main muscles affected: biceps, triceps.)

4 **Effleurage to lower arm**
Using the entire palmar surface of the hand, stroke the lower arm from wrist to elbow in an alternate fashion.
(Main muscle affected: brachialis.)

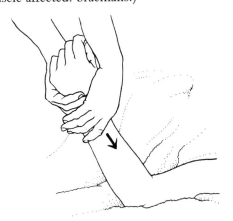

Fig. 4.31 *Effleurage to the lower arm*

5 **Friction circles**
a Friction circle from the wrist to the elbow with a deep push back.
(Main muscle affected: brachialis.)
b Friction circle around the wrist joint using both thumbs simultaneously.

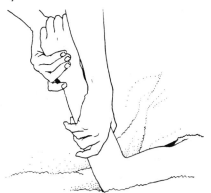

Fig. 4.32 *Friction circles from the wrist to the elbow*

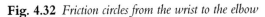

c Friction circle between each metacarpal bone with a deep push back and continue this action down each finger to the tip.

d Effleurage the hand and then turn over so the palm is uppermost.

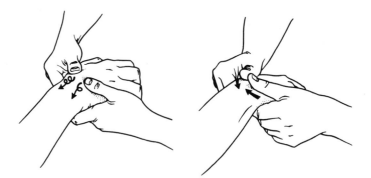

Fig. 4.33 *Friction circles around the wrist*

6 **Friction circles to the hand**
Friction circles across the palm of the hands.

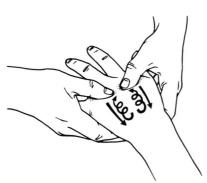

Fig. 4.34 *Friction circles between the metacarpals*

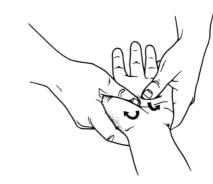

Fig. 4.35 *Friction circles to the palm*

7 **Passive exercise**
Turn the client's hand back to a proline position and grasp the hand in your own, supporting the client's wrist with your other hand, then perform gentle, passive exercises clockwise, anticlockwise, forwards and backwards.

8 **Effleurage the whole arm to finish**
(Main muscles affected: biceps, triceps, brachialis, deltoid.)

POINT TO NOTE

When performing the passive hand and wrist mobility exercises it is very important not to force the joint beyond its natural range.

Chest massage
Preparation
a Gently lower the towel in the area to expose the upper chest area.
b Ensure the client's arms are tucked into the towel unless otherwise requested.
c Apply massage medium to the selected area using effleurage strokes.

Massage sequence

1 **Effleurage to the chest**
Place the entire palmar surface of both hands in the middle of the chest area, then gently work each hand outwards separately, sweeping around the deltoids, over the trapezius, and back over to the starting area.
(Main muscles affected: pectoralis major, deltoid, trapezius.)

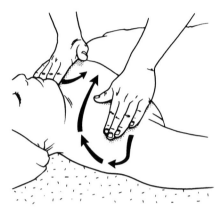

Fig. 4.36 *Effleurage to the chest*

2 **Knuckling of the pectorals**
Clench fists lightly and then knuckle across the front of the pectoral area.
(Main muscles affected: pectoralis major.)

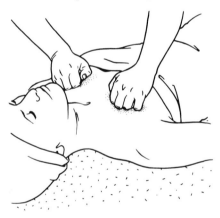

Fig. 4.37 *Knuckling of the pectorals*

3 **Friction circles to the top of the shoulder**
Friction circle a number of times using both thumbs simultaneously in the bicipital groove of the humerus and shoulder area.

4 **Stroking of the deltoids**
a Using the entire palmar surface of both hands, simultaneously stroke around the deltoid area in a clockwise direction and then in an anticlockwise direction.
(Main muscle affected: deltoid.)
b Effleurage the chest area.

5 **Reinforced ironing**
Using double hand pressure, effleurage across the pectoral area in a figure of eight.
(Main muscles affected: pectoralis major, deltoid, trapezius.)

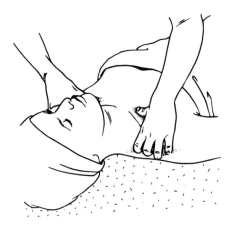

Fig. 4.38 *Friction circles to the shoulders*

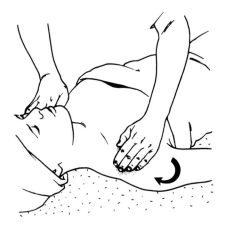

Fig. 4.39 *Stroking of the deltoids*

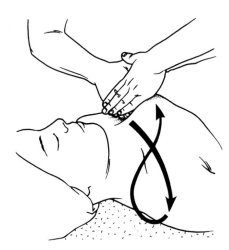

Fig. 4.40 *Reinforced ironing*

6   **Effleurage to the chest area to finish**

GOOD PRACTICE

◆ Avoid abdominal massage if the client has just eaten a heavy meal.
◆ Abdominal massage needs to be lighter than massage on other parts of the body.
◆ Advise the client the abdominal massage may stimulate bowel and/or bladder action.
◆ Clients who are menstruating may prefer this area to be left out of the sequence.

Abdominal massage

Preparation

a Place a rolled towel or small pillow under the client's knees to relax the abdominal wall. Remove the towel in the abdominal area keeping other parts of the body well covered for warmth.

b Apply the selected massage medium to the area by first warming it on your own hands and then applying it to the client's abdomen following the effleurage pattern.

c Ensure that your posture is good, with a straight back and stand with your right thigh towards the couch but facing forwards as in walk-standing position.

Massage sequence

1 **Effleurage to the abdomen**

Place the entire palmar surface of both hands on the abdomen and keeping fingers together, glide hands down towards the symphysis pubis, then glide under to the upper lumber spine where hands should meet and then glide lightly back on to the front of the abdomen.

(Main muscles affected: rectus abdominis, external obliques, internal obliques.)

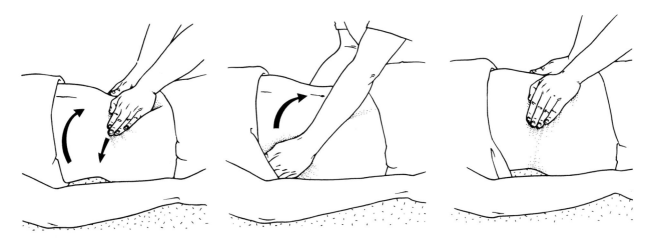

Fig. 4.41 *Effleurage to the abdomen*

2 **Deep stroking of the abdomen**

Place the palmar surface of both hands on the middle of the abdomen and then stroke in a circular motion following the direction of the colon.

(Main muscle affected: rectus abdominis.)

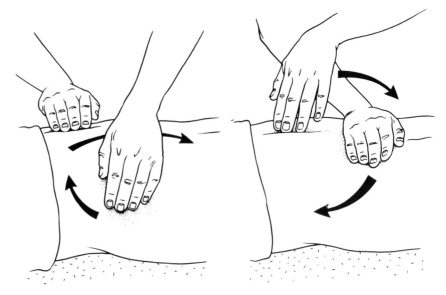

Fig. 4.42 *Deep stroking to the abdomen*

3 **Wringing of the external obliques**
   a Still standing adjacent to the couch with the hands parallel, pick and lift the tissues and squeeze gently in a wringing action.
   b Glide both hands across the abdomen and repeat to the other side.
   (Main muscles affected: external obliques.)

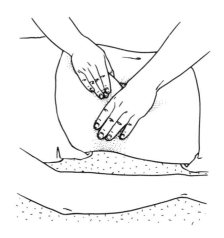

Fig. 4.43 *Wringing to the external obliques*

4 **Skin rolling to the external obliques**
   a Still standing in the same position with hands parallel, slide down the obliques and then feed the tissues through your fingers and thumbs in a rolling motion.
   b Glide both hands across the abdomen and repeat to the other side.
   (Main muscles affected: external obliques.)

5 **Effleurage to the abdomen to finish**
   (Main muscles affected: rectus abdominis, external obliques, internal obliques.)

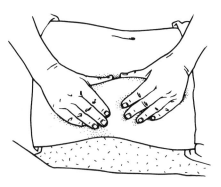

Fig. 4.44 *Skin rolling to the external obliques*

At this point in the massage routine you are now ready to ask the client to turn over so that she is lying prone on the couch. This needs to be done as quickly and discreetly as possible with the least disruption to the client. Lift the towels slightly and ask the client to gently turn over. Re-arrange the towels neatly.

Back of the leg and buttock massage

Preparation

a Remove the towel from the back leg area exposing the leg and gluteal area, but keeping other parts of the body well covered for warmth.

b Place a small rolled towel under the client's ankle for support.

c Apply the selected massage medium to the area by first warming it on your own hands and then applying it to the client's leg from ankle to buttocks using effleurage movements.

d Ensure your posture is good with a straight back.

Massage sequence

1 **Effleurage to the back of the leg and buttock**
Place the entire palmar surface of both hands on the Achilles tendon area of the ankle. With one hand leading, keep fingers and thumbs together and glide the hands along the entire leg to the gluteal area, glide hands around the gluteal, lightly returning down to the ankle.
(Main muscles affected: soleus, gastrocnemius, hamstrings, gluteals, adductors, abductors.)

2 **Deep wringing to the hamstrings and gluteals**
a Slide the hands to the interior aspect of the thigh and then with hands parallel, pick and lift the tissues and squeeze gently in a wringing action. Work the entire hamstring and gluteal areas.
b Effleurage the hamstrings and gluteals.
(Main muscles affected: hamstrings, gluteals, adductors, abductors.)

3 **Alternate palmar lifting of the hamstrings**
a Starting with hands on either side at the top of the thigh, use the entire palmar surface of both hands to gently compress the

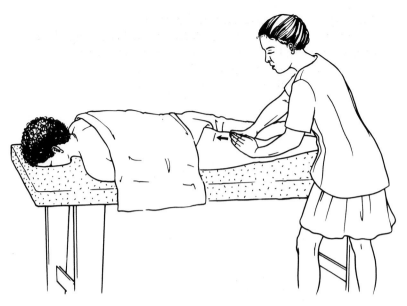

Fig. 4.45 *Effleurage to back of the leg and buttock*

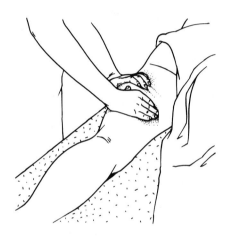

Fig. 4.46 *Deep wringing of the hamstrings and gluteals*

tissues against each other, lifting from side to side. Keep repeating until the back of the knee is reached and then slide back to repeat the sequence.

b Effleurage the hamstrings area.

(Main muscles affected: hamstrings, adductors, abductors.)

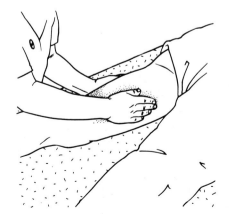

Fig. 4.47 *Alternate palmar lifting of the hamstrings*

4 Hacking to the hamstrings and gluteals
a Using the ulnar border of both hands, briskly but lightly hack the hamstring and gluteal areas in a rhythmical pattern.
b Effleurage the hamstring and gluteal areas.
(Main muscles affected: hamstrings, gluteals, adductors, abductors.)

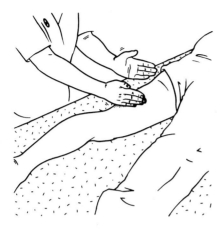

Fig. 4.48 *Hacking to the hamstrings and gluteals*

5 Cupping to the hamstrings and gluteals
a Holding the fingers and palms of the hands in a concave position, briskly but lightly cup the hamstrings area.
b Effleurage the hamstrings and gluteals.
(Main muscles affected: hamstrings, gluteals, adductors, abductors.)

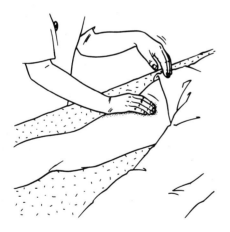

Fig. 4.49 *Cupping to the hamstrings and gluteals*

6 Beating to the hamstrings and gluteals
a Using lightly clenched fists, palms down, lightly beat the hamstrings and gluteals.
b Effleurage the hamstrings and gluteals.
(Main muscles affected: hamstrings, gluteals, adductors, abductors.)
7 Pounding to the gluteals
a Using the ulnar border of lightly clenched fists gently pound the gluteal area.
(Main muscles affected: gluteals.)

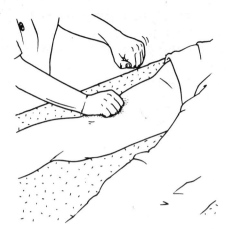

Fig. 4.50 *Beating to the hamstrings and gluteals*

    b Effleurage the gluteal area.
    c Effleurage the entire leg.

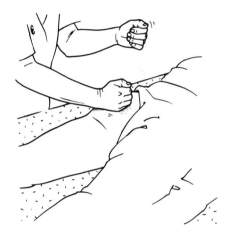

Fig. 4.51 *Pounding to the gluteals*

8   **Deep wringing to the gastrocnemius and soleus**
    a Slide the hands to the interior aspect of the calf, and then with hands parallel, pick and lift the tissues and squeeze gently in a wringing action.
    b Effleurage the gastrocnemius and soleus.
    (Main muscles affected: gastrocnemius, coleus.)

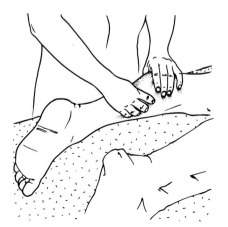

Fig. 4.52 *Deep wringing to the gastrocnemius/soleus*

9 **Alternate palmar lifting to the gastrocnemius and soleus**
   a Starting with the hands on either side at the top of the lower leg, use the entire palmar surface of both hands to gently compress the tissues against each other and lift from side to side. Keep repeating until reaching the ankle, then slide back to repeat the sequence.
   b Effleurage the gastrocnemius and soleus.
   (Main muscles affected: gastrocnemius, soleus.)

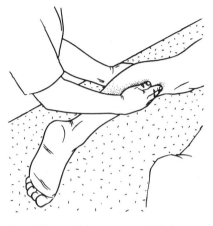

Fig. 4.53 *Alternate palmar lifting to the gastrocnemius/soleus*

10 **Light hacking to the gastrocnemius and soleus**
   a Using the ulnar border of both hands, briskly but lightly hack the gastrocnemius and soleus areas in a rhythmical pattern.
   b Effleurage the gastrocnemius and soleus.
   (Main muscles affected: gastrocnemius, soleus.)

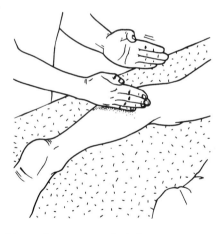

Fig. 4.54 *Light hacking to the gastrocnemius/soleus*

11 **Light cupping to the gastrocnemius and soleus**
   a Holding the fingers and palms of the hands in a concave position, briskly, but lightly and gently, cup the gastrocnemius and soleus areas.
   b Effleurage the gastrocnemius and soleus.
   (Main muscles affected: gastrocnemius, soleus.)

12 **Digital stroking to the calcaneal (Achilles) tendon**
   a Using all the digits of one hand, gently stoke the area.
   (The other hand can be placed on the calf for support)

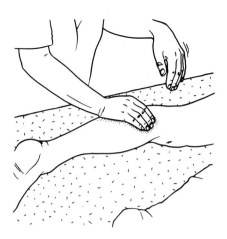

Fig. 4.55 *Light cupping to the gastrocnemius/soleus*

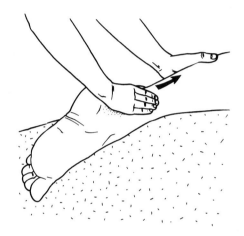

Fig. 4.56 *Digital stroking to the calcaneal tendon*

13 **Effleurage the entire leg to finish**
(Main muscles affected: soleus, gastrocnemius, hamstrings, gluteals, adductors, abductors.)

POINT TO NOTE

On the lower leg area do not perform the beating movement as the muscles are more superficial.

Back Massage
Preparation

a Unless the couch has a breathe hole facility, place a support cushion, rolled towel or similar under the client's forehead to ensure that the neck is straight.

b Remove towel from the back area keeping other parts of the body well covered for warmth.

c Apply the selected massage medium to the area by first warming it on your own hands and then applying it to the client's back area.

d Ensure that your posture is good with a straight back and stand with your right thigh towards the couch but facing forwards.

Massage sequence

1 Effleurage to the back area

Place the entire palmar surface of both hands either side of the spine in the lower lumbar region. Glide up the back area and over the deltoids firmly, then return back to the lumbar area with a light stroke.

(Main muscles affected: trapezius, deltoids, obliques, latissimus dorsi, serratus anterior.)

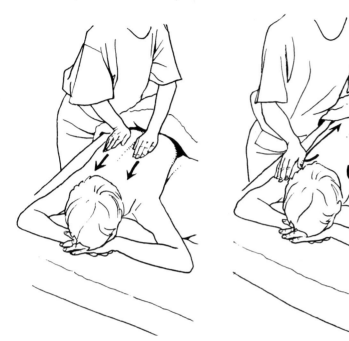
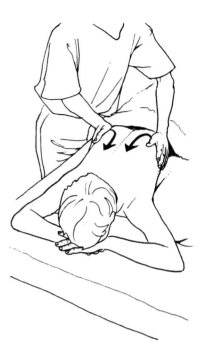

Fig. 4.57 *Effleurage to the back*

2 Wringing of the upper trapezius and deltoid

a Slide both hands to the right side of the client's back in the external oblique area. Then with both hands parallel pick and lift the tissues and gently squeeze in a wringing action. The pressure can be increased over the upper trapezius and deltoid area to suit the client.

b Effleurage the back.

(Main muscles affected: trapezius, deltoids, obliques, latissimus dorsi, serratus anterior.)

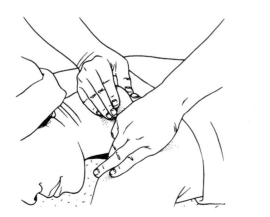
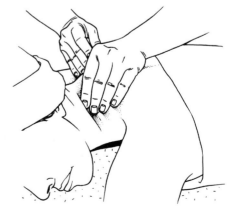

Fig. 4.58 *Wringing to the upper trapezius/deltoid*

3 **Light hacking of the trapezius and deltoids**
   a Using the ulnar border of both hands, briskly but lightly hack the trapezius and deltoids in rhythmical pattern.
   (Main muscles affected: trapezius, deltoids, obliques, latissius dorsi, serratus anterior.)
   b Effleurage the back.

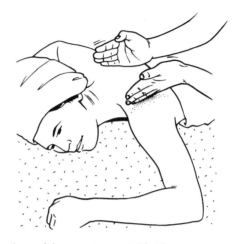

Fig. 4.59 *Light hacking of the trapezius and deltoids*

4 **Light cupping of the trapezius and deltoids**
   a Holding the fingers and palms of the hands in a concave position, briskly but lightly cup the trapezius and deltoids.
   b Effleurage to back.
   (Main muscles affected: trapezius, deltoids, obliques, latissimus dorsi, serratus anterior.)

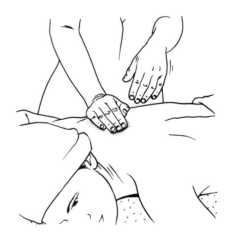

Fig. 4.60 *Light cupping of the trapezius and deltoids*

POINT TO NOTE

Do not apply any tapotement movements over the spine.

5 **Friction circles along the erector spinae muscles**
   a Starting at the sacrum, place both thumbs either side of the
   spine. Working upwards gently, perform friction circles until
   reaching the seventh cervical vertebrae. Gently work into the area,
   then return with index and middle fingers down either side of the
   spine.
   b Effleurage the back.
   (Main muscle affected: erector spinae.)

USEFUL INFORMATION
Tapotement movements
are often omitted from
the back massage routine.

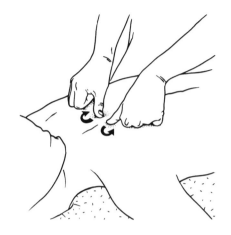

Fig. 4.61 *Friction circles along the erector spinae*

6 **Deep wringing of the trapezius**
   a Slide the hands to the trapezius area and then with the hands
   parallel, pick and lift the tissues and squeeze gently in a wringing
   action.
   b Effleurage the back.
   (Main muscles affected: trapezius.)

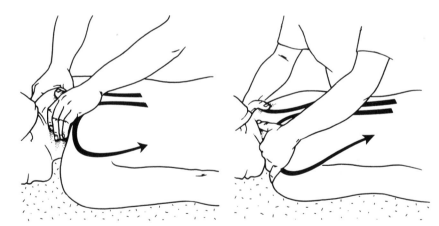

Fig. 4.62 *Deep wringing of the trapezius*

7 **Friction circles across the trapezius**
   Using the thumb digits, gently perform friction circles across the
   entire trapezius area working on any nodules of tension.
8 **Deep stroking of the trapezius**
   a Place the palmar surface of both hands either side of the neck.
   Firmly stroke down either side of the spine to the thoracic region,
   then glide out across the scapulae and up and over the deltoids to
   the starting position.

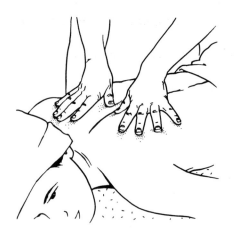

Fig. 4.63 *Friction circles across the trapezius*

b Effleurage the back.
(Main muscles affected: trapezius, deltoids, obliques, latissimus dorsi, serratus anterior.)

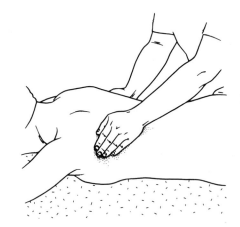

Fig. 4.64 *Deep stroking of the trapezius*

9 **Deep stroking of the spine to finish**
a Place the entire palmar surface of one hand in the cervical region and using alternate hands, gently stroke down towards the lumbar area.

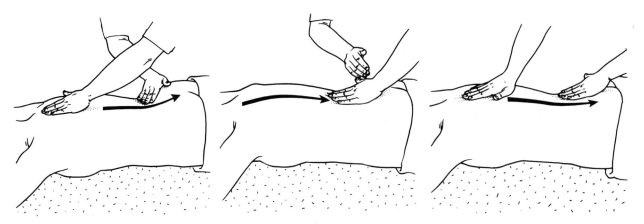

Fig. 4.65 *Deep stroking of the spine*

b Repeat the action a number of times, getting progressively lighter to finish.
(Main muscle affected: erector spinae.)

This is the end of the basic massage sequence.

 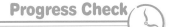

1 Describe briefly how you would prepare a client for massage treatment.
2 Why should abdominal massage be lighter than massage on other parts of the body?
3 Carry out a massage treatment and state the key muscles affected in each area.

Adaptation of massage to suit the individual's requirements

Having mastered the basic principles of rate, rhythm and pressure for the introductory massage routine, a good therapist will develop their skills and knowledge to design a massage suitable for their client's needs.

It is extremely beneficial to take treatments from other therapists, attend short training courses, read trade journals and attend exhibitions, all of which will enable the therapist to enhance their own techniques.

There are many reasons why a client may request a massage, among some of the most popular are:

- Stress.
- Muscular aches and pains.
- Weight loss.
- Poor muscle tone.

Massage for stress and relaxation
The majority of people at some time in their lives will suffer with stress through pressure of everyday living, e.g. it is amazing how tense many drivers become particularly sitting in heavy traffic. Stress has many different physiological and psychological effects on the body: it is often responsible for causing tension in our muscles which if left untreated will eventually affect our posture and may even affect our general state of health. As one of the main benefits of massage is relaxation, it is extremely beneficial for most people provided they are not contra-indicated to the treatment.

There are many forms of massage available to clients, all of which will vary in time and price depending on the type of establishment the client visits and its location.

One hour body massage
The therapist can use the petrissage and effleurage movements from the introductory massage routine along with any other they have learnt from further study, demonstrations or from other therapists to devise an

individual programme for their client. This may also include lymph drainage movements if the therapist feels they are appropriate to the client's needs. They will need to carry out a consultation and ensure there are no contraindications to the massage.

Therapists may choose to alter the order of treatment depending on their own and client's preferences, e.g. many holistic massage therapists commence on the client's back, spending a great deal of time here as this is an area prone to tension. They then move on to the backs, then fronts, of the legs and quite often may effleurage both legs at the same time. The arms and chest areas are next, followed by a face and scalp massage. Note that massage of the abdomen is often omitted.

Half hour body massage

The majority of health spas, as part of their package, offer a half hour massage and therefore the therapist must learn to adapt a one hour routine without making the client feel rushed. Rate and rhythm need to remain fairly constant and pressure altered to suit the client. Some clients prefer to have the time spent on certain areas rather than the whole body, e.g. legs, arms and back. Always establish during the consultation with the client their preferences and any areas of tension. New clients will look for the therapist's professional advice or quietly accept the treatment they are offered. It is far more rewarding for the therapist to discover problem areas which will enable them to give the client a more beneficial treatment rather than make small talk which can often become repetitive.

Back massage

Many salons' and spas' price lists will include a half hour back massage. This can prove to be a very popular treatment as a lot of people at some time in their life will suffer from tension in the shoulders and/or back. This can often be the first massage that clients experience. Over the years people have tended to feel inhibited about exposing their body without first knowing the salon and therapist. In many countries, whether through religion or culture, body treatments are not as popular. The therapist needs to establish a professional ethos that is reassuring to the client and embodies their culture.

During the consultation the therapist needs to establish any particular problems the client may have, e.g. tension in the lower back, along with their likes and dislikes in aromas, sound, colour, temperature and pressure. This will enable the therapist to ensure that the treatment room and product selection will assist more fully in relaxation of the client. The massage techniques selected will help relieve tension in the problem area and will include mainly effleurage and petrissage movements and in particular, deep thumb frictions to the trapezius and erector spinae muscles.

GOOD PRACTICE

Ensure the client is comfortable throughout the treatment. Consider:

- supports under the ankles, knees, chest and head when needed
- comfortable room temperature
- appropriate lighting
- suitable couch/client covering
- appropriate therapeutic music
- correct pressure.

Apprehensive clients

Often clients attending for their first treatment are apprehensive and will tend to talk to overcome their fears. The therapist needs to be reassuring and encourage the client to relax to ensure maximum benefit is gained. The introduction of therapeutic music and essential oils either in the massage medium or in the aroma of the room may help.

It is important to establish the cause of the client's concern so that the therapist is conscious of their dilemma. Generally it can be assumed that the client is apprehensive as they do not understand fully what the treatment involves and/or they are nervous of exposing their body and feeling vulnerable. The therapist should bear this in mind by considering how she/he would feel semi-naked in unfamiliar surroundings with a total stranger who is fully dressed! The therapist should ensure they fully explain the treatment to the client and allow them time to get on to the couch and cover themselves before commencing.

GOOD PRACTICE

- Always state clearly which items of clothing the client should remove.
- Inform the client which way to lie on the couch.
- Always respect a client's privacy and when working on a female's back use a small hand towel to cover the side of their breasts.

Massage for muscular aches and pains

The therapist must first ascertain whether there are any underlying medical conditions which would contraindicate the client from treatment.

Having carried out a thorough consultation and where necessary having gained approval from the client's GP (this should be a note that the client has brought from their general practitioner) the client should be given a heat treatment, such as sauna, steam or infra-red heat lamp, to relax the muscles prior to the massage. The therapist may even decide to use the infra-red heat lamp during the massage to increase the heat within the tissues, thus aiding relaxation.

As muscular tension can cause aches and pains, the therapist should devote more time to particular problem areas using deep kneading and calming effleurage movements. The increase of warmth to the tissues brought about by the increase in blood and lymph circulation will assist in soothing the client's aches and pains.

Massage for weight loss

It is a popular misconception that massage alone can induce weight loss. Weight loss is brought about by diet and exercise. However if introduced as part of a planned treatment and home care programme alongside diet, exercise and electrical treatments, massage can prove to be extremely beneficial.

There are many reasons why a client may be overweight, e.g. it may be hereditary, as a result of over eating or lack of exercise. Whatever the reason the fact that the client has sought help indicates a determination to address the problem. Many people address the issue themselves or seek assistance through therapists or weight loss groups. The therapist must decide with the client the best plan of action to suit their individual needs and constraints such as time and finances available. They must also ensure that there are no underlying medical conditions such as hormone imbalance, e.g. an underactive thyroid gland can cause obesity.

Once a thorough consultation has been carried out and medical approval has been sought (where necessary), the therapist can use her/his knowledge and skills to devise a suitable treatment plan including diet, exercise, electrical treatments and a stimulating massage routine which should include petrissage (skin rolling, wringing and picking up) and tapotement movements (hacking, cupping, pounding and beating) on the areas of excess fat. It may prove beneficial to include manual treatments for stretch marks as often when people lose weight they tend to gain stretch marks. If the client suffers from cellulite the therapist could also include manual treatments for cellulite in the treatment programme (see Chapter 7).

Massage for poor muscle tone

The causes of poor muscle tone are many:

- natural ageing
- lack of exercise
- after rapid weight loss which may be caused through such things as illness or stress, or may be self induced.
- after pregnancy.

To tone poor muscles the therapist would need to recommend exercises to increase the strength of the muscles. These could be supported by salon electrical treatments for muscle tone and a stimulating massage routine incorporating mainly petrissage movements to increase the client's blood and lymph circulation. Once again the therapist could also offer manual treatments and home care products for stretch marks. (See Chapter 7.)

Massage for men

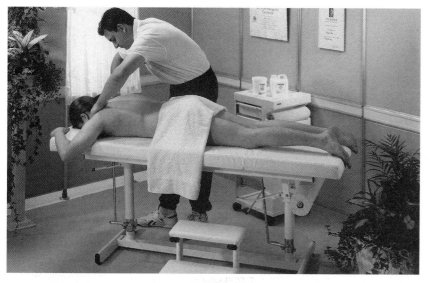

Fig. 4.66

Generally speaking males have more muscle bulk than females, unless of course the female client is a body builder. As the muscles are stronger and firmer, there is a tendency for males to have less subcutaneous (fatty) tissue. The massage movements need to be performed with a greater depth of pressure on men than on women. The type of movements used will obviously depend on the client's reason for treatment but would usually include petrissage (kneading, wringing and picking up), tapotement (hacking, cupping and pounding) and deep effleurage movements. If the massage is for relaxation then the tapotement movements would be omitted. As men usually have much more body hair than women it is important to ensure that the massage medium selected gives enough slip for ease of movement. Generally male massage does not include working on the inner thighs, abdomen or gluteal areas.

ACTIVITY

Select a client, perform a detailed consultation, devise an appropriate massage routine and justify your choice of movements.

Types of massage

Aroma massage

Aroma massage is generally for relaxation and uses ready-blended essential oils as the massage medium. It has become increasingly popular over the last few years and is practised by many beauty therapists. The massage routine incorporates mainly effleurage and petrissage-type movements and is often enhanced by the use of therapeutic music.

The oils used in aroma massage are generally in a diluted concentration compared to those used by a qualified aromatherapist.

GOOD PRACTICE

Ready-blended aroma oils should only be used by qualified massage therapists.

Aromatherapy

This type of massage is a specialist treatment which should only be offered by qualified aromatherapists. It uses plant extracts (essential oils) blended with a carrier oil to form a therapeutic treatment medium to suit the individual client's needs. The massage itself is the method used to transport the essential oils into the client's body and generally consists of effleurage movements.

The last decade has seen a great advance in the recognition of complementary treatments such as aromatherapy. Some aromatherapists work in hospitals under the direction of medical staff and a number of local health authorities have nurses trained and qualified in aromatherapy. For further information see Chapter 11.

Deep tissue massage

Deep tissue massage is considered to be a method of connective tissue massage. It involves a stroking technique which is used to stimulate the release of histamine from what are known as mast cells found within connective tissue. It increases the circulation in the surrounding area, and may produce a generalised flushed appearance and an erythema.

Lymph drainage

This type of massage involves working on the lymphatic system. True lymph drainage massage incorporates superficial effleurage and petrissage movements. Its aims are to relieve congestion within the tissues and increase the drainage of lymph to the lymph nodes. Generally clients come for treatment for specific problem areas rather than having a whole body treatment.

Multi-type massage

Multi-type massage originated in the Far East where it has been practised for many hundreds of years. It involves two therapists working in unison on the one client. It has recently become a fairly popular at a number of international spas. It involves a great deal of training to ensure the therapists are emotionally in tune and that their rate, rhythm and pressure are equal.

Oriental massage

Oriental massage has its origin in the Far East. It has been practised for centuries and is growing in popularity throughout the western world. Oriental massage is pressure massage using any surface of the body e.g. thumbs, hands, feet, elbows, etc. It can also include gentle stretching and manipulation along with the 'laying on of hands' similar to that used in spiritual healing. The application of pressure is usually based along the meridian lines which are used in acupuncture.

Shiatsu is the Japanese name for oriental massage (*shi* meaning finger and *atsu* pressure). The majority of far eastern countries, such as Thailand and Malaysia, have, over the years, developed their own versions of pressure massage.

One of the main differences in oriental and European massage is that the client does not undress, though the therapist and the client need to be dressed in non-restrictive clothing. The massage is performed with the client either sitting or lying on a low bed or a mattress on the floor. It is also quite common in far eastern countries to see holiday makers receiving oriental massage on the beach!

Sports massage

This type of massage has greatly increased in popularity over the last decade, particularly as more and more people are adopting various sports as part of their leisure activities. The sports person is aware of the benefits of sports massage, which include easing aches and pains, and relaxing the musculo-skeletal system or specific muscles or muscle groups. Through specialised training the massage therapist uses a variety of movements to treat the individual client problem, e.g. deep friction movements are often used to break down scar tissue and adhesions.

ACTIVITY

Perform four massage routines on a selection of clients (male and female), who display different bodily conditions and age ranges. Keep a record of the body conditions noted, age and gender of client, the choice of lubricant and the massage routine devised.

Progress Check

1 Give three reasons why massage treatment may be adapted. Explain each reason.
2 How would you deal with an apprehensive client?
3 Name and briefly describe four different forms of massage treatment.

Key Terms

You need to know what these words and phrases mean. Go back through the chapter to find out.

- Adaptation of massage
- Contraindications
- Creating a welcoming environment
- Effleurage
- Frictions
- Massage consultation and assessment
- Massage mediums
- Petrissage
- Preparation for massage
- Principles of good massage practice
- Tapotement
- Types of massage
- Vibrations

ELEMENTARY SCIENCE

5

After working through this chapter you will be able to:

- list the different states of matter
- state the difference between compounds and elements
- outline the differences between mains and battery electricity
- describe the effects of an electric current
- give examples of different electric currents used in therapy treatments.

It is beneficial for the therapist to have an understanding of elementary science, particularly before studying electrical treatments. A whole book could be dedicated to this subject which many therapists find fascinating and may wish to study at greater depth. There is a variety of books and articles available for further research to assist in performing effective electrical treatment programmes.

Forms of matter

Matter is anything that occupies space and possesses mass.

All substances can exist in three different physical states:

- Solid.
- Liquid.
- Gas.

Solids have a definite shape and distinct boundaries, e.g. ice, hair. The particles in a solid are packed closely together and remain in a definite position.

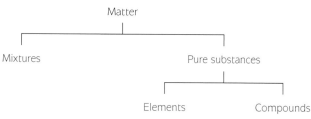

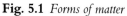
Fig. 5.1 *Forms of matter*

Liquids have a definite volume and take up the shape of their container. The particles in a liquid are closely packed but have a certain freedom to move around.

Gases take up both the shape and volume of their container. The particles in a gas have large spaces between them and move freely (this is why we can smell perfume vapour from a bottle across a room).

All matter is composed of minute particles. In solids these particles are in definite positions, they vibrate in position but do not move from one part of the solid to another. The state of a substance depends on the energy that the substance contains. The solid state has a minimum energy content. When a solid is heated the internal energy is increased and particles vibrate more vigorously until it melts to form a liquid.

The state of matter is affected by temperature and pressure, e.g. if a solid such as ice is placed in a hot temperature, it heats beyond its melting point and becomes a liquid. Water, when heated beyond its boiling point becomes steam, a gas. This *change of state* from liquid water to gaseous steam is utilised in the salon environment when the therapist uses a steam cabinet.

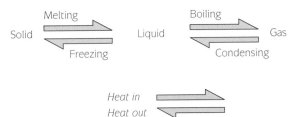

Fig. 5.2 *Changing states*

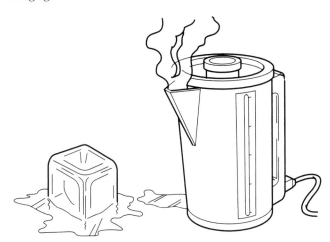

Fig. 5.3 *The three states of water: ice, water, steam*

Atoms

Matter is made up of small indivisible particles called *atoms*, which cannot be created or destroyed.

For a variety of reasons, atoms can be attracted to each other to form *molecules*. A molecule is defined as the smallest part of an element or compound that can exist alone. Under normal conditions, elements which are gases rarely exist as single atoms, the atoms join together in pairs to form molecules, e.g. nitrogen gas.

Nitrogen atom + Nitrogen atom = Nitrogen molecule

Atomic structure

An atom is a particular of matter with clouds of *electrons* (which can be considered as concentric rings or shells) revolving around a small, dense mass of *protons* and *neutrons*, which form the *nucleus* of the atom.

- ⬥ Electrons have a negative electrical charge.
- ⬥ Protons have a positive electrical charge.
- ⬥ Neutrons have no electrical charge.

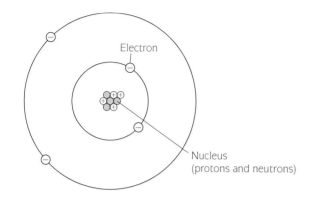

Fig. 5.4 *An atom*

In atoms the positive and negative charges are equal, as they contain equal amounts of electrons and protons, therefore making them neutral.

Electrons fill the shells around the nucleus in a systematic manner. The first shell holds 2 electrons, the second shell holds 8 electrons and the third holds 18.

Elements are held together by forces called bonds. The ease of making or breaking these bonds is referred to as *chemical reactivity*.

The ionic bond is formed by the complete transfer of one or more electrons from one atom to another resulting in the formation of charged particles called *ions*.

An ion is an atom or molecule which has gained or lost electrical charge. The addition of an electron makes the atom or molecule negatively charged, i.e. it has gained the negative charge of one electron, and is known as an *anion*. The atom or molecule losing an electron will become positively charged, i.e. it loses the negative charge of one electron, and is known as a *cation*.

When therapists apply electrical galvanic treatments and products they need to know the relevant electrical charge of the ion in the product in order to perform an effective treatment. (See Chapter 6.)

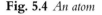

POINTS TO NOTE

- ⬥ Anions are negatively charged ions.
- ⬥ Cations are positively charged ions.

Elements and compounds

An element may be defined as a substance which cannot, by any known chemical means, be split into two or more simpler substances.

Elements are made up of one type of atom which cannot be broken down any further, e.g. atoms of carbon make an element, atoms of oxygen are also an element.

When elements combine chemically together, i.e. *react* with each other, they form a substance. This substance is known as a *compound*, e.g. sodium chloride (table salt) is a compound composed of sodium ions and chlorine ions.

A compound is a pure substance containing two or more elements chemically combined together. Sodium chloride, hydrogen peroxide, keratin, etc. are compounds. Compounds have a fixed composition and their appearance and properties are usually quite different from those of the elements composing them.

When heated, copper nitrate gives off a brown gas and oxygen and leaves a black, solid residue. This indicates that copper nitrate is composed of at least three simple substances. The black solid and the brown gas can be split further. The brown gas (nitrogen dioxide) can be made to yield nitrogen and oxygen. The black solid (copper oxide) can be made to yield copper and oxygen. Copper nitrate is made of copper, nitrogen and oxygen. Copper, oxygen and nitrogen are all elements.

There are over a hundred elements, most of which are present in the Earth's crust either in a free state or combined with other elements in compounds.

> **USEFUL INFORMATION**
>
> Copper oxide and nitrogen dioxide are both compounds.

> **POINTS TO NOTE**
>
> - The constituents of an element, i.e. atoms, cannot be split into anything smaller.
> - A compound can only be split by chemical means into the two or more elements that form the compound.
> - A molecule is the smallest part of an element or compound that can survive alone.

Mixtures

Mixtures contain two or more substances which may be elements or compounds mechanically combined. The constituents of a mixture do not react chemically with each other. A large number of preparations used on the skin are mixtures, e.g. calamine lotion, mascara and cosmetic creams are mixtures of fatty materials and water. A mixture can be separated into its constituents by physical means.

Progress Check

1 List the three states of matter.
2 What two factors can affect states of matter?
3 Describe the atomic structure.
4 State what is meant by the following:
  a element   **b** compound   **c** mixture.

Electricity

We use the phenomenon and power of electricity every day for heating, lighting, washing, ironing, cooking, etc. We use it to look after our appearance (shavers, hair dryers, etc.) and for entertainment (television, video, radio, etc.), but how much do we know about it?

Electricity can be defined as the movement of electrons from atom to atom. The moving electrons create an electrical charge which can be classed as either *dynamic* or *static*.

Electric circuits

An electric circuit can be defined as the path of a electric current linking the electrical appliance to the electricity supply. To create a circuit two ingredients are required:

- a device capable of supplying electricity, e.g. a battery or a generator (mains)
- a complete path of conducting materials in which electricity can flow.

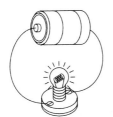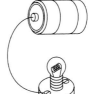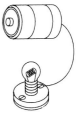

a An electrical circuit must be made from a complete path of conducting material

When the switch is open the circuit is *broken*. No current flows and the bulb does not light

When the switch is closed the circuit is *made*. Current flows and the bulb lights.

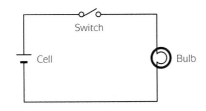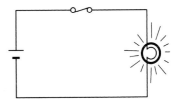

b Switches – 'making' and 'breaking' a circuit

Fig. 5.5 *Electric circuits*

A circuit is made mostly of metals, but sometimes water containing dissolved acids, alkalis or salts can form part of a circuit.

Electric current

Electric current is the name given to a flow of electricity; it tells us the number of electrons passing a fixed spot in the circuit each second. Electric current is measured in amps (A).

Electrical pressure

This is a measure of the ability of a battery or generator to drive the current around a circuit. Electrical pressure is measured in volts (V).

Electric power

This is a measurement of the power used to run a piece of electrical equipment. Electrical power is measured in watts (W).

Electric cells and batteries

An electrical cell consists of:

- a plate of a reactive metal, e.g. zinc
- a plate made of an unreactive conductor, e.g. graphite, carbon
- a solution or paste, called the *electrolyte*, containing acid, alkali or salt.

A chemical reaction between the metal plates and the electrolyte produces electricity.

A battery consists of several cells joined together.

POINTS TO NOTE

- For a current to flow you require a potential difference (p.d.), i.e. there must be an area lacking in electrons and one with an excess of electrons connected by a conductor in order for current to flow.
- The resistance of a conductor refers to its opposition to the low of current. The unit of measurement used for resistance is the ohm (Ω).
- Ohm's law states that the current flowing through a metal conductor is directly proportional to the potential difference (p.d.) across the conductor provided that its temperature remains constant.

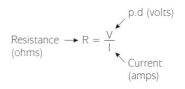

$$\text{Resistance} \rightarrow R = \frac{V}{I}$$

p.d (volts)

Current (amps)

Fig. 5.6 *Ohm's law*

The differences between mains and battery electricity

1 Batteries need replacing or recharging.
2 Mains pressure, or voltage, is much higher than most batteries. In the United Kingdom the mains voltage is 240 volts.

3   Battery equipment is usually portable.
4   Battery circuits conventionally have the current flowing from the positive terminal to the negative terminal all the time. This flow of current is in *one direction only* and is known as *direct current* or DC. An example of the application of DC current in therapy treatments is galvanic treatment (see Chapter 6).
5   The mains circuit produces an *alternating current* or AC (sometimes referred to as sinusoidal current) by continually reversing the polarity (direction of flow) of the current. An example of the application of AC in therapy treatments is high frequency treatment (see Chapter 6).

USEFUL INFORMATION
Ohm's law states that the electrical current will double if the voltage doubles, providing that the temperature remains constant and the resistance of the circuit remains the same.

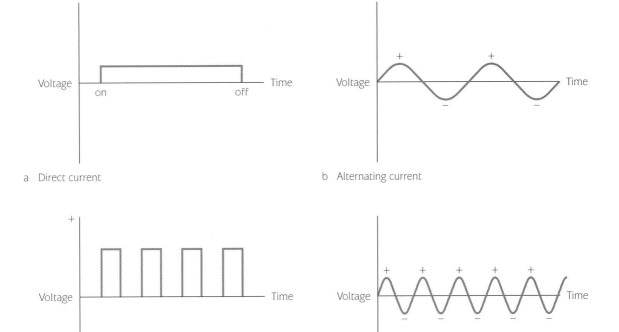

a   Direct current

b   Alternating current

c   Interrupted direct current (as used in NMES)

d   High frequency alternating current

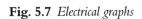

Fig. 5.7 *Electrical graphs*

Earthing electrical appliances

Electrical appliances are earthed to protect the user from possible shock or electrocution.

Note. Appliances need not be earthed if:

- they have an all plastic body
- they are double insulated.

Fuses

There are two types of fuse:

- **Cartridge fuses**. These are placed in plugs to protect the cable of the appliance from overheating.
- **Wire fuse/circuit breaker**. These protect the wiring of the building from overheating.

In order to ensure the correct size of fuse and electrical cable diameter are selected for an electrical appliance, the current (measured in amps) must be calculated using the following equation:

$$\text{Watts} = \text{Amps} \times \text{Volts}$$

or

$$\frac{\text{Watts}}{\text{Volts}} = \text{Amps}$$

Progress Check

If an appliance is rated at 1000 W (1 kW) and the supply is 240 V, what current is drawn by the appliance?

POINTS TO NOTE

To use any electrical appliance on the mains supply it has to be connected with a plug. It is important to note the colouring of the wires in a plug. In the UK the colours are:

- Brown = Live
- Blue = Neutral
- Green and yellow = Earth

The effects of an electric current

Heating effect

Heat is produced if you use:

- large currents
- thin wires
- resistance wires.

The heating effect can be used to good purpose in therapy, for example in the sauna stove and infra-red lamp element.

The chemical effect

The addition of salts, acids and alkalis (*electrolytes*) makes water a good conductor of electricity. An application of this effect in therapy treatments is the use of saline solution on the skin to enable conduction of an electric current, e.g. in neuro-muscular electrical stimulation.

If direct current supplies are used, chemical effects occur at the electrodes. An example of the application of this effect in therapy treatments is galvanic iontophoresis which describes the absorption of ions into the skin.

Magnetic effect

A current passing through a coil of wire (*solenoid*) causes the coil to behave as if it were a magnet, i.e. one end behaves like a north pole the other end like a south pole. If such a coil has a central iron core, the coil behaves as a much stronger magnet. The arrangement is called an *electromagnet*. This is magnet which can be switched on or off as it only acts as a magnet when current is flowing in the coil.

An electromagnet supplied with alternating current will keep reversing its polarity. This is the basis on which an AC motor operates.

An example of the application of electromagnets in therapy treatments are mechanical massagers.

Electromagnetic waves
Wave motion
A wave motion is a disturbance travelling through a medium. Two sets of waves using the same medium can either reinforce or cancel each other out. This is known as *interference* and it can be used to prove that any type of electromagnetic radiation (i.e. heat, light, ultra-violet) consists of waves.

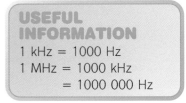

USEFUL INFORMATION
1 mm = 1/1000 m
1 μm = 1/1000 000 m
1 nm = 1/1000 000 000 m

Wavelength and frequency
The *wavelength* is the distance between corresponding points on successive waves. It can be measured in metres (m), centimetres (cm), millimetres (mm), micrometers (μm) or nanometres (nm)

The *frequency* is the number of waves that pass any fixed point in a second. It is measured in hertz (Hz), kilohertz (kHz) or megahertz (MHz).

The higher the frequency, the shorter the wavelength.

USEFUL INFORMATION
1 kHz = 1000 Hz
1 MHz = 1000 kHz
= 1000 000 Hz

POINTS TO NOTE

- The frequency of the mains electricity supply (AC) is 50 Hz.
- A transformer alters the voltage of an AC electricity supply but not the frequency.
- A capacitor charges with electricity and stores it until it is discharged. (A capacitor can be considered as acting as a spring, collecting power as it is compressed and then slowly releasing it as required.)
- Rectifiers change AC to DC as they allow the current to flow through them in one direction only. If a rectifier is used, then a capacitor is needed in the same circuit to smooth the current out.
- The inductance of a coil will oppose the flow of AC current. This type of coil is known as a choke.
- A potentiometer (often referred to as a 'pot') is used to control the intensity of currents. (The control knob on many beauty therapy appliances, e.g. galvanic or NMES, is a potentiometer.)
- The frequency of a high frequency machine will depend on the values of the capacitor and the coil.

Costing of electricity
Electrical costs are based on the number of *units* used. The scientific name for a unit is a *kilowatt-hour*. To calculate the number of units the following equation is used:

$$\text{Units} = \frac{\text{Watts} \times \text{Hours}}{1000}$$

To calculate hours we transpose the formula thus:

$$\text{Hours} = \frac{1000 \times \text{Units}}{\text{Watts}}$$

Examples

1. How long will a 750 watt appliance operate for on 1 unit of electricity?

$$\text{Hours} = 1000 \times \frac{\text{Units}}{\text{Watts}}$$

$$= 1000 \times \frac{1}{750}$$

$$= 1\tfrac{1}{3} \text{ hours} = 1 \text{ hour } 20 \text{ minutes}$$

2. Calculate the cost of using a 3000 watt convection heater for 5 hours at a cost of 7.18p per unit.

$$\text{Units used} = \text{Watts} \times \frac{\text{Hours}}{1000}$$

$$= 3000 \times \frac{5}{1000}$$

$$= 15 \text{ units}$$

$$\text{Cost} = \text{Number of units used} \times \text{Cost per unit}$$

$$= 15 \times 7.18$$

$$= 107.7\text{p}$$

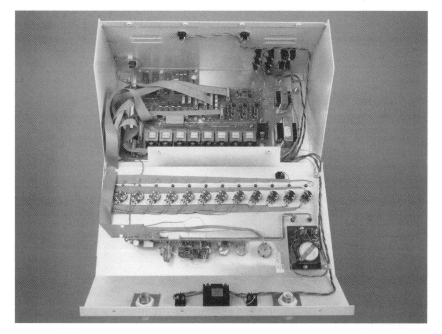

Fig. 5.8 *Inside of a dynatone machine*

ACTIVITY

Research and compare the differences in the manufacturing of galvanic and high frequency machines.

1   Give a definition of electricity.
2   Give an example of:
     a   a conductor
     b   an insulator.
3   What is:
     a   an anion
     b   a cation.
4   State the two components required for the flow of electricity.
5   Explain what is meant by the following terms:
     a   alternating current
     b   direct current
     c   volts
     d   ohms.
6   What effect do the following have on an electric current:
     a   a capacitor
     b   a rectifier
     c   a transformer?

Key Terms

You need to know what these words and phrases mean. Go back through the chapter to find out.

- Atoms
- Compounds
- Earthing
- Effects of an electric current
- Electric cell
- Electric current
- Electric pressure
- Electrical circuits
- Electricity
- Electromagnetic waves
- Elements
- Fuses
- Gases
- Liquids
- Mixtures
- Solids

6

ELECTRICAL EQUIPMENT FOR FACE AND BODY TREATMENTS

After working through this chapter you will be able to:

◊ identify the different types of electrical treatment for the face and body

◊ list the contraindications to electrical treatments

◊ describe the effects of electrical treatments

◊ understand the preparation required for a variety of electrical treatments

◊ competently carry out a variety of electrical treatments for the face and body on clients.

Electrical equipment

A variety of equipment is manufactured internationally to meet the demands of the fast expanding beauty industry. The majority of companies produce a full range of electrical equipment, however some specialise in one area. Each company offers equipment at differing prices according to the development and design on offer and the back-up services available.

When selecting equipment, the therapist should carefully consider the treatments that can best be offered within the salon along with their available budget. Once these have been decided on it is wise to attend exhibitions, read trade journals and liaise through professional associations with other therapists before deciding which manufacturers items to purchase. If possible it is advisable to visit and view equipment showrooms to compare choice, range and availability of equipment.

There are a number of key questions that should be considered before any decisions are made:

◊ Is the therapist to offer salon-based or home visiting services?

◊ Where is the equipment to be used and stored?

◊ How much space is available for equipment presentation and storage?

◊ Would a multi-purpose unit be more beneficial if there is a shortage of storage space? (A multi-purpose unit could also be used as a point of sale for other treatments. However if it is the only piece of equipment, what happens when it breaks down or has to be serviced?)

◊ If the equipment has to be carried in and out of cupboards, is it light-weight?

◊ How are the electrodes stored – with the machine in a purpose-designed area or separately? How will this suit the salon environment?

◊ What is the durability of the equipment? How often will the equipment need servicing? Where will this occur – on or off site? How long will it take? What will it cost?

- What training is offered by the company? Is this included in the price? Where will it take place?
- What back-up services are offered by the company? Do they provide training manuals, telephone support? Do they charge for these services?
- What is the reputation of the company? Are they long standing? Do they attend the major international exhibitions? Are they active in more than one country?
- If purchasing from overseas, always check that equipment is compatible for use in the UK, e.g. check the wiring and voltage, repair and replacement of accessories, etc.
- Ensure items of equipment have been manufactured in accordance with current European directives (EU countries only) and are CE labelled.

Two of the major points that therapists do tend to consider when choosing electrotherapy equipment are the aesthetic appearance and the overall cost but these should not be the only points that are considered!

POINT TO NOTE

If the equipment is not under a guaranteed service warranty, take out a service contract with a local electrician who is familiar with beauty equipment. Ask the manufacturer or the local wholesaler if they can recommend one.

Having purchased equipment, the therapist will want to use it to its maximum potential for the benefit of their clients. The services should be marketed well and full use of existing and passing clientele should be made including displaying information on the new services in the reception area, perhaps offering a discount for a course of treatments and an open evening to demonstrate the treatment and explain its effects.

Electrical treatments are generally given as a course. When used on the body, face, neck and décolleté a number of treatments are often combined together to gain the maximum benefit for the client. If the aim is for figure improvement, home care advice on diet and exercise should be given, and if it is to improve the skin condition, home care advice on the use of professional skin care products should also be given.

Care of electrical equipment

1   Hygiene is of the utmost importance so the machine and accessory items must be kept clean. (Check cleaning instructions before using solvents. Alcohol-based products are **not** recommended for cleaning plastic surfaces/cases, but sun-bed cleanser for acrylic Perspex is often suitable.)
2   Leads and plugs should be regularly checked to ensure there are no loose wires.
3   The equipment should be serviced regularly (portable appliance tested – PAT).
4   The therapist should ensure that all machines are maintained in good working order and kept in a safe place and that they are familiar with its operation.

Safety precautions to be observed when using electrical equipment

1　Ensure the correct care and maintenance has been given to the equipment. (Look for any signs of wear and tear, etc.)
2　Check the machine is placed on a sturdy trolley or where the equipment has its own built-in trolley, ensure the castors are firmly in place and that it is easily accessible for use. Never push trolleys or items on wheels, always pull.
3　Do not place water near or on top of the unit. Do not attempt to operate the machine with damp hands.
4　Make sure that there are no trailing leads that the client or other therapists (including yourself) could trip over.
5　Ensure that the machine is working correctly before applying to the client. Carry out simple self tests.
6　Ensure all accessory items, including products, are at hand before greeting the client.
7　Do not allow the client to touch any machine unless you specifically direct them to do so.
8　Test the equipment on yourself, explaining the procedure, its effects and sensation the client will experience.
9　Check for contraindications and where necessary test the client for skin sensitivity.
10　Before commencing the treatment, ensure all dials are at zero and that the machine is switched off.

Skin sensitivity test

When using electrical currents that pass through the body it is paramount that a skin sensitivity test is carried out to check the accuracy of the client's sensation in the area to be treated. It is usually performed by firstly testing the client's interpretation of different temperature extremes, by placing hot and cold water in glass containers, such as test tubes, and touching the area to be treated intermittently; then the client's sensation of touch is tested using a harsh and smooth surface, such as the pointed tip of an orange wood stick and the other end wrapped in cotton wool. Both these tests should be carried out with the client's view obstructed.

ACTIVITY

Research the number of equipment manufacturers available through your local wholesalers or main centres or electrotherapy supply. Compare their ranges, prices and back up services on offer.

Mechanical massagers

There are three types of mechanical massager available to the therapist, audio sonic massagers, percussion massagers and gyrators. These can be chosen according to the desired effects of treatment and the space available for storage within the salon.

Audio sonic

An audio sonic massager is generally used to help relieve nodules of tension in the muscles. It is a small, hand-held vibrator that emits sound

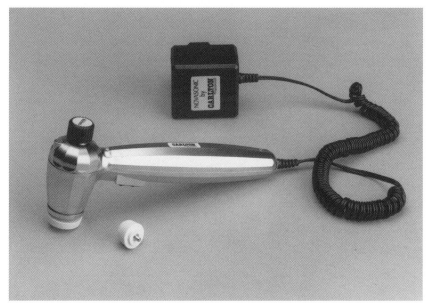
Fig. 6.1 *Audio sonic equipment*

waves which produce a humming noise. These waves will penetrate 6 cm or more into the body's tissues and as the effects penetrate deep down it is ideal for sensitive skins. The action of the massager appears very gentle as it does not move up and down on the skin. It can only be used in small areas at a time due to its size.

The audio sonic is shaped like a small hammer. The external applicator head is directly attached to an internal electromagnetic coil or vibrator, whose action causes the applicator to move 'in and out' at frequencies in the audio spectrum, e.g. 30–20 000 Hz. The adjustable knob on the back or top of the unit is designed to restrict the distance that the applicator travels, thereby controlling the intensity of the massage application. A rocker on/off switch makes or breaks the electric circuit.

Fig. 6.2 *Ball massage head*

The are generally two massage head attachments sold with the unit:

- Ball massage head – used to intensify the actions of the vibrations in small areas.
- Plate massage head – used to evenly apply the vibrations over the largest possible area.

Fig. 6.3 *Plate massage head*

Percussion

The percussion type of mechanical massager is a small, hand-held unit which comes with a variety of massage heads, creating similar effects to manual percussion massage movements. A number of percussion vibrators have an intensity adjustment dial to enable the therapist to increase or decrease the vibration produced according to the depth or tissue being treated, they all have a main switch for turning the unit on or off. Percussion vibrators are generally used on the fine tissues of the face, neck and shoulders.

Different heads supplied are:

- Sponge head – used for gentle stimulation of the tissues.
- Spiky head – a rubber head used to create a more stimulating tapotement effect.

- The intermittent alternating current causes the electromagnet of the vibrator to create an intermittent magnetic effect on the iron bar magnet within the unit which vibrates creating a tapping effect in the massage head attachments.
- The current alternates at 50 Hz releasing a tapping effect every half cycle (100 taps per second are emitted).
- If using audio sonic, a heat treatment such as sauna or steam bath may be given to relax the tissues prior to treatment.

Contraindications
to audio sonic and percussion

- System conditions.
- Skin disorders/diseases.
- Bruised areas.
- Recent scar tissue.
- Highly vascular conditions.
- Varicose veins.
- Thrombosis or phlebitis.
- Over bony areas.
- Recent fractures.

Effects of audio sonic and percussion

- Increases blood circulation.
- Aids desquamation.
- Increases metabolism.
- Promotes relaxation through warming the tissues.

Reasons for using audio sonic

- Where use of other massagers such as percussion is contra-indicated due to skin sensitivity.
- To help break down nodules of tension and relieve tightness in muscle areas, e.g. the trapezius.
- For clients suffering with arthritis to create heat in the tissues which may help ease their aches and pains.

Reasons for using percussion

- To stimulate blood circulation and sebaceous flow in dehydrated or dry skins.
- To produce warmth in the tissues to promote relaxation.

Preparation for audio sonic and percussion treatment

1. Observe general safety precautions for using electrical equipment.
2. The machine is placed on the stable trolley.
3. The machine is checked and tested to ensure it is working correctly.
4. The products required for treatment are selected and placed on the trolley.

Audio sonic and percussion treatment

1   Client is greeted at reception and escorted to treatment area.
2   Consultation is carried out to check for any contraindications and to explain the effects of the treatment.
3   Client removes their jewellery and is helped onto the couch.
4   The therapist ensures the client is warm and comfortable and prepared for treatment.
5   The appropriate massage head for the desired effects is selected and fitted firmly to the unit.
6   A suitable product medium is selected and applied to the area to be treated, e.g. talcum powder for oily skin and cream for dry.

Method

1   Check massage head is firmly attached.
2   Ensure that the unit is switched off and the mains lead is plugged in to the mains.
3   Machine is tested on the therapist in front of the client.
4   Massage heads are cleaned with appropriate disinfecting fluid.
5   The unit is switched on by turning the main switch (on/off).
6   The adjustment dial is altered as necessary.
7   Apply the massage head to the treatment area working in a methodical manner throughout the treatment either using circular movements or working in straight lines. Treatment time will vary between 5–15 minutes according to the area being treated and the effect required.
8   The unit is removed from the client's skin, the machine is switched off and where needed the massage head changed and the treatment routine completed.

GOOD PRACTICE

♦ Remember to avoid applying directly to bony areas such as the zygomatic arch or frontal bone when working on the face or vertebral column on the back.
♦ The therapist may apply the vibrator indirectly over more sensitive bony areas by placing the massage head on to their hand and working across the area to reduce the stimulation achieved.

POINTS TO NOTE

♦ Avoid very bony areas.
♦ Ensure the tapping action is not too strong as this can lead to bruising.
♦ Do not use too close to the ears.

9   The medium used is removed and further treatment may be given if appropriate, e.g. massage.
10   The client is helped from the couch, the record card completed, appropriate home care and further salon treatment advice is given, along with samples of the skin care products used if applicable, and their next appointment is confirmed.
11   The therapist tidies the treatment area and cleans the massage heads used with hot water and wipes them with disinfectant.

ACTIVITY

With a colleague perform on each other an audio sonic and percussion massage treatment. Discuss the physiological and psychological effects.

Gyrators

This is the most widely used mechanical massager and is commonly found in health spas and salons offering body treatments. It creates a much deeper massage effect within the tissues than the audio sonic and percussion vibrators. It is ideal for large muscular areas of the body and sometimes preferred by men with large muscle bulk to manual massage. There are a number of makes of electrical massage apparatus but the specific 'gyratory' action distinguishes this equipment.

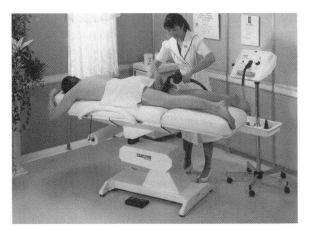

Fig. 6.4 *Gyratory massage*

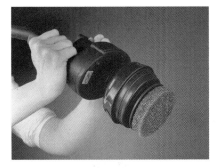

Fig. 6.4a *Guidance control handle*

The trademark G5™ is synonymous when describing gyratory massagers – the French manufacturer Monsieur Henri Cuiner created the very successful range of G5™ massagers over 30 years ago and the trademark derived from G for Gyratory and 5 from the number of accessory heads. Gyratory massagers are usually best used on a free-standing base with castors as this enables easier use and movement of the long flexible drive shaft, which runs from the body and motor of the unit, into which alternative massage heads can be attached.

A rotary electric motor inside the unit causes the crank and peg to fit into the massage head of the machine creating a gyratory (eccentric) movement.

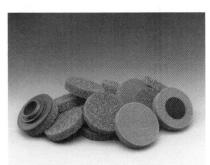

Fig. 6.4b *Disposable sponge heads*

There are a variety of massage head applicators available, the traditional ones tend to be made from rubber or polyurethane. The most commonly used or 'standard' accessory heads are:

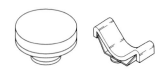

Fig. 6.5 *Round and curved sponge massage heads*

◊ Round and curved sponge heads – used to create an effleurage effect. The curved head is used on curved areas of the body, e.g. arms, shoulders and legs. Used at the beginning and end of treatment. Increases blood circulation and produces hyperaemia in the area being treated. It also promotes relaxation.

- Single and double ball heads – used to create a deep petrissage effect on large muscle bulk, e.g. trapezius and gluteals.
- Egg box head (4 half domed head) – used to create a deep petrissage effect on fatty tissues, e.g. quadriceps and gluteals.
- Multi-pronged head – used to create a deep petrissage effect on fatty tissues.
- Spiky or brush heads – used to create stimulating tapotement effects.

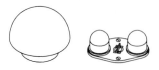

Fig. 6.6 *Single and double ball massage heads*

Fig. 6.7 *'Egg box' massage head*

Fig. 6.8 *Multi-pronged massage head*

Fig. 6.9 *Brush massage head*

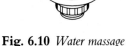

Fig. 6.10 *Water massage head*

A hand-held unit is ideal for the therapist who offers a home visiting service or in a salon that has little storage space. This can operate on the same principles as the larger, heavy-duty, free-standing gyrator (but an electrical motor is housed directly in the body of the unit and no drive shaft is attached). Traditionally small, less powerful hand-held massagers are usually two handed and the massage heads are larger and often fit over the massage plate.

Effects of gyrators
- Increases blood circulation.
- Aids desquamation.
- Increases metabolism.
- Promotes relaxation through warming the tissues.
- Repeated electrotherapy pressure massage may help the more efficient dispersal of fatty deposits, particularly when the client is on a weight-reducing diet and exercise programme.

Contraindications
to gyratory massage

- Skin disorders/diseases.
- Infected acne conditions.
- Bruised areas.
- Cuts and abrasions.
- Recent scar tissue.
- Sunburn.
- Sensitive and fine skin.
- Loose crepey skin.
- Oedema.
- Glandular swelling.
- Highly vascular conditions.
- Varicose veins.
- Thrombosis or phlebitis.
- Over bony areas.
- Very hairy areas.
- Over the abdomen during menstruation and pregnancy.
- Epilepsy.*
- Diabetes.*

* Only to be carried out with medical consent.

GOOD PRACTICE

A heat treatment such as sauna or steam may be given to relax the tissues prior to treatment. It is important that the area to be treated is sufficiently warmed before petrissage type massage is applied.

Reasons for using gyrators

- To help break down nodules of tension and relieve tightness in muscle areas, e.g. the trapezius.
- For general relaxation.
- For improvement of poor circulation.
- To assist as part of a weight reduction programme for spot areas, e.g. quadriceps and gluteals.
- To assist in the improvement of the texture of dehydrated and dry skins.

Preparation for gyratory treatment

1 Observe general safety precautions for using electrical equipment.
2 The machine is placed on a stable trolley where necessary.
3 The machine is checked and tested by the therapist to ensure it is working correctly.
4 The products required for treatment are selected and placed on the trolley.

Gyratory treatment

1 Client is greeted at reception and escorted to treatment area.
2 Consultation is carried out to check for contraindications and to explain the effects of the treatment.

3   Client removes their jewellery and is helped onto the couch.
4   The therapist ensures the client is warm and comfortable.
5   The appropriate massage head to begin the treatment is selected and fitted correctly to the unit.
6   A suitable medium is selected and applied to the area to be treated if necessary, e.g. talcum powder.

Method

1   Check massage head is correctly attached and will not loosen during treatment.
2   Ensure unit is switched off and mains lead is plugged in.
3   Machine is tested on the therapist in front of the client.
4   Clean massage heads are selected.
5   The unit is switched on by turning the main switch (on/off).
6   If the unit has a variable speed control this is adjusted accordingly.
7   Apply the massage head to the treatment area working in a methodical manner.

With the effleurage heads, follow the contours of the client's body and the direction of the venous return.

To create a kneading effect to the tissues the therapist selects a petrissage-type head. This is applied in a circular motion allowing the kneading of the tissues. It is important to lift and support the client's tissues towards the head.

For a desquamating, stimulating effect the therapist selects a tapotement-type head and works in circular movements supporting the client's tissues with their hand.

The treatment is always completed with the effleurage head.

The treatment time will vary according to the area being treated and the effect required, e.g. spot reduction or full body massage treatment. In some cases only a few massage heads will be selected, particularly if performing a full massage routine.

8   The medium used is removed (if appropriate) and further treatment may be given if indicated, e.g. neuro-muscular electrical stimulation.
9   The client is helped from the couch, the record card completed, appropriate home care advice given, e.g. diet and exercise, along with further salon treatment advice and the next appointment is confirmed.
10   The therapist tidies the treatment area and cleans the massage heads with hot water and detergent and then, according to the massage head used, wipes with a suitable disinfectant.

ACTIVITY

Describe suitable gyratory massage treatment programmes for the following clients and conditions:

a 30-year-old active male for relaxation
b 45-year-old female office worker with hard fat deposits on thigh areas.

Progress Check

1 Give six examples of questions that a therapist should consider before purchasing electrical equipment.
2 List the general safety precautions that should be observed when using electrical equipment.
3 Describe how a skin sensitivity test is carried out.
4 a What are the three types of mechanical massager available for salon use?
   b Give three reasons for using each type of massager.
   c List four common contraindications for the three types of mechanical massage.
5 Describe the preparation and treatment for one type of mechanical massage.

Vacuum suction massage

This treatment is used by therapists to assist in the movement of lymph fluid to the main lymph nodes, thus aiding the removal of waste products in the body. It also increases the efficiency of the circulatory system. It is generally given as part of a course of treatments and often combined with other treatments such as manual massage dietary home care advice depending upon the area of the client being treated and the effect required. Treatment of the body using vacuum suction is often used for spot reduction in specific areas such as the thighs and buttocks rather than a full body treatment.

In order to perform this treatment effectively it is essential that the therapist has a knowledge and understanding of the lymphatic system (see Chapter 1).

Vacuum suction machines can be purchased for facial or body treatments. However the majority of manufactures produce mainly body or combined face and body units. These units generally consist of an electrically driven vacuum pump, a mains switch control, a gauge (which registers the amount of 'negative' or 'reduced' pressure produced) and a control dial for increasing or decreasing the amount of pressure required to treat the different tissues of the face and body. Accessory items to the unit are plastic tubing and an assortment of different sized ventouses or cups, which are generally made from Plexiglas or clear Perspex for the body and glass for the face. Some cups have a small hole in the side which the therapist places their finger over to maintain the pressure in the cup or to release the pressure when they want to. If there is no hole in the side of the cup the therapist has to release the pressure by gliding their finger under the cup. Some machines also have an outlet for blowing air out of the unit which can be attached via a nozzle to a bottle which will emit a fine spray. These can be used for a variety of preparations such as rose water for refreshing the client's skin.

POINT TO NOTE

The gauge on a vacuum suction machine registers the height of mercury on a sphygmomanometer. This was incorporated into the unit by manufacturers to meet the tuition requirements of some examining bodies who state the approximate measure that should be registered during use. The majority of therapists judge the intensity required by the percentage of tissue in the ventouse and how it actually feels to the client.

Most vacuum suction machines available offer the therapist the single cup method of application. The multi-cup systems can be used for the body area enabling the therapist to work with a number of cups at the same time, thus reducing the treatment time. The method of application for this treatment is different but the effects achieved are the same. However these systems are not widely used in the salon environment.

The most widely used method of vacuum suction is referred to as the gliding cup method where by the therapist glides the chosen ventouse in a selected pattern and direction towards the nearest lymph nodes. Some units are designed to offer an additional pulsating action where intermittent pressure levels within the ventouse lift and drop the skin and body tissues as the therapist glides towards the lymph nodes. This method produces a gentle tapping effect on the skin producing stimulation in the area of treatment.

In body therapy treatments the therapist may select the gliding cup method for general lymph drainage, the pulsating gliding cup for further stimulation of the tissues along with lymph drainage or the static cup method for spot treatment in areas of fatty deposits, e.g. the thighs.

The static method can be used to lift the tissues in a specific area and generally involves the multi-cup method of application, but can be performed by the therapist with a single cup outlet. The therapist selects the appropriate size cups and applies to the treatment area ensuring the cups are moved around the area to prevent over stimulation and possible bruising. After treatment the gliding cup method is used to drain the lymph to the nearest node.

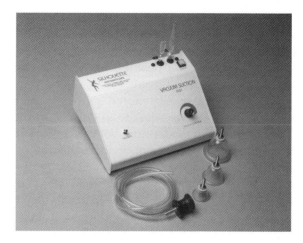

Fig. 6.11 *Vacuum suction machine*

USEFUL INFORMATION

As the tissue is released from the vacuum cup it falls and contracts, the contraction of the veins and lymph vessels forces their fluids on from the treated area.

Vacuum applicators

- **Lymph drainage.** This ventouse can be used for most vacuum treatments. It has a flat, thin head and is useful for working in the fine facial expression lines.
- **Facial cups.** These vary in size and are generally used for general cleansing or lymph drainage.
- **Comedone applicator.** These have a small, round opening which is used over the site of comedones, exerting even pressure on the surrounding issues.
- **Body cups.** These vary in size depending on the amount of adipose tissue in the area being treated.

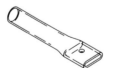

Fig. 6.12 *Lymph drainage applicator*

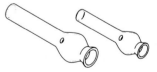

Fig. 6.13 *Facial cups*

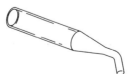

Fig. 6.14 *Comedone applicator*

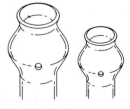

Fig. 6.15 *Glass body cups*

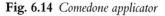

The larger the diameter of the ventouse, the greater the reduced pressure will be at the same setting of depression.

Contraindications

to vacuum suction massage

- Skin diseases/disorders.
- Bruised areas.
- Cuts and abrasions.
- Varicose veins.
- Highly vascular conditions.
- Recent scar tissue.
- Sunburn.
- Sensitive or fine skin.
- Loose, crepey skin.
- Epilepsy.*
- Diabetes.*
- Any glandular swelling.
- Infected acne conditions.
- Bony areas.
- Very hairy areas.
- Thrombosis and phlebitis.
- Oedema.
- Heart conditions.*

* Only to be carried out with medical approval.

Effects of a vacuum suction massage treatment

- Increases blood circulation.
- Increases lymph circulation thus aiding removal of toxins and waste products.
- Aids desquamation.
- Improves general skin texture.
- Stimulates metabolism.
- Promotes cellular regeneration.
- Scar tissue may be softened.
- May help in the utilisation and movement of fatty cells when combined with diet and exercise.

Reasons for using vacuum suction treatment

- To assist in reducing cellulite.
- To assist in reducing areas of oedema (non systemic).
- For sluggish lymph circulation in specific areas, e.g. legs.
- To assist in a weight loss programme combined with diet, exercise and other salon treatments.
- To stimulate dry skin. The treatment time would be approximately 8–12 minutes.
- For deep cleansing very oily skins. The treatment time would be approximately 10–15 minutes.
- As a general skin cleanser on all but sensitive skin types. The treatment time for this would be approximately 5–8 minutes.

* The vacuum pump inside the unit is driven by an electric motor which produces suction in the ventouse by reducing the amount of air available thus causing the client's skin to be drawn up into the cup.
* The degree of reduced pressure produced by the vacuum pump can be increased or decreased according to the density of the client's body tissue by altering the intensity control allowing more or less air to leak which affects the amount of vacuum produced.

General preparation for vacuum suction treatments

1 Ensure the unit is switched off and connect the mains lead.
2 The therapist selects the size ventouse required for the treatment area and attaches it to the plastic tubing which connects onto the outside of the unit.

Preparation for facial vacuum suction treatment

1 Observe general safety precautions for using electrical equipment.
2 The machine is placed on a stable trolley.
3 The machine is checked and tested by the therapist to ensure it is working correctly.
4 The products required for treatment are selected and placed on the trolley.

Facial vacuum suction treatment

1 Client is greeted at reception and escorted to treatment area.
2 Consultation is carried out to check for contraindications and to explain the effects of the treatment.
3 Client removes their jewellery which is kept safely by the therapist until the end of the treatment.
4 Client is helped onto the couch and their clothing and hair protected accordingly.
5 The therapist ensures the client is warm and comfortable.
6 The skin is cleansed with appropriate products.
7 A steam treatment may be given to soften the tissues.
8 A suitable product medium is selected and applied to the client's face and neck.

Method

1 A suitable ventouse is selected to suit the treatment area and the desired effects.
2 Check ventouse is correctly fitted.
3 Ensure mains lead is plugged in to mains supply and that all switches are off and all dials are at zero.
4 Machine is tested on the therapist in front of the client.
5 Check ventouse is re-cleaned with appropriate disinfecting fluid.
6 The unit is switched on by turning the main switch (on/off).

7 The intensity dial is adjusted to achieve the appropriate reduced pressure in the ventouse.

8 The cup is held in a perpendicular way to apply the ventouse to the skin. Remember not to draw more than 20% of the skin and tissues up into the cup.

9 Following the contours of the client's face and neck glide the cup slowly, to allow time for the effects of the treatment to be achieved, to the nearest lymph nodes.

10 The suction in the ventouse is released before the cup is removed from the skin by the therapist releasing their finger from the hole on the side of the cup or where there is no hole, by the therapist gliding their finger under the cup.

11 Following the pattern shown in Fig. 6.16, repeat the sequence to each area 4–8 times depending on the skin reaction.

12 If the desired effect of the treatment is to loosen stubborn comedones the appropriate cup is used in small circular movements over the problem areas which tend to be the nose, upper lip and chin.

13 The product medium is removed and either further treatment such as massage and/or a face mask may be given or the skin is toned and moisturised with appropriate products.

14 The client is helped from the couch, the record card completed, appropriate home care and further salon treatment advice is given along with samples of the skin care products used and the next appointment is confirmed.

15 The therapist tidies the treatment area and washes the cups and tubes used in hot water and detergent and then soaks them in an appropriate disinfectant.

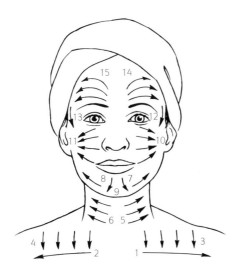

Fig. 6.16 *Direction of flow to the lymph nodes of the face neck and décolleté*

USEFUL INFORMATION

In some Far Eastern countries it is common practice for therapists to perform the vacuum suction massage in conjunction with a steam treatment. This causes an erythema much more quickly due to the heat of the steam.

POINTS TO NOTE

● The loosening of blockages can be combined with the general cleansing treatment.
● When using the comedone applicator, cotton wool may be placed in the top of the ventouse to prevent waste matter entering the plastic tubing.

Body vacuum suction treatment

1 Client is greeted at reception and escorted to treatment area.
2 Consultation is carried out to check for contraindications, to explain the effects of the treatment and decide on the desired effects required from the treatment.
3 Client changes, showers and may have a heat treatment to soften and/or another salon treatment, e.g. a mechanical massage.
4 Client is helped on to the couch.
5 The therapist ensures the client is warm and comfortable.
6 A suitable product medium is selected and applied to the treatment area.

Method

1 Suitable ventouse(s) are selected to suit the treatment area and the desired effects.
2 Check ventouse is correctly fitted.
3 Ensure mains lead is plugged in to mains supply and that all switches are off and all dials are at zero.
4 Machine is tested on the therapist in front of the client.
5 Check ventouse is re-cleaned with appropriate disinfecting fluid.
6 The unit is switched on by turning the main switch (on/off).
7 The mode of use is selected, e.g. pulsating method or static cup.
8 The intensity dial is adjusted to achieve the appropriate reduced pressure in the ventouse(s).
9 The cup is held in a perpendicular way to apply the ventouse to the skin. Remember not to draw more than 20% of the skin and tissues up into the cup.
10 **a** If using the gliding cup method the contours of the client's body are followed gliding the cup slowly (to allow time for the effects of the treatment to be achieved) to the nearest lymph nodes. The pattern shown in Fig. 6.17 indicates the movement sequence for working on the body with the gliding cup. The sequence is generally repeated to each area 4–8 times depending on the skin reaction.
b If using the spot treatment static or pulsating cup method, the appropriate size ventouse for the amount of adipose tissue is applied to the area. The suction in the ventouse is released before the cup is removed from the skin by the therapist releasing their finger from the hole on the side of the cup or, where there is no hole, by the therapist gliding their finger under the cup and placing it in another area.
Note. Trainee therapists sometimes combine the two methods of use, e.g. firstly using the gliding cup to loosen the tissues and stimulate the blood circulation prior to using the multi-cup spot treatment, which may help to loosen fatty deposits, before completing the treatment with the gliding cup to drain toxins and waste to the nearest lymph nodes.

11 The oil is removed and further treatment may be given, e.g. massage.

12 The client is helped from the couch, the record card completed, appropriate home care and further salon treatment advice is given and the next appointment is arranged.

13 The therapist tidies the treatment area and washes the cups and tubes used in hot water and detergent and then soaks them in a disinfectant.

> ### USEFUL INFORMATION
>
> Although traditional body vacuum suction is not the most common salon treatment, there is an increasing use of pressure massage equipment which promotes lymph drainage and new aspiration devices (such as Cellu M6 and Celluloss) incorporate the basic principles and direction of flow of body vacuum.

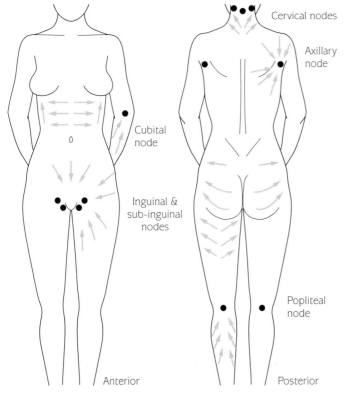

Fig. 6.17 *Direction of flow to the lymph nodes of the body*

POINTS TO NOTE

- When applying the multi-cup static or pulsating method, a rocking action is used to roll the cups onto the skin at the same time to ensure the suction in the cups is equal.
- Care must be taken not to use too high a reduced pressure in the ventouse or to pull the cup off without releasing the pressure or to work in an area too long as all these can lead to dilated capillaries and bruising of the skin.

GOOD PRACTICE

Drain to the lymph node, not over it.

ACTIVITY

Plan a course of body vacuum suction treatments for a client with sluggish lymph circulation. Clearly outline the treatment objectives, describe the consultation, treatment methods and products to be used along with the client home care advice. Evaluate and justify your findings on the effectiveness of the programme.

Electrotherapy treatments

Therapists use the term electrotherapy to refer to electrical treatments where low currents are passed through the client's body for their therapeutic effects.

The three main electrotherapy treatments used by therapists are:

- High frequency.
- Neuro-muscular electrical stimulation (NMES), sometimes referred to as electrical muscular stimulation (EMS).
- Galvanic.

High frequency

The term high frequency traditionally applies to the high frequency apparatus used to stimulate blood flow and uses a rapidly alternating electrical current in the region of 100 000–250 000 hertz. It is a high voltage, but low current treatment. As the pulses of the current are short, they do not stimulate motor points to contract muscles – instead they pass directly into the skin via the electrode applicator at the point of contact producing warmth in the tissues which creates a heating effect. The therapist can apply high frequency in two ways depending upon the client's skin condition. Each method creates different effects on the tissues:

- Direct method.
- Indirect method (often referred to as the Viennese massage).

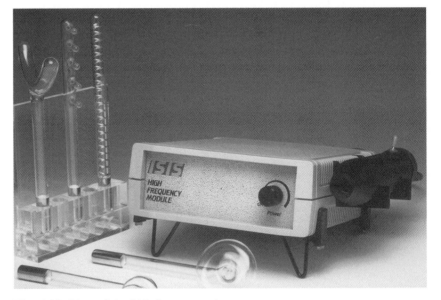

Fig. 6.18 *Isis modular high frequency unit*

POINT TO NOTE

High frequency is most popularly used on the face. However, it can be used in the same way on the body.

High frequency equipment may vary in general appearance as manufacturers develop equipment to appeal to therapists from an aesthetic and economical view but the basic operations of the equipment will be similar. There are generally two main control switches: the on/off switch and the intensity control. A mains lead connects the unit to the power supply. A flex leads from the unit to the handle which is used to house the glass electrodes. There is a variety of electrodes that the therapist can select to use depending upon the method of application and the area to be treated and the desired effects.

Electrodes

The glass electrodes have metal conducting caps (ends) which connect with the metal plate found in the handle allowing the current to flow from the machine to the electrode. The electrodes fit firmly into the holder but not tightly, otherwise the therapist would be unable to change electrodes.

- **Large head surface electrode (large mushroom).** This is used for facial and body work when using direct high frequency. It can also be used for 'sparking' treatments to intensify the current by using only on a side edge lifted on and off the skin with small movements.

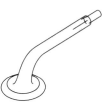

Fig. 6.19 *Large head surface electrode*

- **Small head surface electrode (small mushroom).** Used for direct high frequency. This electrode is useful for working on small, difficult areas such as the nose. It can also be used for sparking.

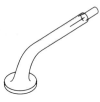

Fig. 6.20 *Small head surface electrode*

- **Roller electrode.** Used for face and body direct high frequency treatments. It rolls easily over the skin and can be used without gauze or a sliding medium.

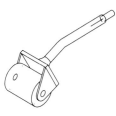

Fig. 6.21 *Roller electrode*

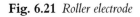

- **Neck electrode**. Used for direct high frequency application to the neck area or other curved areas of the body, e.g. arms.
- **Sparking electrode**. Used for application of direct high frequency for sparking to specific areas and cauterising individual pores. Care should be taken to use a low current with this electrode.
- **Rake electrode**. Used for direct frequency to the scalp area.
- **Intensified saturator electrode**. This electrode is used for indirect high frequency and is known as a saturator. It usually contains a metal spiral running through the inside of the glass which intensifies the effect and ensures that only a low current is required to give maximum effect.

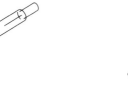

Fig. 6.22 *Neck electrode*

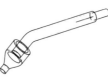

Fig. 6.23 *Sparking electrode*

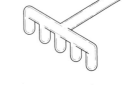

Fig. 6.24 *Rake electrode*

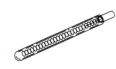

Fig. 6.25 *Intensified saturator electrode*

POINT TO NOTE

Within each electrode is sealed a small quantity of inert gas, usually argon. As the current flows through the gases a coloured glow is produced. The electrodes glow either blue–violet if they contain argon or red–orange if they contain neon.

Contraindications

to high frequency

- Cuts or abrasions to the skin in the area to the treated.
- Skin diseases or disorders.
- Highly vascular conditions.
- Sensitive skin.
- Highly nervous clients.
- Excessive metal in the area of application, e.g. plates or fillings.
- Swellings in the area.
- Very hairy areas.
- Sinus blockages.
- Heart conditions.*
- Epilepsy and diabetes.*
- Circulatory conditions.*
- Pregnancy.*
- Asthmatics.*

* Only to be carried out with medical approval.

The indirect method

This method of applying the high frequency current involves creating a circuit of current which flows from the saturator to charge the client. The therapist massages the client, thus discharging the current from the client's face to the therapist's massaging finger or hand.

Effects of indirect high frequency

- Increases circulation.
- Increases metabolism.
- Warms and relaxes the tissues.
- Improves the skin texture.
- Improves the moisture balance of the skin.
- Calms the sensory nerve endings.

Reasons for using indirect high frequency

- To improve dry or dehydrated skins.
- To improve tired skin.
- To help improve fine lines.
- To help relax the tissues.
- To help improve poor circulation.

Preparation for indirect high frequency treatment

1 Observe general safety precautions for using electrical equipment.
2 The machine is placed on a stable trolley.
3 The machine is checked and tested by the therapist to ensure it is working correctly.
4 The products required for treatment are selected and placed on the trolley.

Indirect high frequency treatment

1 Client is greeted at reception and escorted to treatment area.
2 Consultation is carried out to check for contraindications and to explain the effects of the treatment and skin sensitivity test is carried out.
3 Client removes their jewellery which is kept safely by the therapist until the end of the treatment.
4 Client is helped on to the couch and their clothing and hair protected accordingly.
5 The therapist ensures the client is warm and comfortable.
6 The skin is cleansed with the appropriate products.
7 A suitable product medium is selected and applied to the client's face and neck, e.g. massage or nourishing cream.

Method

1 Ensure mains lead is plugged in to mains supply and that all switches are off and all dials are at zero.
2 The therapist tests the machine in front of the client and reassures them where necessary about the buzzing noise it makes.
3 Talcum powder is applied to the client's hands to absorb any perspiration.
4 The saturator is wiped with disinfectant and placed firmly in the holder.
5 Depending upon the apparatus used the saturator is held firmly by the client at the free end, taking care not to hold over the point of electrode insertion into the handle. The handle can also usually be

held by the client with their second hand but check the intended use with the manufacturer as in some cases this is not advised and the handle is supported by a towel.

6   The therapist places one hand in contact with the client's skin and begins to massage using small circular effleurage movements whilst with the other hand turning the intensity dial slowly, to suit the client's tolerance.

7   Place the other hand on the opposite side of the client's face and without losing contact, massage using both hands. The therapist should feel warmth in their fingers.

8   The treatment time will vary between 8 and 20 minutes depending upon the client's skin condition.

9   At the end of the treatment the therapist keeps one hand in contact whilst using the other to turn the intensity dial to zero before switching off the machine.

10   The cream is removed and either further treatment such as a face mask may be given or the skin is toned and moisturised with appropriate products.

11   The client is helped from the couch, the record card completed, appropriate home care and further salon treatment advice is given along with samples of the skin care products used and the client's next appointment is confirmed.

12   The therapist tidies the treatment area and cleans the electrode used by carefully wiping with hot water and then disinfectant. Special care must be taken not to wet the metal and connector of the saturator. All electrodes should be dry before being stored for later use.

POINTS TO NOTE

- The intensity dial may need to be reduced when progressing to areas of finer skin, e.g. the forehead.
- The intensity of the current in the tissues will be increased when lifting one hand off the skin during the massage.
- Tapotement movements such as tapping will intensify the current in the area being treated.
- In the past, talcum powder was used as a medium to create a stimulating effect, but its drying effects are not beneficial for a dry or dehydrated skin.

GOOD PRACTICE

- Care should be taken when working around the hairline as sensation will usually intensify because hair is a conductor of electricity.
- Contact must not be broken. If the circuit is completely broken and then remade without turning the intensity dial to zero, the client may feel a stronger tingling sensation which may make them apprehensive of further treatment. However if the therapist wishes to intentionally create a stimulating effect on the skin they can slowly lift the fingers slightly off the skin and return them.
- Rings must not be worn by the client on the hand that holds the saturator (and preferably not at all).
- Care must be taken to ensure any belts with metal buckles are kept away from the saturator or removed.
- The client or therapist must not touch any metal conducting material whilst the indirect high frequency treatment is in progress, e.g. couch, trolley, etc.

Direct high frequency

This method of application of the high frequency current uses glass electrodes which are placed in direct contact with the client's skin. The current is dispersed at the point of contact with the client and as the effects are concentrated around the electrode, they are superficial.

Effects of direct high frequency

- Increases metabolism.
- Warms and relaxes the tissues under the electrode.
- Improves the skin texture.
- Improves the moisture balance of the skin.
- Calms the sensory nerve endings.
- Produces ozone which has an anti-bacterial, germicidal effect on the surface of the skin. This effect can be intensified with sparking.

Reasons for using direct high frequency

- To improve the condition of seborrhoeic or oily skins.
- To improve the condition of oily areas, e.g. T-zone, blemished skin on any area of the body.
- To aid the healing of pustule-prone skins by using sparking on the skin.
- To destroy bacteria through the creation of ozone through sparking.
- To stimulate secretion in a dry skin by treating the skin for a few minutes, e.g. 3–4 minutes.

Preparation for direct high frequency treatment

1. Observe general safety precautions for using electrical equipment.
2. The machine is placed on a stable trolley.
3. The machine is checked and tested by the therapist to ensure it is working correctly.
4. The products required for treatment are selected and placed on the trolley.

Direct high frequency treatment

1. Client is greeted at reception and escorted to treatment area.
2. Consultation is carried out to check for contraindications and to explain the effects of the treatment.
3. Client removes their jewellery which is kept safely by the therapist until the end of the treatment.
4. Client is helped onto the couch and their clothing and hair protected accordingly.
5. The therapist ensures the client is warm and comfortable.
6. The skin is cleansed with the appropriate products.
7. A suitable medium is selected and applied to the client's face and neck, e.g. oxygenating cream and gauze.

USEFUL INFORMATION

The application of the direct high frequency electrode creates warmth on the skin and converts the stable oxygen molecules in the oxygenating cream to unstable ozone molecules (which have a germicidal effect).

Method

1 Ensure mains lead is plugged into mains supply and that all switches are off and all dials are at zero.
2 The therapist tests the machine in front of the client and reassures them where necessary about the buzzing noise it makes.
3 The selected electrodes are wiped with disinfectant and stored safely for use.
4 The electrode is placed firmly in the holder.
5 The therapist either places the electrode in contact with the client's skin and moves it around using small circular movements whilst turning the mains control switch on and the intensity dial up to suit the client's tolerance, or places their finger in contact with the electrode before turning the machine on then the intensity dial up and placing both finger and electrode in contact with the client's skin before removing the finger.
6 The treatment time will vary depending upon the client's skin condition, e.g. oily skin 8–15 minutes, dehydrated skin 3–4 minutes.
7 At the end of the treatment, or between changing electrodes, the therapist must keep the electrode in contact with the client's skin whilst turning the intensity dial to zero and switching the machine off before removing the electrode from the skin, or place their finger on the electrode before lifting it off the client's skin and turning the intensity dial to zero and switching the machine off. Some units have a secondary on/off switch directly on the handle to assist with an easier change over of electrodes, etc.

Note. When sparking to create a germicidal effect which may destroy bacteria, the electrode is lifted off the skin. The distance created between the electrode and the skin should only be a few millimetres, causing the current to 'jump' from the electrode to the client's skin thus creating a spark which in turn produces ultra-violet rays which destroy bacteria. The germicidal effect is created by the ionisation of the oxygen in the air which creates ozone. Controlled quantities of ozone help promote the healing of pustules and papules. Pores are constricted when the sparks stimulate the skins nerve endings.

8 The selected medium is removed and either further treatment such as a face mask may be given or the skin is toned and moisturised with appropriate products.
9 The client is helped from the couch, the record card completed, appropriate home care and further salon treatment advice is given along with samples of the skin care products used and the client's next appointment is confirmed.
10 The therapist tidies the treatment area and claims the electrodes used by carefully wiping with hot water and then disinfectant. Special care must be taken not to wet the metal end connector of the saturator. The electrodes are stored dry for later use.

POINTS TO NOTE

♦ With high frequency the current disperses into the client's body at the point of contact.
♦ As the effects are concentrated around the electrode they are superficial, but care must be taken when sparking not to over-treat as this can lead to over desquamation and drying of the skin during subsequent days.

1   Give four examples of vacuum applicators and in each case briefly outline their purpose.
2   List ten contraindications to vacuum suction.
3   State four reasons for giving a vacuum suction treatment.
4   Describe a high frequency current.
5   Name and describe the two different treatments that can be given using the high frequency machine.

Neuro-muscular electrical stimulation (NMES)

This treatment is referred to by many different names such as electrical muscle stimulation (EMS), faradic (after the original type of current used for muscle stimulation), or by manufacturers' trade names, e.g. Slendertone™ and Ultratone™. It is used to improve and maintain muscular tone and is a passive form of exercise as the client lies and relaxes whilst the machine emits electrical impulses to stimulate the muscles' motor nerves to bring about muscle contraction. To be more effective the treatment has to be part of a course to develop the full effect within the muscles. It is extremely beneficial for clients who do not enjoy physical exercise or who are contraindicated to strenuous exercise or for those wishing to tone particular muscle groups, e.g. abdominals for postnatal mothers.

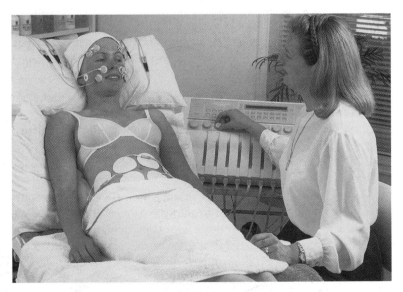

Fig. 6.26 *Neuro-muscular electrical stimulation*

POINT TO NOTE

A course of NMES treatment will improve the client's shape and inch loss will usually be noted.

NMES machines use an interrupted direct current of a low frequency and relative very small pulse width which is released into the body via a conductive electrode which is connected to the faradic unit via electrical leads. The majority of machines offer the therapist the facility to use the equipment on both face and body by using different electrodes and by varying the parameters of the current. Machines, however, are available for just face or body. Faradic treatments have been extremely popular for figure improvement programmes particularly when combined with other salon treatments such as gyratory massage and galvanic along with home care advice on diet and exercise. In recent years there has been great technological advancement by equipment manufacturers who have developed and adapted faradic currents to develop more specialised salon treatments for figure improvement (see Chapter 7).

NMES units generally have the following controls:

◆ A mains switch for turning the unit on or off. This is often combined with a timer.
◆ A safety aspect on most modern machines is a reset feature which prevents the machine working if any of the electrode outlet dials are not at zero.
◆ Intensity dials for each electrode outlet. As these dials are increased, so is the intensity of the current flowing through the electrodes.
◆ Contraction (surge or stimulation period) and relaxation dials which enable the therapist to select the appropriate times to suit the area of the body being treated and the existing condition of the client's muscle.
◆ A pulse sequence, wave form or phasic control. On the majority of equipment only two types are found; mono-plastic and bi-plastic. Mono-plastic emits pulses flowing in one direction only. Bi-phasic emits pulses flowing in both directions; back and forth or negative to positive then positive to negative. The other selections available either on this dial or as a separate mode dial are:

Mono-phasic on a regular basis. Pulses are emitted as per the machine setting, e.g. contracting for 2 seconds and relaxing for 2.5 seconds.
Bi-phasic on a regular basis. Pulses are emitted as per the machine setting.
Mono-phasic and bi-phasic on an irregular basis. With this setting the machine is programmed to alter the pattern of the set contraction and relaxation time. This is particularly useful when a client is a little apprehensive of the treatment and tends to automatically tighten their muscles when they expect the contraction to occur. It is also useful to add variety to the treatment for a regular client.

◆ A frequency dial. This enables the therapist to select the number of pulses per second emitted from the machine to stimulate the motor points. Traditionally for superficial muscles, such as those of the face, 120 is used whereas for work on larger muscles between 60 and 90 is used. However the most recent research has shown a wider application of frequency is beneficial, especially when recreating passive exercise most closely similar to physical activity.

USEFUL INFORMATION
The relaxation time is never less than the contraction time.

- A pulse width. This changes the actual width (i.e. the length of time it stays in the muscle) of each pulse emitted. The higher the setting of this dial the longer the time and therefore the greater is the effect to the muscle. For facial muscles a lower setting is usually used, e.g. 80 μs, whereas on the large body muscles a higher setting is required, e.g. from 160 μs upwards and if the client has a lot of adipose tissue the dial may be started at a higher setting still, such as 240 μs. (μ is the abbreviation for millionth or micro, hence here this means a time base in microseconds which are very quick.)
- Some machines have master output control which can increase the percentage intensity of current to all the electrodes in use without turning them up individually.
- Pulse ramp envelope control. Usually only available on more specialised units, this controls the configuration of pulses in the contraction time. It is adjusted to enable more comfortable, effective contractions.
- Sequential programming. Some specialist units offer the facility to create your own sequential treatment where frequency, contraction, relaxation and pulse width can be pre-programmed and altered at regular intervals and stored in the memory.

GOOD PRACTICE

Care must be taken not to over work the muscles.

Electrodes

There is a wide variety of electrodes available for use with faradic-type machines. To enable the current to flow to stimulate the muscles a positive electrode (anode) and negative electrode (cathode) are needed.

The most widely used modern faradic electrodes for application of the current to the body are rubber pads which are impregnated with an electrical conductor, such as carbon, on one side. These pads can vary in shape and size but are used in pairs to enable the current to flow from one to the other.

For facial treatments there are three types of electrode available for use:

- Facial block electrode (dual head). The most popular type manufactured and used houses the anode and cathode in its insulated holder. They vary in form and in use, e.g. some have an in-built intensity control to adapt the current easily, the distance between the anode and cathode may be fixed or if the electrode has a stylus the therapist can alter the distance between these. They are ideal for stimulating a number of motor points which are situated closely together on the face.
- Mushroom electrode (disc electrode). A metal disc in the electrode must be covered in several layers of lint to protect the client. The *indifferent electrode* is protected with a foam pouch and is placed in contact with the client's body by either lying it under the shoulder or, as with some machines, by using a wrist clip. The mushroom head is placed on the motor point of the muscle, acting as the *active electrode* and completing the electrical circuit.

USEFUL INFORMATION

The mushroom electrode is not particularly used in salons but has traditionally been used by colleges.

- Mask electrode. This houses a variety of electrodes inside to stimulate all the muscles of the face at the same time. This would not be used on claustrophobic clients.

Types of padding

The selection of the padding method for treatment will be dependent on a number of things:

- The phase control to be used. With bi-phasic the current is even from the positive and negative electrodes whereas with mono-phasic the current is stronger from the negative electrode.
- The areas to be treated and the number of pairs of electrodes available, e.g. if there are a large number of muscles to stimulate there may be insufficient electrodes to use the longitudinal method and therefore split padding may have to be used.
- Manufacturers' instructions. These should always be followed carefully as the manufacturers will recommend the most suitable type of padding to gain maximum benefit from their machine.

Longitudinal padding

Modern longitudinal padding involves placing the anode and cathode on to the top and bottom motor points of the same muscle, e.g. rectus abdominus, triceps, rectus femoris, etc., bringing about a smoother, even contraction. This term was used to describe the padding of the origin and insertion of a muscle whereby the current had to flow via the motor point to bring about a contraction. Modern longitudinal padding usually refers to the placing of the electrodes on to a muscle with two motor points.

Dual or duplicate padding

This type of padding involves using the anode and cathode of a pair of pads on one or two muscles on one side of the body and then placing another pair on the adjacent muscle group, e.g. the obliques, rectus abdominus, adductors, abductors, etc.

Split padding

With this type of padding a pair of pads is split and placed on the same muscle group on opposite sides of the body, e.g. gluteus maximus, pectorals, etc.

- With split padding you cannot alter the intensity if one side is weaker than the other.
- With split padding the bi-phasic mode must be selected.

ACTIVITY

With a colleague carry out three different body NMES treatments using the different methods of padding. Discuss the effectiveness and comfort of each method.

Contraindications

to NMES

- Disorders of the nervous system.
- Disorders or injury of the muscular system.
- Loss of skin sensation.
- Recent scar tissue.
- Broken bones.
- Hypersensitive skins.
- Heart conditions.
- Pacemakers.
- High or low blood pressure.*
- Thrombosis or phlebitis.
- Highly apprehensive clients.
- Epilepsy.*
- Diabetes.*
- Migraine sufferers.
- Cuts and abrasions.
- Highly vascular conditions.
- Metal plates, pins, bridges, IUD or if the client has an excessive amount of fillings.
- Over bony areas.
- Pregnancy.**

* Only to be carried out with medical approval.

** Exclude the abdomen.

Effects of NMES

- Stimulates the nerves and causes muscle contraction which acts as a passive form of exercise to strengthen and tone muscles.
- Increases blood circulation.

Reasons for using NMES

- To strengthen and tone poor muscles, e.g. abdominal and pectorals of postnatal mothers.
- To improve the contours of the face and body, e.g. platysma, abdominal, gluteals.
- To assist in tightening muscles after weight loss.
- To assist in improving a client's posture by stretching and toning shortened muscles, e.g. pectorals in kyphosis.

Preparation for NMES treatment

1   Observe general safety precautions for using electrical equipment.
2   The machine is placed on a stable trolley.
3   The machine is checked and tested by the therapist to ensure it is working correctly.
4   The products required for treatment are selected and placed on the trolley.

NMES treatment

1   Client is greeted at reception and escorted to treatment area.
2   Consultation is carried out to check for contraindications and to explain the effects of the treatment. A skin sensitivity test is carried out on the area to be treated.
    Note. If performing a body treatment, the client's measurements can be noted prior to treatment.
3   Client removes their jewellery, showers and may have a heat treatment to relax the muscles prior to treatment and/or an additional salon treatment, e.g. gyratory massage.
4   Client is helped onto the couch.
5   The therapist ensures the client is warm and comfortable.
6   The skin is free of grease as this would act as a barrier to the current and prevent a good contraction.
7   The therapist tests the machine in front of the client.
8   If treating the body, elasticated straps are wrapped and firmly secured around the area to be treated.
9   Having considered the client's needs and the machine being used, the therapist selects an appropriate method of padding, dampens the electrodes with warm water or conductive gel and places them firmly in contact with the client's skin.

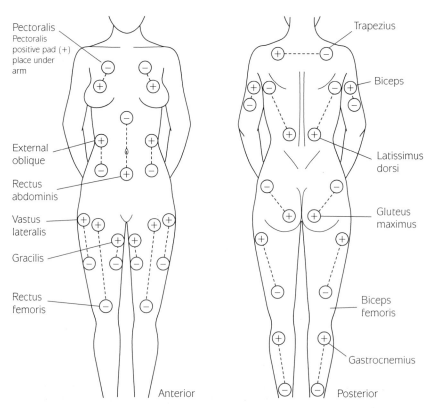

Fig. 6.27 *Example of faradic padding on the biphasic mode*

Method

1   Ensure mains lead is plugged in to mains supply and that all switches are off and all dials are at zero.
2   The therapist selects the appropriate treatment time, contraction and relaxation period, the mode, pulse sequence and width.
3   If performing a facial treatment the therapist dampens the facial electrode and places it firmly in contact with the treatment area.
    Note. If using the mushroom electrode, the therapist first places the indifferent electrode firmly in contact with the client's skin (behind the shoulder or strapped to the wrist). If using a mask electrode it is firmly strapped around the client's face and neck and as the electrodes are simultaneously activated by the intensity dial the therapist would check on client sensation and comfort until contractions were achieved. The treatment time would begin at around 8 minutes and build throughout the course of treatments to 15 minutes.
4   The therapist slowly turns up the intensity dial during the contraction time only, checking with the client on how it feels.

GOOD PRACTICE

◆ It is very important to use a good conductive medium.
◆ If working on the body all electrodes need to be turned up individually until the client feels a slight tingling sensation. By doing this it allows the client time to relax and adjust to the treatment before the therapist turns the individual intensity dials to achieve a contraction.

POINT TO NOTE

Some machines allow the therapist to increase the intensity during the treatment to all electrodes by adjusting the master output dial.

When working on the face, neck and décolleté areas it is advisable to contract the muscle 6–8 times before switching the intensity dial off during the relaxation period and moving the electrode to the next muscle. The sequence is then repeated two or three times throughout the course of treatments.

When working on the body the therapist must ensure even contractions are achieved on all the muscles being worked. If a muscle is weaker it will need a lower intensity to a stronger more toned muscle. The treatment time is usually around 20–40 minutes depending upon the treatment effects and condition. It is important to ensure that the client is warm and comfortable throughout the treatment.

5   At the end of the treatment the therapist ensures all dials are switched off before removing the electrodes. It is advisable to turn the intensity control down during the relaxation period.
6   If recommended, further treatment may be given.
7   The client is helped from the couch, the record card completed (if performing a body treatment the client's measurements may be recorded), appropriate home care and further salon treatment

USEFUL INFORMATION

Saline solution used to be applied to the electrodes as a conductor but most manufacturers today feel that there are sufficient mineral salts present in tap water to act as a conductor.

USEFUL
INFORMATION
Faradic pads deteriorate
with use and become less
conductive so will need
replacing regularly.

advice is given (with faradic treatment it is recommended that a client has a minimum of two to three sessions per week for six to eight weeks) along with samples of any skin care products used and the client's next appointment is confirmed.

8   The therapist tidies the treatment area and cleans the electrodes used by carefully wiping with hot water and detergent.

POINTS TO NOTE

Poor contraction of muscles may be due to:

- Any grease left on the skin.
- The electrodes being too dry (they may need re-damping during the treatment).
- The electrodes not being firmly in contact with the skin.
- The intensity selected being too low.
- The pulse frequency and width not being set correctly.
- Trying to stimulate muscles through large quantities of adipose tissue which can act as a barrier to the current.
- Incorrect positioning of the electrodes. It is important to switch the intensity dial to zero before moving the pads.
- Faulty connections on the machine or leads. The leads need regular checking and maintenance.
- Muscle fatigue.

Galvanic treatments

Galvanic treatments have become extremely popular over the last few years. The current brings about chemical and physical reactions within the body and it is commercially used with professional products to improve the client's face and body appearance. There are a wide variety of gels and ampoules manufactured and recommended for different skin types and conditions.

The galvanic machine can be applied with the appropriate products to offer two treatments to the client:

- Desincrustation – this is given to deep cleanse the skin.
- Iontophoresis – this is used to introduce beneficial ingredients into the skin for particular skin types or conditions, e.g. oily, dry or couperose skins.

Galvanic treatment is used on the body to assist in the dispersal of cellulite.

POINT TO NOTE

The range of products available include gel and ampoule preparations and specially formulated solutions.

The principles of the galvanic treatment for face and body is the same but the application, products used, treatment time, further salon treatment and home care advice are different. The machines use a direct current of a low voltage. They can be purchased for face or body work individually or combined in a face and body unit or in a combined unit with another electrical treatment such as high frequency. This last combination is commonly found in salons as these two treatments are popularly used with professional products for improved skin care (see Chapter 7).

Galvanic units consist of:

- A mains control switch which may be connected to a timer
- Outlets for connecting the electrodes which are used in pairs (anode and cathode)
- Intensity dial and milliamp meter for registering the amount of current applied (and directly to indicate the level of the client's skin resistance).
- Polarity switch which is often referred to as 'normal' or 'reverse' where 'normal' indicates that the internationally accepted law of colour coding applies (red = positive, black - negative).

It is extremely important that the therapist reads and follows the manufacturer's instructions as although there is a standard understanding that the red wire of an electrode is positive and the black lead is negative, most manufacturers have adapted their machines to enable the therapist to reverse the polarity of the leads at the flick of a switch which could easily cause confusion if the manufacturer's instructions are not read.

The therapist must fully understand their unit and if terms such as 'normal' and 'reverse' are indicated, know accurately how this refers to the polarity of the leads and outlets. Usually this is a simple point to clarify, but it should not be assumed as manufacturers vary in the use of terminology and presentation, i.e. some units have separate outlets for the anode and cathode and others are coupled.

The intensity of the output is measured in milliamps (mA) and can be registered on either:

- a moving coil meter, i.e. a gauge with an arm
- a LED (light emitting diode)
- a LCD (liquid crystal display).

For facial therapy treatment, intensity settings are low and indicated by the product directive and the type of skin being treated. Ranges between 0.2–0.6 mA are common, but individual sensory responses are an important factor to be considered along with manufacturer's instructions.

For body therapy the following calculation can be used to work out the maximum milliamps current setting for a pad size:

Manufacturer's recommended maximum = 0.05 mA per square centimetre

Pad size = 11×11 cm = 121 cm^2

Maximum current setting = 121×0.05 = 6.05 mA

Terminology referred to in galvanic treatments

- Anode = positive electrode.
- Cathode = negative electrode.

USEFUL INFORMATION

The type of product, its viscosity, etc., will determine the most appropriate method of application. Each product will list the most active ingredients for a specific purpose, i.e. products for couperose skins tend to contain a vasoconstrictor such as horse chestnut.

USEFUL INFORMATION

Galvanic machines contain:

- A rectifier – changes the alternating current to a direct current.
- A capacitor – smoothes out any irregularities in the direct current.
- A transformer – reduces the voltage of the alternating current given out at the mains supply.

- Active electrode = the electrode in contact with the client's face during facial treatment.
- Indifferent electrode = the electrode held by the client to complete the electrical circuit.
- Anions = negatively charged ions, used in professional products which determine the polarity of the active electrode.
- Cations = positively charged ions.
- Anaphoresis = the flow of anions to the anode.
- Cataphoresis = the flow of cations to the cathode.

The galvanic treatment operates on the basic principle that like poles repel and opposite poles attract (see Fig. 6.28). The products selected are repelled into the skin by the active electrode which must be of the same polarity as the product.

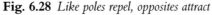

Fig. 6.28 *Like poles repel, opposites attract*

POINT TO NOTE

The polarity of the active electrode is determined by the product used so care should be taken to read the manufacturer's instructions. The majority of products tend to be 'negative to positive' but the actual time for which the negative or positive poles are used will once again vary depending on the type of treatment being given and the manufacturer's instructions.

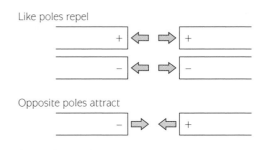
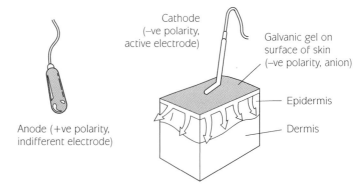

Fig. 6.29 *Anaphoresis*

Electrodes

There is a variety of electrodes available for use on the face.

Types of active electrode:

- Metal rollers.
- Metal ball – single/double prong.
- Tweezer or flat head electrode.

Tweezers or flat head electrodes are usually covered with either dampened gauze, lint or cotton wool, according to the manufacturer's instructions or worked over a gauze masque soaked in active solution.

Types of indifferent electrodes:

- Metal bar. Some companies recommend that the electrode is covered in a dampened sponge pouch.
- Flat plate. These are generally supplied with a sponge pouch which is dampened before application.

Body electrodes

- Galvanic pads. These come in pairs, having a positive and negative electrode, and should be supplied with sponge pouches which are designed to protect against galvanic burns. The sponges are dampened prior to use and the active side of the galvanic pad is placed face down. Several layers of a lint wadding can be used instead but care must be taken to ensure an even contact is made.

  Note. It is important to check that the sponge or lint layers do not dry out during treatment.

USEFUL INFORMATION

Some conductive electrodes are conductive on both sides. This is not recommended for safe body application. If these are to be used care must be taken to insulate the top of the pad before securing with elasticated straps.

POINT TO NOTE

During a facial treatment the active cathode removes the body's sebum and in doing so lowers the skin's resistance to the current; it may therefore be necessary to reduce the intensity of the current during treatment.

GOOD PRACTICE

- Sponge pouches must be thoroughly washed after use with warm water and detergent then soaked in a suitable disinfectant and thoroughly rinsed.
- Sponges will deteriorate with wear and tear and must be replaced as needed.

Contraindications

to galvanic treatment

- Loss of skin sensation.
- Recent scar tissue.
- Infectious skin diseases or disorders.
- Broken bones.
- Hypersensitive skins.
- Heart conditions.
- Pacemakers.
- Low blood pressure.
- Epilepsy.*
- Diabetes.*
- Migraine sufferers.
- Cuts and abrasions.
- Highly vascular conditions.
- Metal plates, pins, bridges or an excessive amount of fillings.
- Pregnancy.*

* Only to be carried out with medical approval.

Effects of galvanic treatment

Effects at the cathode

The cathode produces an alkali effect on the skin by bringing about a chemical reaction between sodium ions and the hydroxyl ions of water to produce sodium hydroxide which is an alkali, thus creating the following effects:

- Breaks down the acid mantle.
- Relaxes the pores.
- Increases the blood circulation – vasodilation occurs.
- Hyperaemia.
- Warmth in the tissues.
- Brings about saponification – the emulsifying and removal of sebum.
- Creates a softening and drying effect on the skin.
- Stimulates nerve endings.
- Moisture is temporarily drawn to the cathode.

Effects at the anode

The anode produces an acidic effect on the skin by bringing about a chemical reaction between the chloride ions and hydrogen ions present in tap water to produce hydrochloric acid and oxygen, thus creating the following effects:

- Restores the acid mantle.
- Tightens the pores.
- Hardening of the skin.
- Creates warmth in the tissues.
- Reduces circulation.
- Soothing effect on the nerve endings, if used for a short time.

ACTIVITY

Research the variety of products available for use with galvanic equipment. Consider their size, cost, ingredients and usage.

POINTS TO NOTE

- Care should be taken when using galvanic treatments, particularly with treatment to the body as if too high an intensity of current is used or the duration of the treatment is too long or skin sensitivity has not been accurately diagnosed or insufficient insulation is used, it may cause a galvanic burn which can be a mixture of a chemical and over-heating reaction.
- Galvanic burns are extremely painful and take a very long time to heal. They generally appear under the cathode and will initially look red and will later turn grey and weep.

GOOD PRACTICE

- The therapist should always remain with a client during galvanic treatments and check on their comfort continually.
- It is essential for all galvanic treatments that a good and even conduction is maintained at all times and is achieved by a moist working surface and even pressure of working electrodes and uninterrupted contact.

Reasons for using galvanic treatment

- To deep cleanse the skin.
- To introduce active ingredients to benefit the client's skin condition.
- To assist in dispersing cellulite.

Preparation for galvanic treatment

1 Observe general safety precautions for using electrical equipment.
2 The machine is placed on a stable trolley.
3 The machine is checked and tested by the therapist to ensure it is working correctly.
4 The products required for treatment are selected and placed on the trolley.

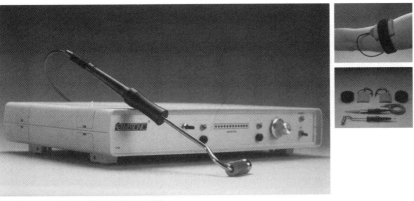

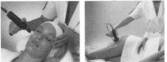

Fig. 6.30 *Galvanic machine*

Galvanic treatment to the face and neck

1 Client is greeted at reception and escorted to treatment area.
2 Consultation is carried out to check for contraindications and to explain the effects of the treatment. A skin sensitivity test is carried out on the area to be treated.
3 Client removes their jewellery.
4 Client is helped onto the couch and their clothing and hair protected.
5 The therapist ensures the client is warm and comfortable.
6 The skin is cleansed with suitable products and if using a cream-based product the therapist must ensure that there is no residue left on the skin which would act as a barrier to the current.
   Note. A vapouriser can be used to soften the skin and lower the client's skin resistance. There is also a variety of conductive lotions available that may be used.
7 A suitable medium is selected and applied to the client's face and neck, e.g. desincrustation gel or active ampoule. It is usually recommended that ampoules are applied with a gauze masque rather than directly onto the skin.

Note. The type of product selected for facial work will influence the type of electrode used, e.g. metal roller and ball electrodes tend to be used with gels whereas the other electrodes tend to be used with ampoules.

Method

1 Ensure mains lead is plugged in to mains supply and that all switches are off and all dials are at zero.
2 The therapist tests the machine in front of the client and explains its use.
3 The selected electrodes are wiped with disinfectant and prepared for use according to manufacturer's instructions.
4 The therapist ensures the electrodes are correctly fitted and that the correct polarity for the product being used is selected.
5 Depending on the type of indifferent electrode being used, it is either given to the client to hold firmly or is placed under the client's shoulder or clipped to the client's arm.
6 The therapist places the selected active electrode in contact with the client's skin and moves it around using small movements whilst turning the mains control switch on and the intensity dial up according to the manufacturer's instructions. Do not begin treatment on the forehead or around the eyes.
   Note. The client is advised that they may get a metallic taste in the mouth if they have fillings whilst working around the mouth and nose area. Some clients feel a slight warmth in the tissues, others don't feel any reaction, but do not be tempted to increase the milliamp intensity beyond recommended levels as blood vessels can dilate and if there is insufficient product on the skin a galvanic (chemical) burn could result. Ensure that the machine is working correctly and any manufacturer's instructions for equipment/product are being followed.
7 The therapist moves the active electrode slowly over the client's face and neck in a methodical pattern. The treatment time will vary according to the type of treatment being given, the skin condition and the manufacturer's instructions, so it is essential that the therapist studies these carefully. Carlton Professional recommend the following for use with their products and equipment:

   Desincrustation – 15–20 minutes negative to positive.
   Iontophoresis – 5–7 minutes negative to positive.

   The positive polarity is generally used for the final 2–3 minutes.

   It is important that the therapist keeps the active electrode moving and in contact with the skin whilst turning the intensity dial to zero before removing the electrode from the skin to reverse the polarity.
8 At the end of the treatment the therapist ensures all dials are set to zero and switched off before removing the electrodes.
9 The selected medium is removed and further treatment, such as facial massage or direct high frequency, may be given or the skin is toned and moisturised.
10 The client is helped from the couch, the record card completed, appropriate home care and further salon treatment advice is given, along with samples of the skin care products used and the client's next appointment is confirmed.

11 The therapist tidies the treatment area and cleans the electrodes used by carefully wiping with hot water and disinfectant.

Galvanic treatment to the body

1 Client is greeted at reception and escorted to treatment area.
2 Consultation is carried out to check for contraindications and to explain the effects of the treatment. A skin sensitivity test is carried out on the area to be treated.
3 Client removes their jewellery, showers and may have a mild heat treatment to relax the tissues prior to treatment and/or an additional salon treatment such as gyratory massage.
4 Client is helped onto the couch.
5 The therapist ensures the client is warm and comfortable.
6 The therapist ensures the skin is free of grease as this would act as a barrier to the current.
7 The therapist tests the machine in front of the client and checks all leads are providing a working circuit.

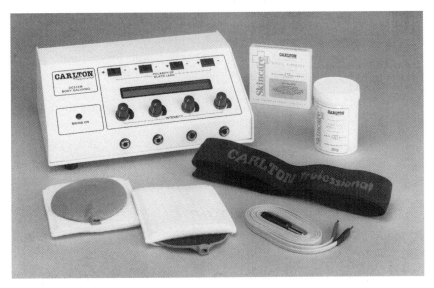

Fig. 6.31 *Super galvanic equipment*

POINTS TO NOTE

Prior to treatment mild sudation is recommended, but not any excessive sweating.

Method

1 Ensure mains lead is plugged in to mains supply and that all switches are off and all dials are at zero.
2 Elasticated body straps are wrapped firmly around the area to be treated. The therapist applies the selected product, e.g. cellulite gel or ampoule to the skin/sponge pouch and places the insulated electrodes according to manufacturer's instructions. (If the electrodes are conductive on both sides ensure the top surface is insulated before fixing with elasticated strapping). In treatment for cellulite the stronger, active, cathode pads are placed on the main cellulite areas whilst the anode is generally placed parallel or opposite.

Electrical Equipment for Face and Body Treatments **199**

3 The therapist ensures the electrodes are correctly fitted and that the correct polarity for the product being used is selected.

4 The intensity dials are turned up individually until either the client feels a slight tingling sensation, or until the maximum output recommended is reached.

5 The treatment time may take up to approximately 20 minutes according to the client's tolerance. The polarity is generally reversed for the last 3–5 minutes of the treatment.

6 At the end of the treatment, or in between changing polarity, the therapist must turn the intensity dial to zero before switching off the machine and removing the insulated electrodes from the skin.

7 The selected medium is removed and further treatment such as NMES may be given. Care should be taken in any subsequent pad and product placement to avoid over irritation or stimulation.

8 The client is helped from the couch, the record card completed, appropriate home care and further salon treatment advice is given and the client's next appointment is confirmed.

Note. For treatment of cellulite it is recommended that the client has a minimum of 2–3 sessions per week with a total number of 12 treatments before a significant difference can be seen.

9 The therapist tidies the treatment area and cleans the electrodes used by carefully wiping with hot water and then disinfectant.

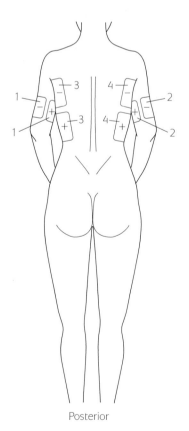
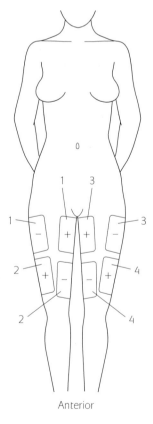

Posterior   Anterior

Fig. 6.32 *Example of galvanic padding*

- For treatment of cellulite, diet and exercise should be combined with body galvanic treatments.
- The client's cellulite condition can often appear worse before improvement is seen due to the redistribution of fatty fluids in the area.
- Body galvanic treatment helps to relax and loosen the adipose tissues and waste elements that bring about cellulite. It is not effective as a treatment on its own.

ACTIVITY

1 Identify three clients with differing skin conditions, design individual treatment programmes for them using electrical equipment. Carry out the treatments keeping a record of the products and equipment used, duration of each treatment, home care and clients' views and evaluate the effectiveness of the programmes.
2 With a colleague design and carry out a programme, including the use of electrical equipment, to assist with figure improvement. Keep a record of the treatments and home care and evaluate the effectiveness of the programme.

USEFUL INFORMATION
Ozone is produced when the vapour passes over the high pressure mercury lamp which turns the available oxygen to ozone.

Vapourisers

For years vapourisers have been used to prepare a client's skin for further treatment, such as prior to a cleansing face mask or galvanic treatments. The warmth of the vapour relaxes the tissues and softens the skin. It may also induce slight perspiration which has a cleansing action on the skin and the warmth will stimulate the sudoriferous glands thus assisting in the elimination of waste. There are a variety of vapourisers available including mobile free standing units with a height adjustment facility and portable machines that are easily transported and sit on a sturdy trolley or table top. Usually distilled water is placed inside the unit and is heated by the internal heating element until a fine spray of vapour flows through the vapour jet. Most manufactures have designed units with a safety device; either a device to warn the therapist that the water level is low, or a cut-out switch to prevent the unit boiling dry. Most vapourisers have an optional ozone switch enabling the therapist to combine vapour with ozone which has an anti-bacterial effect on the skin and is therefore particularly beneficial for congested skins or after extraction work has been carried out. Vapourisers are used for differing lengths of time and from different distances from the skin according to the desired effect and overall treatment programme.

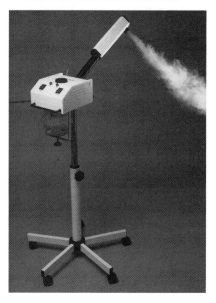

Fig. 6.33 *Vapouriser*

Contraindications

to using a vapouriser

- Highly vascular conditions.
- Sunburn.
- Acne rosacea.

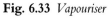

Brush cleansing

Brush cleansing machines are used to aid the desquamation of the skin and to aid cellular regeneration by stimulating the skin's blood circulation. They can be used to give a deep cleansing of the skin, to aid in the removal of peels or masks or to give a stimulating massage. The units are supplied with a variety of massage heads allowing the therapist to select the appropriate head according to the client's skin type and the desired effects of the treatment. The machines have a mains on/off

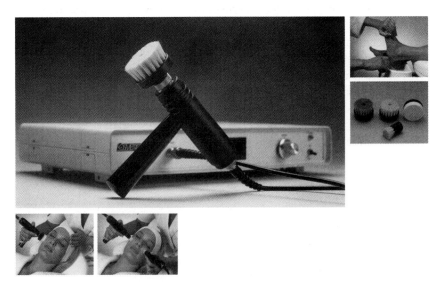

Fig. 6.34 *Brush peeling machine*

switch and a variable speed control and some incorporate a directional control to enable the therapist at a turn of a dial to ensure the skin is being lifted rather than pulled down. If the machine is being used for cleansing or massage, suitable water-based foaming products should be used to facilitate the action of the massage heads. The circular, rotating heads should be applied to the skin dampened and flat to the skin, i.e. making a right angle between skin and handle.

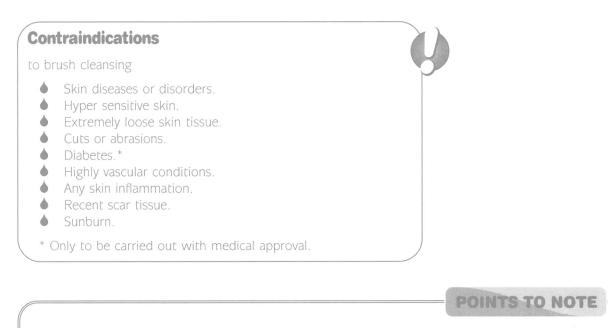

Contraindications

to brush cleansing

- Skin diseases or disorders.
- Hyper sensitive skin.
- Extremely loose skin tissue.
- Cuts or abrasions.
- Diabetes.*
- Highly vascular conditions.
- Any skin inflammation.
- Recent scar tissue.
- Sunburn.

* Only to be carried out with medical approval.

POINTS TO NOTE

- Brushing can be used for lymph stimulation massage. The direction of the massage head should be 'lifting' the skin.
- Treatment time is on average 5–7 minutes.

Progress Check

1 State the different types of electrical treatments for:
  a the face   **b** the body.
2 Describe the general effects of the following treatments:
  a neuro-muscular electrical stimulation
  b desincrustation
  c iontophoresis
  d vapourisers
  e brush cleansing.
3 List four contraindications for each of the following treatments:
  a neuro-muscular electrical stimulation
  b facial galvanic treatments
  c vapourisers
  d brush cleansing.
4 Describe the electrical currents used in the following treatments:
  a neuro-muscular electrical stimulation
  b galvanic
5 Explain the following terms:
  a anode   **b** cathode   **c** anion   **d** cation.

SPECIALISED SALON TREATMENTS FOR FIGURE AND SKIN IMPROVEMENT 7

After working through this chapter you will be able to:
- identify the different specialised treatments available
- describe the benefits of the specialised treatments.

As with all specialised salon treatments, it is essential to research the companies' products and equipment, the effects, potential market and growth of the treatments. It is important to note that with these specialised salon treatments the therapist must undertake all necessary training from the manufacturer/agent concerned.

Manual treatments

Manual cellulite treatments
A number of professional skin care companies offer specialised manual treatments that aim to reduce and improve the appearance of cellulite. They normally work in two ways, either by the action of the product itself or the massage techniques used.

Products
There are certain ingredients, in particular plant extracts and essential oils, that are known to have an effect on cellulite. Examples of these include:

- Essential oil of rosemary – this has a tonic effect and is anti-toxic.
- Essential oil of sandalwood – eliminates toxins and decongests.
- Essential oil of patchouli – this has a regenerative effect and is healing.
- Essential oil of lavender – this has a healing and diuretic effect.
- Seaweed – acts as a diuretic
- Horsetail extract – tonic action on the tissues.

Massage techniques
These often incorporate specialised movements that help in lymphatic drainage and compression-type movements as the circulation is reduced in these areas and needs improving if the effective elimination is going to take place.

For any of the cellulite treatments to be successful they need to be given in courses with proper home care advice. The client should be encouraged to look at their diet and eliminate convenience-type foods, too much salt, sugar, tea, coffee, etc., and to look at their lifestyle; in particular smoking, alcohol consumption and exercise.

The client must be able to attend the clinic at least two to three times a week for a course of treatments lasting from 20 to 30 minutes on average. The client must also be prepared to invest in products to be used at home in between salon visits and to use them daily.

Example of a cellulite treatment

1 Perform a detailed consultation, checking the area for any contraindications.
2 Prepare the client for treatment ensuring comfort throughout.
3 Uncover the area and clean with specialised toning product.
4 Apply exfoliating cream evenly to the treatment area, remove when dry using circular movements. Support the skin as required.
5 Wipe area with toner to remove any residual cream.
6 Apply cellulite treatment oil and massage the area using lymphatic drainage movements and compression techniques.
7 Apply specialised cellulite gel/serum and work into the area.
8 Often some form of heat is next applied to the area to help the absorption of the products; it may be in the form of cellophane sheeting, a warm poultice or a thermal blanket.
9 Remove the thermal medium and any traces of residual product.
10 Apply cellulite cream and massage into area.
11 Recommend home care advice and book the next treatment.

Products for home care

Home care normally consists of using some kind of cellulite serum/gel and cream which needs to be applied daily, preferably morning and at night, and usually following a brisk circulatory massage.

Stretch marks

These treatments aim to reactivate the dermis and increase the localised circulation. Success of the treatment will depend on regular salon treatment (2–3 times per week) over a course of 12–20 on average. The client will also need to purchase home care products to be used in between salon visits.

Common ingredients used in stretch mark treatments include plant extracts and essential oils. For example:

- Hops – have a firming and tightening effect.
- Ginseng – aids cellular stimulation and has an anti-ageing effect.
- Horsetail – restores elasticity in fibres and collagen of the skin.
- Essential oil of mint – tones, firms and increases circulation.

Example of a stretch mark treatment

1 Perform a thorough consultation, checking the area for any contraindications and make sure that the stretch marks are at a stage where they will respond to treatment.
2 Wipe over the area with toner and exfoliate to remove dead skin cells to allow easier absorption of products.
3 Next stimulate the area to be treated with either a body brush, body mitten, specific equipment or even brisk effleurage-type movements.
4 Apply a specialised stretch mark gel/solution and work it into the area briskly.
5 A stimulating product is applied and massaged into the area. The massage sequence should be quite brisk and include pinching-type movements.
6 Thermal equipment/product can be applied to allow the active solutions to penetrate more thoroughly.
7 Remove any residue of products.

8   Finally prescribe the most appropriate products for the upkeep of the skin at home and book the next treatment.

Skin improvement treatments

One of the latest advances in skin improvement has been the development of skin renewal treatments. On the surface it may seem that nothing is new, peeling products have been used for a long time – even as far back as Egyptian times. As recently as 1927 chemical peels were used to dissolve dead skin tissue. However in the last few years two substances have been generating media interest. They are retinoic acid and alpha hydroxy acid (AHA).

Retinoic acid

Retinoic acid is Vitamin A and was originally developed as a formulation for the treatment of acne vulgaris. It was found to speed up the natural shedding of the epidermis and recent trails have shown it to be very effective (if used in low concentrations) on sun damage, ageing, fine lines and wrinkles and pigmentation. However it does need to be used for six months and once discontinued, stops working. There can be side effects however and a lot of people develop residual inflammation as the treatment reduces the thickness of the stratum corneum.

This is not performed as a salon treatment, clients usually obtain the retinoic acid on prescription. Beauty therapists need to take great care with any client using retinoic acid products. In particular avoid waxing, peeling or extracting in areas being treated.

Alpha hydroxy acids (AHA)

These are also sometimes referred to as fruit acids and were developed following the interest in retinoic acid.

They work by causing micro-exfoliation which speeds up the natural exfoliation process of the skin. Some of the ingredients literally digest the surface cells therefore revealing new skin. This is a very important concept in the treatment of the skin as many problems that occur are the result of a build of dead skin cells or *hyperkeritinisation* as it is technically known.

Great care should be taken with the use and administration of these products however as they can be extremely harsh if not used in the correct quantity.

Some key ingredients used in AHA creams are:

- **Lactic acid**. This alpha hydroxy acid occurs naturally in sour milk and dissolves the intercellular cement holding the skin cells together. It also works on follicular skin cells helping dislodge blockages and therefore helping prevent congestion.
- **Glycolic acid**. This is used for its small molecular structure as it is able to penetrate quickly and deeply and dissolves the natural moisturising factor of the skin. It can cause more irritation than lactic acid.
- **Salicylic acid**. This stimulates the formation of new epidermal skin cells in the stratum germinativum and has antiseptic properties.
- **Bromelain**. This is a pineapple derivative and is a fruit enzyme that digests surface skin cells.

- **Papain**. This comes from the papaya fruit and is an enzyme. It again digests the surface skin cells.
- **Citric acid**. This is derived from citrus fruits and is also a fruit enzyme that digests the surface skin cells.
- **Plant and flower extracts**. Examples include orange flower, aloe vera and cornflower. They are added for their soothing and hydrating properties.

Buffers

Alpha hydroxy acid treatments have a buffer added to make them less aggressive in reaction on the skin. Plant extracts and enzymes are used as buffers and they have the effect of altering the pH of reaction.

AHA treatments exist in two forms; a concentrated strength for use by the therapist in the clinic and a lower concentration for the client to use at home daily between salon visits. The combination of the professional and the home care products will achieve the most rapid improvement in the appearance of the skin and as a general guide most manufacturers recommend a course of at least six salon treatments to be taken once a week initially with the daily use of home care products.

Example of an AHA facial treatment

1 Perform a detailed consultation checking the area for any contraindications.
2 Remove the eye and lip make-up with a suitable product making sure there is no residue left on the skin.
3 Next cleanse the face and neck with an appropriate cleanser at least twice and again thoroughly remove.
4 The special fruit acid solution is applied to the skin and left on according to individual manufacturer's instructions.
5 After the correct time the product is removed very thoroughly, usually with sponges and copious amounts of warm water, making sure no residue is left.
6 Extractions can now be performed where necessary.
7 The skin is massaged with a special soothing product to help calm the skin and reduce irritation.
8 A soothing mask is applied.
9 A special toner is applied often by means of a 'spray' action.
10 Finally a protective cream is applied to filter ultra-violet rays and nourish the skin.
11 To conclude the treatment the therapist explains the relevant homecare and retail advice and confirms the date of the next appointment.

POINT TO NOTE

Some clients may feel mild tingling or itching whilst having AHA treatments and the skin may even be pink for a short time afterwards. This is a normal reaction and must be clearly explained to the client. However, in extreme cases an abnormal reaction may occur in which case treatment should be discontinued.

GOOD PRACTICE

Many manufacturers recommend some form of patch testing of products before commencing treatments and also a preparation product for the client to use at home prior to embarking on the course.

Body wraps

Body wraps have been used in the professional beauty market for a number of years in varying forms. Most are marketed as a 'slimming treatment' as body tissues are compressed and slight fluid loss will result in inch loss together with a slight weight decrease. Body wraps offer other benefits such as cleansing the skin, tightening loose tissue, detoxifying the body, revitalising and helping improve cellulite and stretch marks.

Body wraps normally consist of three principles:

- Specialised products that contain active ingredients designed to be absorbed by the skin and aid in the elimination process. Example of key ingredients most commonly used are seaweed – used for its diuretic effect, mineral extracts – used to nourish the skin and oceanic clay which acts as a poultice to draw toxins from the body.
- A wrapping medium – these can be almost like elastic bandages or even be some form of plastic or rubber sheeting.
- Thermal activity. This can be in the form of a heat treatment – infra-red lamps or a thermal blanket – and is designed to keep the client warm as the wrapping medium and products cool. Some manufacturers suggest exercises to keep warm and to help with toning the body at the same time.

Most body wrap treatments are designed to be taken in courses attended regularly together with home care products and diet and exercise advice.

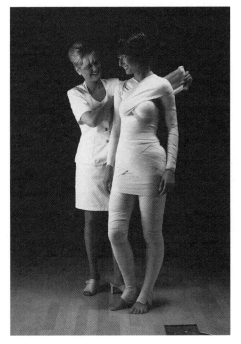

Fig. 7.1 *Universal contour wrap*

Example of a body wrap treatment

1   A detailed consultation is carried out with the client checking for any contraindications and the client is weighed and measured.
2   Specific measurements are marked to show the client exactly where the tape measure was placed.

3   The wrapping medium is prepared, in particular bandages are normally soaked in a special 'clay' solution. (This should be done before the client arrives).

4   The client is then wrapped in the bandages/wrapping medium and most manufacturers suggest that the bandages are applied upwards in line with venous return. Particular attention should be observed to wrapping the back so as to offer lumbar support.

5   Extra amounts of the product are sometimes added for specific areas.

6   Once all the bandages/wrapping medium are in place, check with the client that they feel comfortable.

7   A thermal device is used to keep the client warm while the bandages cool. During treatment time it also induces relaxation. Some manufacturers recommend gentle exercise or the use of a toning table. (In this case the client will normally wear some form of protective tracksuit)

8   After approximately one hour the bandages/wrapping medium are removed and the client is remeasured. Whereas some manufacturers recommend taking a shower to remove traces of product left on the skin, some products will have been completely absorbed and a shower is not necessary.

9   Finally, recommend homecare and retail products necessary for the maintenance of the treatment and confirm the next treatment.

POINT TO NOTE

It is extremely important to receive proper training in the application of body wrapping as the technique for applying the bandages requires particular skill and should only be carried out after completing a manufacturer's recommended course.

Progress Check

1   Give an example of a manual cellulite treatment.
2   What is the main purpose of a stretch mark treatment?
3   Give three factors that should be considered when performing an AHA treatment.
4   What are the main benefits of a body wrap treatment and how often should it be performed?

Toning tables

Toning tables may appear to be a relatively new concept in figure correction; however early models have existed since the 1930s when they were produced for physiotherapy and rehabilitation purposes. Modern tables have quickly established themselves in the professional beauty market. They normally consist of a motorised bed-type unit with various movable sections. It is possible to purchase them in two forms; either as individual units or as a multi-function unit.

Individual units are tables designed to work on one specific area of the body and would normally be part of a group of approximately six or seven units which the client uses in a treatment session lasting approximately one hour. The obvious advantage of having individual units is that more than one client can be using the tables simultaneously. The main drawback is that a lot of space is needed because each unit measures approximately 8 × 1.1 m (6.5 × 3.5 ft). This normally means that if the salon is going to purchase individual units either it is very large, or is going to specialise in toning tables and figure correction treatments generally. This type of toning table is very popular with health spas.

Multi-function units are beds with all the features of the individual units incorporated into them so the client does not have to move once treatment commences. This type of unit is ideal if space is a problem, but it does restrict the number of clients that can use it in any one day.

The main benefits of toning tables
Toning tables are designed to improve muscle tone, mobility and reduce inches without the use of any kind of weight. They work on the principles of both isotonic and isometric exercise.

Different tables or parts of the multi-function table produce varying movement, rhythm and speed which produces progressive resistance. This in turn strengthens muscle fibres as each fibre is shortened in length improving elasticity. Toning tables also increase body temperature by increasing blood circulation; this also helps in the removal of waste products and toxins.

Types of toning table
- **Circulation table (warm-up and cool-down)**. This produces a gentle vibration which is designed to increase the circulation and relax tense muscles. It should be used at the start and the end of a treatment session. There is normally an arm bar present on this table to help in toning of the upper arms, back and chest.
- **Leg table**. This concentrates on the inner and outer thighs and gluteals, but has a toning effect on the entire leg area.
- **Sit-up table**. This works the abdominal area and it is suggested that 10 minutes on this table is the equivalent to around 80 sit-ups.

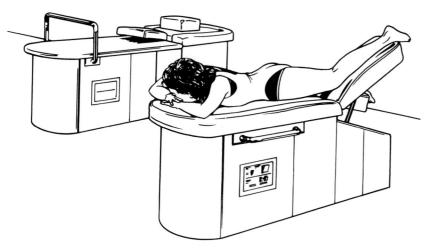

Fig. 7.2 *Toning tables*

- **Stomach/hip table**. This table stretches and lifts the gluteals and works the abdomen at the same time. It will also help to improve overall posture.
- **Twister table**. This table alternately lifts and raises the lower legs.
- **Stretching table**. This table affects the upper body, lifting the rib cage and bust and easing tension in the upper back.

A normal treatment session will last approximately one hour with roughly ten minutes being spent on each table/function. Most beds have a control panel which allows the therapist to adjust the speed of the table according to the health and general fitness of the client.

Electrical treatments

Micro-electrotherapy

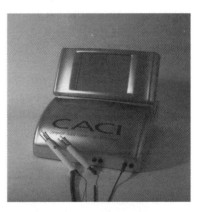

Fig. 7.3 *Micro-current machine*

Micro-current electrotherapy is a staple part of beauty therapy these days, but what is it and how exactly does it work?

Micro-current machines use a modified direct current usually with a low frequency range and relatively long pulse width 'on' time (compared to NMES devices) which is measured in micro-amps (a micro-amp being a millionth of an amp). A micro-amp (μA) is a thousand times smaller than a milli-amp (which is a thousandth of an amp). In beauty therapy the milli-amp is the scale of amplitude usually used for measuring the output ranges of traditional galvanic devices.

As micro-current is so small, the client should feel little, if any, sensation – it is virtually subsensory and it does not stimulate motor points or nerve pathways as does NMES. It bypasses the surrounding structures and enters the belly of the muscle to stimulate the muscle. Micro-current works in harmony with the body's own bio-electrical field.

More than twenty years ago, in the USA, Dr Thomas Wing carried out pioneer work using micro-current to treat sports injuries and Bell's palsy and stroke victims. During his work he discovered that by using micro-current he could realign the damaged muscle tissue to the healthy side of the face. He noted that during these treatments the damaged muscle tissues were actually lifting higher than the healthy side and he realised the beneficial effects this current would have on the cosmetic industry.

From Wing's research, the CACI™ machine (computer-aided cosmetology instrument) evolved and was introduced into the UK for cosmetic work. Once CACI™ was launched around 1993, most other electrotherapy manufacturers added micro-current into their range of equipment.

By using micro-current via cotton-tipped probes or roller bars – which work along the origin and insertion to grab the belly of the muscle – on a healthy muscle where there is no nerve damage, the nerve pathway is clear and the effects obtained are quite significant. It has other healthy effects since it not only works on muscles but also on skin.

The main effects are that:

- Fine lines and wrinkles are softened and reduced.
- It helps to normalise sebaceous secretions so it is good for dull, sallow skin tones, oily skins and sluggish complexions.
- It is extremely beneficial for photo-damaged skin, acne pitting, stretch marks, keloid scarring and cellulite.
- It refines, re-moisturises, rejuvenates and re-texturises skin.

As micro-current uses a modified direct current, it will basically have the same physical and physiological effects of the direct current used in galvanic treatments, but because of the relatively short pulse width 'on' times (compared to galvanic continuous direct current) and usually much lower levels of amplitude these effects are significantly reduced.

- Where the current passes through tissues, stimulation of the metabolism encourages lymphatic and venous drainage.
- Where the electrodes are in contact with the skin there will be the effects of both poles. The negative pole causes deep cleansing; dilation of blood and lymph; exfoliation of the stratum corneum; stimulation of nervous response. The positive pole creates tightening of the pores; firming of the tissues; soothing of the nervous response; and constriction of blood and lymph flow.

Micro-current is generally considered safe, with some top athletes using it to treat muscle and soft tissue injuries. The muscles cannot be harmed, and if a client does not keep up the maintenance, the muscles will never be worse than when the client started their course, they will merely return to the original condition. As the basic principle of treatment is to re-educate muscles, lifting and toning the facial or body contours, a course of treatments is necessary, followed by a monthly maintenance programme. A course of treatment will vary slightly depending on the condition of the client's muscles, but an average course is between 10 and 14 treatments that are carried out preferably two to three times a week for the first few weeks, decreasing to once a week as the lift on the muscle lasts.

There are some conditions that are contraindicated to treatment including epilepsy; skin disorders; pregnancy; recent scar tissue; pacemakers; heat conditions; metal pins and plates in the immediate area; and silicone implants and collagen ridges. It is always wise to ask clients with high blood pressure and spastic conditions for a letter of approval from their GP before considering treatment.

As with all therapy treatments, it is essential to carry out a thorough consultation and prepare a treatment plan for the individual client. This should include personal dietary and medical details and should be reviewed by the therapist. Keeping photographic evidence at varying stages throughout the course is useful since many clients tend to forget the original condition of their muscles as they become more used to their new look. Like all records these must be kept confidential.

Micro-current treatments for the face are very popular but they can also be used on the muscle of the body or for cellulite. An average facial treatment lasts between 60 and 75 minutes.

POINTS TO NOTE

- A micro-current machine has a waveform (whereas traditional galvanic machines do not). The waveform is the 'shape' of the current (as can be seen on an oscilliscope – a special device to visualise and measure electrical current). Most machines produce a selection of waveforms. These are often selected for use according to the client's needs, for example a sharp waveform may be recommended for a client with a severe ageing condition, and a gentle waveform for a younger client with good muscle tone. The waveform is created by interrupting the direct current and controlling the actual build-up, duration and decline of the pulses (see Fig. 7.4).
- The selection of frequency indicates the number of pulses per second emitted from the machine (the number of waves that pass any fixed point in a second) and are measured in hertz (Hz). The higher the frequency, the shorter the wavelength (the intensity shows the strength of the current and is shown in micro-amps).
- Some manufacturers generate the pulses as direct current, then reverse each alternate pulse electronically. Some enable the operator to select the options of pulse, frequency, intensity and waveforms, while others pre-set them.

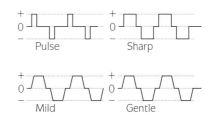

Fig. 7.4 *Waveforms*

Example of a micro-lifting treatment for the face

1 A very detailed consultation is carried out with the client, checking for any contraindications and discussing appropriate products to be used.

2 The skin is thoroughly cleansed ensuring that all traces of the medium are removed.

3 A specialised gel/solution is normally applied. This often contains essential oils and prepares the area for lifting by increasing the circulation and stimulating the lymphatic system. The probes are gently worked over the area.

4 A lymphatic programme is normally applied with the probes being used to follow the direction of lymphatic drainage.

5 A lifting programme is used with the machine being set on a low frequency to work the muscles, stretching and shortening as appropriate.

6 Further programmes may now be used depending on the individual manufacturer's machine. These may include more lifting, working on the lymphatic system or working on softening fine lines and wrinkles.

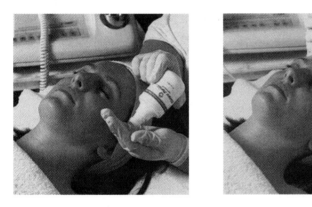

Fig. 7.5 *Facial toning treatment*

7 The treatment is normally concluded by wiping over the area to remove any residue and applying a moisturising product.

8 Relevant home care and future treatment advice should be given.

Treatment time per session for micro-electrotherapy is approximately 45 minutes to one hour.

Note. As with any toning programme it is essential that a course of treatment is given and regular maintenance is given thereafter.

Progress Check

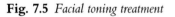

1 List the six classifications of toning table and explain the main purpose of each.
2 State the main effects of micro-electrotherapy treatments.
3 List the contraindication to specialised salon treatments.
4 What safety precautions should be observed when carrying out specialised treatments?

Specialised galvanic, high frequency and NMES treatments

Over the last decade the choice of specialised treatments has made the beauty profession one of the most innovative in existence. Modern therapy treatments have been adapted from straightforward galvanic, faradic and high frequency principles to incorporate advances in technology. Some of these treatments are designed specifically for use on the face but many are for body application. Not all are 'new' however, as some are adaptions of old ideas.

Slimming treatments incorporating iontophoresis, faradic and thermal clay

This treatment is a mixture of faradic muscle stimulation and galvanic current applied in the iontophoresis mode to allow ingredients designed to help with the removal of cellulite penetrate more deeply. The treatment stimulates the circulation, aids lymphatic drainage and increases cellular activity all at the same time as toning the muscles. A special current-conducting clay is applied as this allows the treatment area to be larger and ensures even distribution of the current.

It is recommended that treatment is taken in intensive courses with products used at home in between salon visits.

> **POINT TO NOTE**
>
> Wet, elasticated bandages can replace the use of the clay masque and specially made flexible, conductive, black strapping can be used instead of traditional static electrodes.

Facial treatments incorporating galvanic and high frequency treatments

These treatments are not so new and have been used in salons now for well over twenty years. They work on the principle of combining the beneficial effects of galvanic, normally the iontophoresis mode, with direct high frequency and specialised products to produce a complete treatment that is deeply cleansing, re-hydrating and increases cellular regeneration. The treatment normally lasts about one and a quarter hours and is suitable for most skin types. Cosmetic houses produce specialised products to work with the equipment and an intensive training course is usually necessary to ensure therapists adhere to correct procedures to gain maximum effect. Some manufacturers have taken the treatment a stage further and developed specialised adaptations for the eyes, neck, bust and back areas offering excellent results.

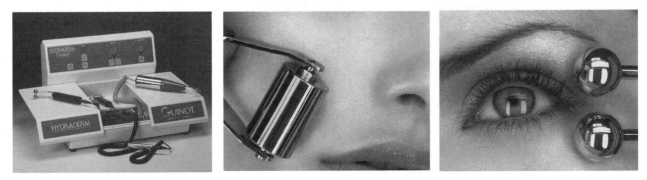

Fig. 7.6 *Hydradermie*

Sequential body toning systems

This is the term used to describe a new range of more sophisticated toning machines that are controlled by micro-processors.

Many combine iontophoresis, infra-red and programmed electro-stimulation over a frequency range of 100–800 Hz. Session times will vary according to individual manufacturers and specific programmes, but on average treatment times are approximately 30–40 minutes. Infra-red is used to warm the area and thus improve the effectiveness of the treatment as current transmission will be maximised. Specialised products are applied to the area together with electrodes to release trapped fatty deposits while at the same time sequential electro-stimulation of the muscles, commencing at the ankles and gradually progressing upwards, increases the lymphatic and circulatory system to help in the dispersal of the accumulated waste products and the mobilised fat. Another key feature of such systems is that the programme can be adapted to meet the individual client's needs.

Treatments should be given in courses of approximately twelve over a one month period for optimum results with a regular maintenance programme thereafter.

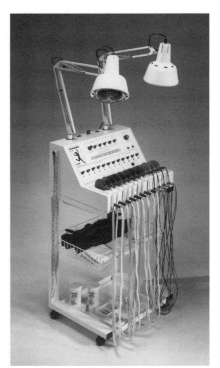

Fig. 7.7 *Sequential body toning equipment*

POINT TO NOTE

Specific sequencing EMS units are specially designed to closely emulate exercise by varied passive stimulation and the range of frequency, 5–70 Hz, is controlled to stimulate most effectively the range of muscle fibre activity. These units use advanced micro-processor control and offer a constantly changing parameter of stimulation. They follow the latest research into electrical muscular stimulation.

Ultra-sound treatments

Treatment with ultra-sound has been in existence for a long time and is traditionally used by physiotherapists. It incorporates wave-type sound energy of a frequency that is just about audible which is transmitted via a flat, disk-shaped applicator to the tissues. It is able to penetrate to a depth of approximately 6 cm depending on the type of tissue. It agitates the cells, releasing toxins and fatty accumulations.

It is an effective treatment not only for muscular tensions, but also for cellulite and related disorders. A specialised coupling cream is normally used in conjunction with the treatment.

Interferential therapy

Interferential current is an alternative type of muscle stimulation to faradic that produces practically no sensation during treatment. The reason for this is that two medium frequency currents are delivered to the treatment area by separate circuits.

Where the two currents meet, a third frequency is produced. This is equivalent to the difference between the two original frequencies. There is no surge or interruption during treatment.

Interferential currents are used in therapy treatments for a number of reasons:

- A constant 'third frequency' will have an analgesic action which will help to reduce pain.
- A variable 'third frequency' will improve localised circulation, lymph drainage and cell metabolism which will help to reduce toxins and waste accumulations.

Progress Check

1 What conditions are treated with specialised galvanic/high frequency/faradic treatments?
2 Give the main benefits of galvanic/high frequency facial treatments.
3 What systems of the body will be affected by a sequential body toning treatment?
4 Describe interferential current.

Specialised slimming programmes

Over the last few years manufacturers have been researching and developing slimming programmes incorporating a variety of heat, vibration, galvanic, faradic and specialised products. A typical treatment can involve:

- Detailed consultation with measurements being taken.
- Pressure massage.
- Heat therapy such as sauna with the use of products that contain ingredients such as seaweed.
- Interrupted direct current on accupressure points (which may help to reduce appetite).
- The client is wrapped in polythene-type sheeting which induces perspiration.
- Vibration and heat from the bed form the next stage of the treatment. The heat is normally derived from infra-red lamps.
- Finally the treatment finishes with a shower and measurements being checked and home care and retail advice given.

Lifting treatments

With advances in micro-current a number of electrotherapy companies have launched new combined units and, in some cases, support products to gain maximum effects. The following are some of the latest on the market.

- Body Sculpture by CACI™ with the Quantum™ system is an all-in-one computerised body care and slimming system incorporating micro-current for lifting and shaping, cellulite body treatments and synchronised lymphatic drainage. The computerised micro-current with pre-set programmes tightens skin and facial muscles, softens fine lines and wrinkles, increases collagen production and improves circulation. Complementing the treatment is the Body Sculpture™ range of products, which includes active collagen ampoules and aloe vera gel.

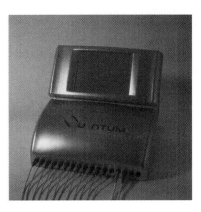

Fig. 7.8 *Body Sculpture™ machine*

◆ Technique Infusion by Silhouette™ incorporates its micro-current systems to infuse a range of concentrated actives such as: collagen (anti-wrinkle mask) to plump up fine lines, replenishing tired tissues; anti-acne mask (containing orris root) to purify and tighten open pores and stabilise the skin's pH whilst reducing the excessive production of sebum; Skin-lite™ mask (containing grape extract) to treat uneven skin tones and pigmentation; vitamin C eye-and-lip pads to improve the skin's elasticity, rehydrating and protecting against free radicals (pollution), softening fine lines and wrinkles and lightening dark shadows.

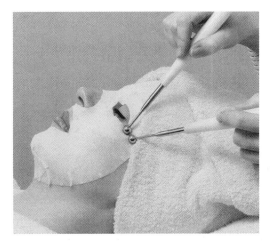

Fig. 7.9 *Technique Infusion™*

◆ Sports Compact 20™ and Super Pro 20™ by Ultratone™ are units for all sports training and beauty therapy applications. Sports 20™ features computerised physio-sequential rotating programmes for body building, strength stamina, speed, flexibility, rehabilitation, oedema reduction, TENS pain reduction and endorphin release. Super Pro 20™ features 41 sequencing programmes, 30 of which are 'multi-area' – delivering different rotating programmes to individual areas during the one treatment – and also includes a hands-free facial micro-current programme for lifting, tightening and toning.

◆ Ultrasound Sonocare by Ella Bache™ incorporates ultrasonic vacuotherapy and ultrasonic vascular drainage. It has an ultrasound transducer with a frequency of 0.6 MHz to optimise penetration of the active ingredients in their gels. The hand-held vacuolyser head has a suction head with an ultrasonic ceramic flange which, through a frequency of 3 MHz, vibrates. The head combines ultrasound waves with suction. Each programme involves six steps: cleansing, exfoliation, Sonocare system (cellular stimulation, muscular toning, and drainage); pulverisation; mask application and application of a day-care product.

◊ The VIP Body System by Scanda Sol™ combines the latest in light therapy with acupuncture to combat cellulite. Infra-red light is applied to break down adipose tissue, then faradic waves are applied to acupuncture points in the treatment area to elongate and contract the muscle.

◊ In Cellular Electrotherapy by Biogénie beaute Concept™, alternating current signals of a harmonious electrical frequency to the dermal tissues permit direct current and sinusoidal signals to pass through the skin without irritation and enable micro-currents to effect specific results at cellular level. Biogénie Visage™, for example, is an 'anti-gravity' massage, using four sinusoidal signals delivered to the skin via sponges soaked with a conductive product and inserted into round electrodes (4 cm diameter). The sculpting massage action lifts, tones and re-energises facial tissues.

Endermologie™

One of the most exciting innovations in the treatment of cellulite is Endermologie™, a treatment developed in the early 1980s by a French engineer, Louis-Paul Guitay, who had suffered muscle and skin damage in a car accident.

This treatment was for burns, to prevent skin contraction and to loosen scar tissues. While conducting these initial treatments, it was discovered that the treatment unexpectedly improved cellulite on patients suffering the condition and this is how it came to be used for aesthetic purposes.

First used in France, then in the USA, it is now recognised worldwide in over seventy countries and has the endorsement of over 3,000 plastic and cosmetic surgeons and dermatologists. Most importantly it has been given approval by the American Food and Drug Administration as the only approved method for cellulite reduction.

So what exactly is Endermologie™? The treatment is a non-invasive, non-surgical procedure used for its toning and aesthetic effects for cellulite and post-operative liposuction. Cellulite does not respond well to diet, exercise and weight loss alone. Proof of this is evident, as pockets of dimpled localised skin can be visible on well-toned and fit people. Affecting women more than men, cellulite is a hormonal condition exacerbated by factors such as pregnancy and the menopause. It is caused by fat stored in the adipocytes, which are fat cells in the hypodermis, swelling and distorting connective fibres and creating the orange peel effect associated with cellulite. This is turn causes the circulation to become sluggish leading to a build-up of toxins, along with congestion, leading to the dimpled effect.

Endermologie™ treatment consists of the Cellu M6™, a hand-held massaging unit that delivers intermittent suction and rolling via two motorised heads to the area being treated as well as the surrounding soft tissues. This patented action of rollers, gentle suctionary stretch and deep massage is applied to the affected areas in a unique way. The fibrous tissues are thus stretched and weakened and this has the effect of minimising the dimpled effect.

Benefits of treatment

It is now thought that during this process of stimulation, collagen is also increased, helping to give the skin a smoother and more contoured appearance. It is worth noting that during the treatment there will be deep stimulation of the blood and lymphatic circulation which will also help in sending oxygen to the affected areas and carrying away stagnant toxic waste.

The treatment programme

The treatment works best if taken in courses, with an initial 14 treatments recommended, each lasting approximately 35 minutes. These should be taken twice a week followed by a maintenance schedule of one or two per month. A very precise 'before' and 'after' photographic record is made, with clients standing in a specific photograph measuring station which has built-in foot markers to ensure consistent positioning of the body and feet on every photograph. This gives totally measurable results to the effectiveness of the programme and is not liable to therapist error with a tape measure or different angle of camera and so on. During treatment, the client wears a special protective body stocking to prevent skin friction and to afford a degree of modesty.

Endermologie™ have developed two machines: the Cellu M6 IP™ is the larger and recommended for medical and sports applications, whilst the Cellu M6™ is the smaller and developed specifically for the beauty industry.

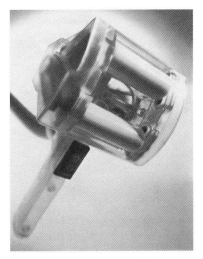

Fig. 7.10 *Endermologie Cellu-M6™*

Example of an Endermologie™ treatment

1   Firstly, a thorough consultation is carried out detailing all medical history and contraindications and so on. During the consultation a photographic measuring session is performed with the client being

led into a special photographic measuring station. The feet are placed on specific foot markers and then the cellulite can be photographed from all angles and at an exact distance.

2 Next, the therapist helps the client into a one-size body stocking and on to the couch for treatment.

3 Treatment commences and the motorised main head is worked over the body in rhythmic patterns from the upper back, down the tops of the arms, across the back over the gluteals and all the way down to the ankles and on the front of the body. A variety of techniques are employed including:

- *sanding*, which is used to revitalise while stimulating the dermis to achieve tissue resurfacing following weight loss or pregnancy or as part of an anti-aging treatment
- *kneading*, which is designed for areas with a high concentration of cellulite especially where it is long established
- *figure-of-eight*, which is specific to cellulite ridden areas and designed to smooth tissue
- *winding* for the beginning and end of a treatment of a particular area which is a smoothing manoeuvre designed to control the newly regained smoothness of the skin
- *bouncing*, a technique that can be incorporated into all other movements except for sanding, which is especially recommended on thick and fatty areas.

4 Once the treatment is finished the client is helped off the couch and to get dressed after any more photographic evidence is recorded.

5 After care advice and follow up sessions are booked in.

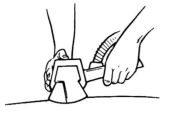

Sanding

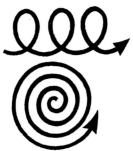

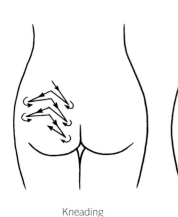

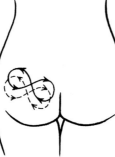

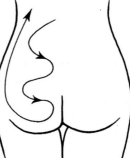

Kneading   Figure of eight   Winding   Bouncing

Fig. 7.11 *Endermologie™ techniques*

Micro-dermabrasion

Micro-dermabrasion is becoming increasingly popular in the beauty therapy industry. It is a skin re-surfacing treatment designed to correct or improve a range of skin abnormalities that originate in the epidermis or superficial layers of the dermis.

The treatment evolved from dermabrasion, which has been used by dermatologists in the medical profession for a very long time. This form of treatment is correctly known as open dermabrasion and uses wire brushes and diamond fraises to deeply remove the epidermis down to the lowest levels; it is very invasive but effective.

Micro-dermabrasion, or closed dermabrasion, on the other hand, is less invasive but will work much more deeply than any exfoliating product or treatment currently offered in the beauty therapy clinic. It can be used to treat stretch marks, post-acne scars, post-surgical scars, wrinkles, hyperpigmentation and inactive keloids.

Micro-dermabrasion equipment consists of a vacuum pump, compressor, crystal canisters and a delivery hand-held unit with pipework. Most systems operate in a similar fashion using a device which allows the projection of a flow of inert corundum crystals onto the skin via a controlled vacuum unit. This is achieved by placing the hand unit onto the skin, which normally has a 3–6 mm diameter hole, so the vacuum automatically generates a flow of crystals towards the skin. When the micro-crystals hit the skin's surface they cause billions of micro-traumas which in turn remove small fragments of skin cells. The micro-crystals and removed skin particles are then simultaneously sucked up towards a disposable flask. It is important to look for a machine that is totally hygienic, that is one which has a disposable container for the contaminated crystals and where the hand-held unit can be sterilised. Machines can be set at different levels to allow for the required depth of abrasion needed. Most machines have about three levels of peeling.

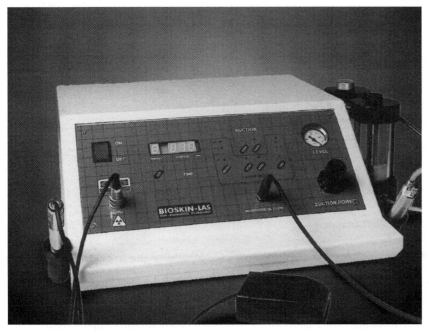

Fig. 7.12 *Micro-dermabrasion machine*

The treatment programme

- Level 1 involves the peeling of the stratum coreum of the epidermis which is suitable for fine lines and wrinkles and as a hydration pre-treatment to improve the penetration of products.
- Level 2 involves peeling more of the epidermis for thicker skins, scar tissue, pigmentation and acne scarring.
- Level 3 involves deep peeling all of the epidermis until blood appears. This is for medical application and only to be carried out by a physician.

The crystals that are used in the treatment are composed of aluminium oxide (corundum) and pointed like diamonds. They are completely non-toxic so totally safe when they come into contact with the skin. Micro-dermabrasion is suitable for most skin types from oily/acne to dehydrated and mature. It can also help with stretch marks. The treatment offers other benefits such as increased circulation, oxygenation of the skin, increased cell renewal, refining open pores and pigmentation and improving the skin's absorption of other products.

Contraindications
to micro-dermabrasion

- Eczema.
- Psoriasis.
- Broken skin.
- Over moles.
- Diabetes.
- Retin A users.
- Keloid scarring.
- Scarring under six months.

After care and home care advice

1 Following treatment, it will be necessary to advise a client to wear a sun block at all times and not to wear make-up for 24 hours afterwards. The client should also be advised that the skin may peel for a few days afterwards (this is because the treatment speeds up cell regeneration) and any flakes of skin can be gently removed with a warm face cloth.
2 Home care products should complement salon treatments.
3 Some micro-dermabrasion equipment incorporates an infra-red laser that emits monochromatic pulsating light. This is designed to speed up healing of the skin following treatment, regenerating the skin's surface through high stimulation of the fibroblast cells which increases the production speed of elastic fibres and collagen, whilst also creating faster absorption of liquids through the capillaries with reduction in swelling. The laser application reduces the number of micro-peeling treatments needed and accelerates the skin's repairing process.

Cosmolight™

A very new and exciting treatment combining holistic as well as technological advancement is Cosmolight™. The system combines a non-coherent pulsating light ranging from 600 to 1200 nm (this means that it is part of the visible and invisible light spectrum but contains no UV properties) with a 'biological resonant wave' to create a holistic therapy that heals or regenerates conditions such as acne, stretch marks, back pain, sports injuries and signs of aging.

Cosmolight™ penetrates the skin up a level of 7 cm and the light is generated by a pure cold light source and gives no sensation of heat. The principal effect is to stimulate the fibroblast cells to speed up collagen and elastin production. Secondly, the biological resonant wave creates a vibratory wave which pulsates at the same rate as the body's blood and lymph systems. This has the effect of dilating the arteries to allow increased blood flow and provide greater nutrition for the newly active light-stimulated skin cells.

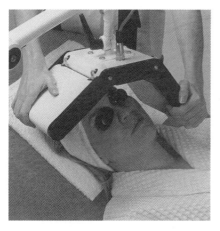

Fig. 7.13 *Cosmolight™*

Example of a Cosmolight™ treatment

1   After a detailed consultation that checks medical history and contraindications, the client is prepared for treatment, for example for a treatment on the face, the area would be thoroughly cleansed and toned.
2   Shields are placed over the eyes to block the light and help the client relax. (The light will not damage the eyes.)
3   The therapist sets the required setting for both the light energy and the biological wave and sets the timer.
4   The three-sided Cosmolight™ light pane, each section about the size of a paperback book, is positioned over the area. The treatment commences.

5   Whilst the client relaxes under the lights, the therapists uses the Cosmolight™ pen, a needle-free acupuncture device, to stimulate meridian points, for example during an anti-ageing treatment the points relating to liver, intestines and bladder would be stimulated to improve lymphatic drainage.

6   After ten minutes, the light panel is removed and the contents of an ampoule are applied, which will contain vitamins, minerals and anti-oxidants. The light panel is then replaced so that it can propel the active ingredients deeper into the skin.

7   After five minutes, the light panel is removed before a second ampoule, specific to the client's needs, is applied, followed by a further five minutes from the light panel.

8   The light pen is then used to work on deeper facial lines, scars or even cold sores.

9   The treatment panel is then placed on the soles of the feet for ten minutes to work on the reflexology points and boost circulation. At the same time, the pen is used to stimulate additional meridian points.

10 After treatment, the client is offered a glass of water to boost detoxification and after-care and home-care advice is given.

Benefits of treatment

As a holistic treatment, Cosmolight™ has the effect of healing and regenerating a variety of conditions both inside and outside the body, including burns, cold sores, cellulite, eczema, psoriasis, fine lines and wrinkles, scars, stretch marks, spots, sports injuries and general aches and pains. It is suitable for clients of all ages and some conditions will show signs of improvement after just one session.

Skin testers

Electronic skin testers for registering the pH of the skin are widely used in the Far East, and are gaining in popularity throughout the world.

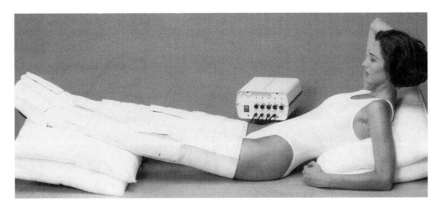

Fig. 7.14 *The flux system of Press-o-therapy™*

Pressure massage

This is the name given to a range of specialist equipment which causes 'pneumatic' compression of the limbs. Pressure is delivered in a rhythmical manner thus simulating the natural pumping action of muscles and aiding lymphatic flow. The treatment primarily affects the vascular system so is excellent for helping many conditions associated with inefficient blood and lymph circulation, including gravitational oedema and the early stages of cellulite.

Treatment times will vary, but an average session will last about 20–30 minutes and can be combined with other salon services such as facials and massage.

Oriental analysis

Arousing a great deal of interest over recent years, Oriental analysis has grown in popularity in recent months. It involves reading a client's face, hands, feet and body to gain a greater insight into understanding the client's well-being, history and personality. It is offered as a postgraduate course for therapists by Eve Taylor at her Institute of Clinical Aromatherapy and is practised worldwide by many of her past students.

ACTIVITY

Research manufacturers who offer the following:

a AHA treatments
b sequential body toning and specific sequencing EMS
c specialised high frequency/galvanic treatments
d body wraps
e micro-electrotherapy treatments.

Key Terms

You need to know what these words and phrases mean. Go back through the chapter to find out.

- Alpha hydroxy acids
- Body wraps
- Cellulite treatments
- Micro-electrotherapy
- Pressure massage
- Specialised galvanic/high frequency/faradic/NMES treatments
- Specialised slimming programmes
- Stretch mark treatments
- Toning tables

8

After working through this chapter you will be able to:
- identify the different types of spa treatment
- list the contraindications to spa treatments
- describe the effects of spa treatments
- understand the preparation required for a variety of spa treatments
- completely carry out a variety of spa treatments on clients.

Hydrotherapy

The therapeutic and social benefits of water have been used by all cultures for centuries. The Romans developed bath houses containing large hot and cool baths. People would progress from the coolest through to the hottest and finish, if they wished, with a cool plunge. Communal bathing was common practice in Roman society. There are only a few of the original Roman baths found today in the United Kingdom. The best and most famous examples are the Roman baths at Bath in England (hence the name 'Bath').

Health spas in European countries such as Austria and Germany have proved highly popular for years. The bathing in and drinking of mineral water along with additional treatment rooms have developed over the centuries and are often recommended by medical practitioners for their therapeutic benefits.

Health hydros and spas have increased rapidly in popularity over the past decade mainly due to the public's growing awareness of stress, health and personal appearance.

Today a common occurrence is for children to go to their local swimming baths with friends and for adults to attend health and leisure clubs for health and relaxation. If you asked a cross-section of children through to adults to list three things they most enjoy on holiday you could be quite certain that the majority of people will include swimming in their list.

POINT TO NOTE

Hydrotherapy means treatment with water in any physical state (i.e. liquid, water vapour, steam, ice).

Heat treatments

Heat treatments are used either as a spa treatment for relaxation or to prepare clients for further salon treatments such as massage. Over the last decade they have grown in popularity and can be found in local council sport centres, health and fitness clubs, health spas and in larger salons offering body treatments. There is a variety of different heat treatments which are continually being added to.

The general effects of heat treatments

1 Increase body temperature.
2 Metabolism is increased as heating of the body accelerates the natural chemical reactions that occur within the body, e.g. burning of energy, production of carbon dioxide. This in turn will increase the demand for oxygen and nutrients within the tissues, therefore increasing the amount of waste produced.
3 Circulation is increased. As the temperature in the body is increased the blood vessels dilate to allow the blood to flow more quickly to the surface thus reducing the body temperature. Other factors which trigger this process, known as vasodilation, are the stimulation of the sensory nerve endings and an increase in the body's metabolism.
4 Blood pressure is lowered as the pulse rate increases, causing the superficial blood vessels to dilate which automatically lowers the blood pressure due to the reduced resistance to the flow of blood through the blood vessels.
5 The heart rate increases to meet the demands of the body on the circulatory system.
6 Perspiration is induced to help cool the body. This aids removal of waste from the body and has a cleansing and softening effect on the skin.
7 The activity of the sudoriferous and sebaceous glands is increased.
8 Muscle fibres are relaxed in preparation for further salon treatment, e.g. massage.
9 Sensory nerve endings are soothed by mild heat.
10 A sense of general relaxation is achieved.

USEFUL INFORMATION
Hyperaemia is the term given to describe the increase in the flow of blood brought about by vasodilation.

POINT TO NOTE

The effects of heat treatments will vary according to the length, temperature and type of treatment given, for example electrically heated under-and over-blankets create a heated environment which can be a very gentle sudation or that of a personal sauna cocoon.

General safety precautions to be observed in the spa area

- Ensure all equipment is serviced regularly.
- Always follow manufacturers' instructions.
- Hygiene is of the utmost importance, so ensure all equipment is maintained and cleaned according to the manufacturer's recommendations.
- Floors in the spa area should be non-slip.
- Spillages should be cleared up immediately.
- Clean towels and gowns must be regularly replenished.
- Dirty laundry baskets should be emptied regularly.
- Soaps, shampoos, body lotions should be replenished.
- Clients must always be checked for contraindications.

In Scandinavia countries, pine log cabins were built by the side of lakes to enable people to take a cool dip in between sessions in the sauna. Today they are commonly found both indoors and outdoors. Saunas produce dry hot air and the pine logs absorb the condensation produced in the sauna.

A sauna resembles a wooden cabin. Saunas are usually made from pine logs or panels which are packed together with insulating material (fibre glass) to prevent heat loss and ensure the heated air remains dry. They contain pine shelving at different heights for resting on. Pine slats (duck boards) on the floor protect clients' feet from heated flooring which could burn them. A thermostatically controlled electric stove, on top of which is a tray of non-splintering stones (coals), is used to heat the sauna. Manufacturers should ensure that the heating capacity of the electric stoves have the correct power rating for the size of the sauna.

When installing saunas the contractors should check that there is sufficient space around the cabin to enable air to circulate. An air inlet is found at floor level and an outlet is found near the top of the cabin. As the power rating for sauna stoves is much higher than for normal household electrical appliances, the sauna stove is fitted directly to the consumer's mains electrical supply. (They cannot be run from a plug socket!) A thermometer should be placed as near as possible to the roof of the sauna to accurately measure the temperature inside the sauna. It is important to have some way for a client to measure time whilst in a sauna so either an egg timer or clock should be in the sauna or a clock on a wall outside which can be seen through the window of the sauna door.

Note. Remember to make sure timers are working correctly.

Water can be ladled onto the coals of the sauna stove. This creates steam and increases the humidity in the sauna, which in turn reduces the rate of the evaporation of sweat from the client's skin making the sauna feel hotter. Hot air does not have the same heat capacity as hot water, therefore the temperature of a sauna does not feel as hot on the skin as water would. The temperature of a sauna can vary between 50–120 °C (the boiling point of water is 100 °C).

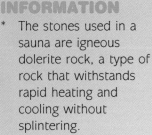

USEFUL INFORMATION

* The stones used in a sauna are igneous dolerite rock, a type of rock that withstands rapid heating and cooling without splintering.
* Birchwood twigs used to be used in Scandinavian countries by sauna users for their suppleness to stimulate the blood circulation by tapping them on the skin.

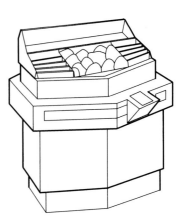

Fig. 8.1 *Sauna stove*

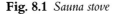

◆ If the air is too dry the body's natural perspiration evaporates quickly, which has a cooling effect on the skin, and signs of dehydration such as tiredness and dry throats can occur.

◆ If the humidity of the air is too high, perspiration produced to assist in the cooling of the body does not evaporate leaving people feeling hot and clammy.

◆ A hygrometer is used to measure humidity.

◆ A comfortable sauna temperature for a new client unaccustomed to a sauna treatment is 60–80°C.

◆ A comfortable sauna humidity is approximately 50–60%.

◆ As hot air rises, a thermometer should be placed near the top of the sauna.

Care of the sauna

1 Hygiene is of utmost importance as although the air in the sauna is too hot for growth of micro-organisms, bacterial infection could be housed and grow in the wooden walls and furnishings of the sauna due to the warm, moist conditions.

2 The sauna should be regularly disinfected by scrubbing the benches and floor with disinfectant products recommended by the manufacturer.

3 Disposable client footwear can be used to reduce the risk of passing contagious foot conditions such as verrucas.

4 At the end of the day, the sauna doors should be left open to allow for a change of air. This prevents stale odours from lingering.

Contraindications

to a sauna

◆ Low and high blood pressure.
◆ Heat conditions.
◆ Thrombosis or phlebitis.
◆ Bronchitis.
◆ Asthma.
◆ Epilepsy.
◆ Dysfunction of the nervous system.
◆ Oedema.
◆ Recent scar tissue.
◆ Severe bruising.
◆ Diabetes.*
◆ Early stages of menstruation.
◆ Pregnancy.*
◆ Heavy colds/fever.
◆ Infectious skin diseases.
◆ Athletes foot.
◆ Verrucas.
◆ Sunburn.
◆ Claustrophobia.
◆ After alcohol consumption.
◆ After a heavy meal.

* Only to be carried out with medical approval.

* The moisture content of the air is referred to as humidity. Relative humidity is the measurement of moisture content as a percentage of the maximum it can hold at that temperature. 100% is the maximum capacity of moisture content in air.
* 60–70% relative humidity is a comfortable humidity for working conditions.
* As the temperature of air increases, so does its capacity for holding moisture, e.g. if the temperature of a salon was 20 °C and the relative humidity measurement was 70%, then raising the room temperature to 100 °C would decrease the relative humidity to approximately 20%.
* The relative humidity in a sauna can be as low as 10%. This causes perspiration to evaporate very quickly, thus causing a cooling effect on the skin so that the sauna does not feel as hot as the actual temperature recorded in the sauna. Water loss is from the whole of the body and it should be remembered that if the temperature is high and the relative humidity is low then there is a danger of dehydration, breathing difficulties and scorching of the lungs.

Effects of a sauna

- Increases body temperature.
- Metabolism is increased.
- Blood pressure is lowered.
- Pulse rate increases.
- Circulation increases.
- Perspiration is induced which aids removal of waste from the body and has a cleansing and softening effect on the skin.
- The activity of the sudoriferous and sebaceous glands is increased.
- Muscle fibres are relaxed in preparation for further salon treatment, e.g. massage.
- A sense of wellbeing is achieved.

Preparation of the sauna

1. Observe general safety precautions.
2. The sauna stove is switched on to allow the temperature of the sauna to build up prior to use. A large sauna will take approximately one hour to heat up whereas a smaller sauna will take approximately thirty minutes.
3. The air vents should be open to allow the air to circulate.
4. A pine bucket filled with water is placed in the sauna with a ladle. Pine fragrance can be added to the water to produce a pleasant fresh smell when used on the coals.
5. Paper towels may be placed on the floor.
6. Showers are checked and appropriate products are made available for clients, e.g. shower gels and caps.
7. Towels are replenished.
8. Throughout the day the laundry basket is emptied and towels, etc. replenished.

Note. Different establishments will offer different services to clients and will outline these to therapists in their induction programme, e.g. towels may be placed in the sauna for clients to rest on, clean bath robes may be placed in the sauna area.

Sauna treatment

1. Client is greeted at reception and taken to a changing area.
2. Consultation is carried out to check for contraindications and to explain effects of treatment.

Note. In health spas a detailed consultation is undertaken on the guest's arrival by a member of their medical staff. The therapists would still explain the effects of the treatment to a new guest.

GOOD PRACTICE

The overall hygiene of the spa reflects on everyone working there so it is paramount that a therapist uses their initiative to refill products, empty laundry baskets, replenish towels and clean areas as needed – **don't** wait to be asked. *Ensuring the work place is kept clean and tidy is part of a therapist's job.*

3   Client removes items such as contact lenses, spectacles and jewellery before showering to remove deoderants, body lotions, fragrances, etc.

4   Client is taken to sauna and advised if it is their first treatment to spend approximately 5–8 minutes on a lower shelf, allowing them time to adjust to the temperature of the sauna. It must be stressed to the client that if at any time they feel light-headed they must come out of the sauna.

5   Therapist informs client of the time and asks them to take a cool shower or use the plunge pool for a short time to cool the body, stop perspiration and tighten the pores which have dilated due to the heat of the sauna and through perspiration. The temperature of the plunge pool/shower should be approximately 15–21°C.

6   The client can return to the sauna for 10–20 minute periods in between taking cool showers or using the plunge pool for up to a total treatment time of approximately 30 minutes.

7   The client should relax after a sauna either in a rest area or by having a further treatment such as a massage and drink plenty of fluids to prevent dehydration.

Vibratory sauna

The vibratory sauna machine looks like an elongated steam cabinet as it allows a client to lie flat inside it. It is manufactured from moulded plastic with a vibrating couch which has a built-in head rest. Control panels on the outside allow the therapist to set the temperature, duration, vibration along with the stereo and fan control for cooling the sauna.

There are control panels situated at a convenient location inside the chamber to enable the client to alter the temperature, music and to operate the fan. During treatment heat is introduced into the sauna whilst the couch vibrates gently, to relax the client's muscles and help reduce stress. The built-in stereo system allows the therapist to play therapeutic tapes and aromatic oils can be used to further enhance the client's relaxation.

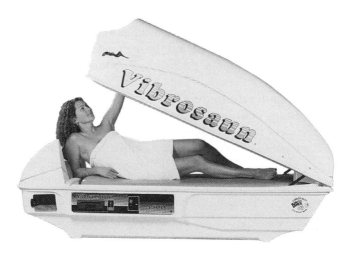

Fig. 8.2 *A vibratory sauna*

Contraindications

to vibratory saunas

- Thrombosis or phlebitis.
- Circulatory conditions.
- Infectious skin conditions.
- Sunburn.
- Pregnancy.*
- Menstruation.
- Heavy colds or fevers.
- After alcohol or a heavy meal.
- Low and high blood pressure.
- Epilepsy.
- Diabetes.*
- Dysfunction of the nervous system.
- Oedema.
- Recent scar tissue.
- Athlete's foot.
- Verrucas.

* Only to be carried out with medical approval.

POINT TO NOTE

The vibratory sauna is a personal treatment, the temperature can be set to suit the individual client.

Effects of a vibratory sauna

- Increases body temperature.
- Increases circulation.
- Heart rate increases.
- Pulse rate increases.
- Blood pressure is lowered.
- Increases metabolism.
- Induces perspiration.
- Relaxes muscle fibres.

Care of the vibratory sauna

The sauna should be cleaned between clients according to the manufacturer's instructions.

Preparation of the vibratory sauna

1. General safety precautions should be observed.
2. Fresh paper towels are placed over the vibratory couch.
3. The sauna should be switched on at the mains. (There is no need to preheat the chamber.)

Vibratory sauna treatment

1. Client is greeted at reception and taken to a changing area.
2. Consultation is carried out to check for contraindications and to explain the effects of the treatment.
3. Client removes items such as spectacles and jewellery prior to showering to remove deodorants, fragrances, body lotions, etc.
4. The client is helped into the cabinet and the therapist switches on the vibratory couch and music.
5. The room lights may be dimmed or the client may opt to wear eye shields.
6. At the end of the treatment, the body is cooled slightly by the fans which automatically cut in.
7. The client is helped out of the cabinet and may take a cool shower prior to resting. The drinking of suitable fluids is recommended.

GOOD PRACTICE

- Some clients are irritated by music so therapeutic tapes should only be used with the client's agreement.
- As clients are all individuals, it is important to establish what types of fragrance they like before selecting aromatic oils.

Progress Check

1. Define hydrotherapy.
2. List the ten general effects of heat treatments.
3. Explain the term 'relative humidity' and its relevance to a sauna treatment.
4. Give four points that should be considered when taking care of the sauna.
5. Describe in detail the preparation, client consultation, treatment and after care advice given for a sauna treatment.
6. State the effects of a vibratory sauna treatment. Also state four contraindications to treatment.

Steam treatments were first used by the Turks and Romans and are sometimes referred to as a Turkish bath. The original Turkish and Roman baths were found in large buildings which contained steam baths of various temperatures, where people met socially for a relaxing bath.

There are two mains types of steam treatment available: steam cabinets, rooms or steam baths. Both enable clients to receive a wet heat or 'moist heat' treatment.

Steam cabinets

Steam cabinets are designed for individual treatment enabling clients to sit in the cabinet with their heads outside so that they can breathe in the normal air of the room.

A modern steam cabinet can be constructed from either metal or moulded fibreglass. The fibreglass model is more expensive but is easier to clean and as fewer towels are needed to protect the client from the heat of the metal they tend to be more popular, even though they tend to be more expensive.

Steam cabinets have an opening for the client's head and a hinged door for easy access to and from the cabinet making them more suitable than saunas for clients who have a tendency to suffer from claustrophobia. Inside there is an adjustable seat which is raised or lowered according to the client's height. Beneath the seat at floor level is a water tank, made from cast iron or aluminium, which is heated by an electrical element. The size of the water tank varies and should be considered when purchasing a steam cabinet. The larger the capacity of the tank the longer it can be used before the therapist needs to refill it. Therefore in a spa where the steam cabinets receive more use, a cabinet with a large water tank would be more beneficial.

To operate the steam cabinet the therapist will find a:

💧 Mains switch on the wall. The cabinet must be fitted directly to the mains electrical supply due to the power rating of the heating element.

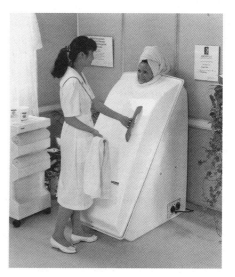

Fig. 8.3 *Steam cabinet*

- Timer switch to set the time for prior heating of the cabinet and the actual treatment time.
- Temperature gauge to set the cabinet to the appropriate temperature.

The timer and the temperature gauge are generally found adjacent to each other on the outside of the cabinet often at floor level near the heating element.

Steam cabinets produce wet heat as the thermostatically controlled water tank heats the water until it boils producing wet steam which mixes with the air inside the cabinet or room creating water vapour (at a lower temperature than the 100 °C required to boil water) at a temperature tolerable to the skin. The highest temperature advised for use in a steam treatment for the body is 45 °C.

The relative humidity of the air inside the steam cabinet or bath is generally around 92–97%. As the air is virtually saturated, the sweat produced by the sudoriferous glands, due to the heating of the body by the water vapour, is unable to evaporate and cool the body and therefore it trickles off the body.

POINT TO NOTE

The body will replace any lost fluids during a heat treatment. It will absorb extra water from the intestines which can lead to constipation or create further problems for those clients who suffer with this condition.

Steam rooms

Steam rooms accommodate a number of clients who may take a treatment at the same time. This type of treatment is becoming more popular in Europe where social attitudes to exposed bodies are far less puritanical than in, say, Far Eastern countries where body treatments are only just beginning to increase in popularity.

The length of time for a steam room to heat up ready for use will depend upon its size. Some are designed for individual use whilst others can accommodate up to eight people. Individual steam 'tubes' provide a mini-steam-room environment which takes up a small amount of space and is easily affordable for salons.

Advantages of using a steam cabinet

For the client:

- Steam cabinets are a more private treatment than the communal steam room.
- The temperature can be adjusted to suit the individual client.
- Clients are able to keep their head out and keep their hair dry.
- It is far more suitable for claustrophobic clients as their head is out of the steam.
- The client is able to breathe in the air in the room rather than steam.

USEFUL INFORMATION

Breathing in hot air of a high relative humidity can cause water-logging of the lungs as the air is cooled and water condensed from it as it enters the body.

For the salon:

- The running costs are much lower than with a steam room as the heating element in a steam cabinet uses far less power.
- The initial financial outlay is much lower.
- The space required to accommodate the cabinet in the salon is much smaller.

Care of steam cabinets and rooms

1 Hygiene is extremely important as moist heat provides an ideal breeding environment for micro-organisms.
2 The steam baths and rooms must be cleaned down with suitable disinfectants recommended by the manufacturers before and after treatment.
3 The doors of the steam bath and room should be left open at the end of the day to allow for an interchange of fresh air, preventing stale odours.
4 Disposable footwear can be used to prevent the risk of cross-infection of contagious foot conditions.

Contraindications
to steam treatments for the body

- Thrombosis or phlebitis.
- Asthma and other respiratory conditions.
- Low or high blood pressure.
- Heart conditions.
- Epilepsy.
- Diabetes.*
- Athlete's foot.
- Verrucas.
- Infectious skin diseases.
- Sunburn.
- Pregnancy.*
- Menstruation.
- Clients on restricted diets who may have a tendency to become light-headed.
- Heavy colds/fevers.
- After a heavy meal or alcohol.
- Claustrophobia.**
- Dysfunction of the nervous system.
- Severe bruising.
- Recent scar tissue.

* Only to be carried out with medical approval.

** Some clients find the steam cabinet less claustrophobic.

POINT TO NOTE

If given approval by a medical practitioner, clients with skin conditions such as psoriasis and eczema may receive wet heat treatments as they may help these conditions.

Effects of a steam treatment for the body

- Body temperature rises.
- Metabolism is increased.
- Circulation is increased.
- Heart rate increases.
- Pulse rate increases.
- Blood pressure is lowered.
- Perspiration is induced.
- Cleansing and softening of the skin takes place.
- Superficial muscles are relaxed.

Preparation of the steam cabinet

1 Observe general safety precautions.
2 The cabinet is cleaned with sterilising liquid.
3 Metal heating trough is filled with water.
4 Towel is placed over seat to protect the client and if using a metal bath, towels must be placed inside to protect the client. Place a towel over the opening in the bath to prevent heat loss.
5 The water tank guard must be in place so as to protect the client from burning themselves.
6 Turn on the mains switch and set the temperature gauge to maximum to heat the bath. Set the timer to allow sufficient time for the bath to heat. (This will vary depending on the capacity of the water tank. Note the manufacturer's recommendations for heating time. A general guide for the time taken for a small tank to heat is approximately 15 minutes.)
7 Once heated, adjusted the temperature gauge to 50–55 °C and check the timer switch does not click off allowing the temperature to fall.

Steam cabinet treatment

1 Greet client at reception and take them to changing facilities.
2 Consultation is carried out to check for contraindications and to explain the treatment and its effects.
3 Client removes items such as jewellery, spectacles and contact lenses and showers to remove deodorants, fragrances, body lotions, etc.
4 The client is helped into the bath. A fresh towel is placed around the client's neck for protection and to prevent heat loss.
5 The timer is set to the appropriate time, generally 15–20 minutes.
6 The therapist should reassure the client throughout the treatment and be at hand should they need them.
7 At the end of the treatment, help the client from the bath and direct them into a cool shower.
8 The use of an exfoliating product is recommended to speed up cellular regeneration and general skin texture.
9 The client should relax after the steam treatment and drink plenty of liquids.

> **USEFUL INFORMATION**
>
> Steam cabinets can be purchased with aromatherapy atomising systems to enable the therapist to infuse the cabinet with selected essential oils to suit the individual client.

> **GOOD PRACTICE**
>
> It is important to look directly at the client's face and not at the client's body when helping them in and out of baths and showers. Imagine how you would feel if a fully clothed person stared at your naked body!

Floatation treatments

There are two types of floatation treatment; *wet floatation* and *dry floatation*.

Wet floatation tank

These are made from moulded fibreglass and can vary in size. They are generally rectangular, shaped like a small room, with a door opening outwards on the side of the tank. Inside the interior colour is usually blue and there is approximately 12 inches of warm, saturated salt water heated to body temperature on the floor surface, which will allow everyone to float. A small interior light illuminates the tank enabling the client time to climb in and settle before switching it off. The switch control is in easy reach on the side wall.

The tanks are often found in health spas and leisure centres and are situated in a separate room with access to a shower. Clients are advised to shower to remove any body creams, etc., and to apply petroleum jelly to any cuts preventing the brine (salt water) from entering any abrasions and causing a stinging sensation. It is suggested that no clothing is worn in the tank. Ear plugs are provided and often a neck cushion, which can be very reassuring to the weak or non-swimmer who believes they cannot float. A small step at the side of the tank allows the client to climb easily into the illuminated tank and a pull bar allows easy closure of the door. The client can take their time to adjust to the warm, slightly restrictive environment before switching off the interior light. There is usually an intercom system which enables the therapist to check the client is comfortable, play therapeutic music and reassure the apprehensive client that someone is at hand should they need them. The tanks generally have a small, round ventilation hole which also allows the client to be phased into total darkness by first switching of the interior light and using a delay switch to turn the lighting off in the outer room (light can still enter the tank from the outer room through the door frame and the ventilation hole). This is extremely beneficial for apprehensive clients. The client lies on their back, the neck supported if they wish by a neck cushion, allowing the brine water to support their body thus relaxing all superficial muscles and releasing tension in the body. If the client wishes, therapeutic background music is played and after the client has had sufficient time to drift off, the music quietly ends allowing a peaceful and tranquil period before the music is quietly reintroduced, slowly bringing the treatment to an end.

Afterwards the client needs to shower to remove the brine from their skin and hair using professional products that could also be sold to them by the therapist.

Health spas book an hour treatment. Out of this the client would spend 40–45 minutes in the floatation tank.

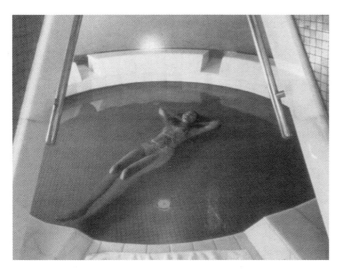

Fig. 8.4 *Wet floatation*

After a beneficial treatment the exhilarating, uplifting experience of 'walking on air' brought about by the total relaxation of mind and body can make this an almost addictive treatment.

Care of the floatation tank

1   The tank must be free of debris such as oils, scum, loose hairs, etc.
2   The inside of the tank, above the water line, must be cleaned a minimum of once a week or as necessary.
3   The water in the tank must be filtered between uses and the temperature checked.
4   The level of the water has to be checked between clients.
5   The pH of the water should be 7.6. This should be checked on a daily basis.
6   The level of bromine must not be higher than 2 p.p.m. and must be checked a minimum of once a week.
7   The tank must be tested either by an independent laboratory or by the Environmental Health Department.

Contraindications

to wet floatation

- Claustrophobia.
- Highly nervous clients.
- Severe cuts/abrasions.
- Recent scar tissue.
- Infectious skin diseases.
- Severe eczema/psoriasis.
- Plantar wart (verruca).
- Tinea pedis (athletes foot).
- After alcohol consumption.
- Heart conditions.*
- Epilepsy.*
- After a heavy meal.

* Only to be carried out with medical approval.

Effects of a wet floatation treatment

- Warms the body tissues aiding relaxation.
- Relaxes muscles through the buoyancy of the water.
- Eases aches and pains.
- A general feeling of wellbeing is achieved.

Preparation of the wet floatation tank

1 Observe general safety precautions.
2 Check the tank and shower areas are clean.
3 Ensure the level and temperature of the water are correct.

Wet floatation treatment

1 Greet client at reception and take them to changing facilities.
2 Consultation is carried out to check for contraindications and to explain the effects of the treatment.
3 Client removes items such as jewellery, spectacles and contact lenses, and may shower.
4 Client protects any minor skin abrasions with petroleum jelly and inserts ear plugs.
5 Client enters floatation tank, closes door and in their own time switches off the interior light.
6 If the client wishes, the therapist can play piped music during the floatation time.
7 At the end of the treatment the therapist would advise the client to shower to remove the salt from skin and hair.
8 The client should rest in a relaxation room and drink fluids as required.

Dry floatation tank

Dry floatation tanks were originally developed in Austria and have been extremely popular there for many years. They are made of a stainless steel frame containing a tank of water which can be thermostatically controlled, into which a duck board is set which can be lowered to suspend the client in water with no pressure points. The water tank is sealed by a flexible membrane, the tank is clad in upholstered panels which make it appear rectangular in shape, similar to a bath tub.

The client lies on the raised bench which is protected by paper roll. Protective paper sheeting may be placed over the client. The therapist pushes a control button to lower the board thus suspending the client's body weight, protected by vinyl, in warm water, the temperature of which remains constant.

The dry tanks are mainly found in health spas in treatment rooms with easy access to a shower. The dry floatation method can be used in a number of treatments some of which involve coating the body in various ingredients for different effects, e.g. mud can be used for its exfoliating and softening effects, a mixture of hay softened with its own juices and eucalyptus essential oil is said to be beneficial for sluggish lymph circulation and respiratory conditions and milk and essential oils can be used for softening the skin and has therapeutic benefits. The floatation can be given on its own for the therapeutic benefit of releasing tension in the body and for relaxation.

Once the client is suspended in the dry floatation tank the therapist switches on gentle therapeutic music, dims the lights and places an alert button within easy reach of the client. The client is then left to relax for approximately 40 minutes.

The therapist will check on the client's comfort after 5–8 minutes, remaining close at hand outside the door throughout the duration of the treatment and returning to the room at the end. The control button is pressed which slowly raises the board under the client's back and brings them back to the top of the tank, the vinyl cover is removed and the client is helped off. If a specific treatment such as mud has been used the therapist will have to place protective covering on the floor between the tank and the shower.

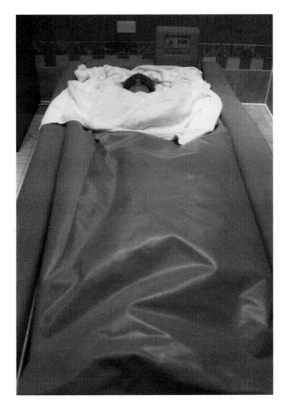

Fig. 8.5 *Dry floatation*

Care of the dry floatation tank
The tank should be cleaned with a sterilising liquid recommended by the manufacturer.

Contraindications

to dry floatation

- Infectious skin conditions.
- Severe respiratory conditions.
- Heavy colds/fevers.
- Heart conditions.*
- Diabetes.*
- Epilepsy.*

* Only to be carried out with medical approval.

Effects of a dry floatation treatment

💧 Aids relaxation.
💧 Relaxes muscles through the buoyancy effect of the water.
💧 Eases aches and pains.
💧 A general sense of wellbeing is achieved.

Note. If specific treatments are used in conjunction with dry floatation then the specific benefits from these can be added to the above list.

Preparation for a dry floatation treatment

1 Observe general safety precautions.
2 The vinyl sheeting must be clean, dry and protected as necessary.
3 The board is raised to the top of the tank and the temperature control switch is turned to pre-heat the water.

Dry floatation treatment

1 Greet client at reception and take them to changing facilities.
2 Consultation is carried out to check for contraindications and to explain the effects of the treatment.
3 Client removes items such as jewellery, spectacles and contact lenses, etc., and may shower.
4 The client lies on top of the tank and the therapist covers them.
5 The therapist presses a switch which lowers the board.
6 The lights are dimmed and music played to suit the individual client.
7 At the end of the floatation time the therapist raises the board and helps the client up.
8 If specific treatments such as mud baths have been given, the client showers to remove the products for their body.
9 The client should relax in a rest room and drink fluids as needed.

Progress Check

1 List four contraindications for each of the following treatments:
   a steam cabinet   **b** wet floatation   **c** dry floatation.
2 For each of the following treatments describe two effects:
   a steam room   **b** wet floatation.
3 Describe how a steam cabinet operates.
4 State the advantages for the client and salon of using a steam cabinet.
5 Explain the preparation, consultation, treatment and after care advice given for a dry floatation treatment.

Foam baths

Foam baths are far more likely to be found in a health hydro offering a variety of spa treatments than in a beauty salon where the costs of purchase, installation and running could prove too high an expense. However modifications to a general household bath can transform it for use as a foam bath.

Foam baths found in health hydros are found in the spa area and resemble a household bath in appearance. A perforated, plastic duck board is found at the bottom of the bath which will allow compressed air to be forced through the hundreds of tiny holes into the bath water. Only a small quantity of water is needed, approximately 10–15 cm to cover the duck board. The water is heated to between 37–43 °C depending on the individual client. Concentrated foam essence such as seaweed is added to the water prior to the compressor being switched on. The compressor pumps air to beneath the duck board where it will force its way through the perforated holes to aerate the water. The compressor is left on until the foam created by the aeration of the water and foam essence reaches the top of the bath. The client lies in the foam in a semi-reclined position with their head resting on the back of the bath, outside of the foam.

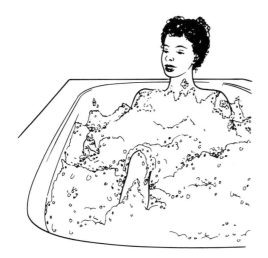

Fig. 8.6 *Foam bath*

POINT TO NOTE

Foam is made up of approximately 10% water and 90% air.

Care of the foam bath

The bath should be cleaned between client use with a sterilising fluid recommended by the manufacturer.

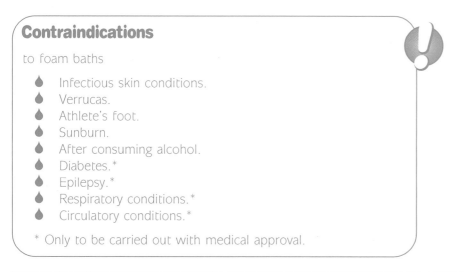

Contraindications

to foam baths

- Infectious skin conditions.
- Verrucas.
- Athlete's foot.
- Sunburn.
- After consuming alcohol.
- Diabetes.*
- Epilepsy.*
- Respiratory conditions.*
- Circulatory conditions.*

* Only to be carried out with medical approval.

Effects of a foam bath

- Induces perspiration.
- Raises body temperature.
- Induces circulation.
- Muscle fibres are relaxed.

Preparation of the foam bath

1. The bath is cleaned and filled with sufficient warm water to cover the duck board.
2. A selected concentrated foam essence is added to the water, e.g. seaweed.
3. The compressor is switched on to aerate the water.
4. Once the foam reaches the top of the bath the compressor is switched off. The foam bath is now ready for use.

Foam bath treatment

1. Client is greeted at reception and taken to changing facilities.
2. Consultation is carried out to check for contraindications and to explain the effects of the treatment.
3. Client removes items such as contact lenses, spectacles and jewellery prior to showering to remove fragrances, deodorants, body lotions, etc.
4. Client is helped into the bath.
5. Treatment time is generally around 15 minutes.
6. Client is helped from the bath.
7. A warm shower may be taken using exfoliating products for cellular regeneration.
8. The client should relax in rest area and drink fluids as required.

Aerated baths

There are many types of aerated bath to be found in health spas, hydros and clubs, and they can also be found in hotels and individual homes. They vary in size, shape and price. The simplest form is a normal household bath with an air pump outside which pumps air into the water.

Aerated baths were developed in France. They are filled with water and air is forced into the water either through a hose or through holes in a duck board in the bath. Essence may be added to aerated baths for their individual properties. Treatment time would last approximately 15 minutes.

Hydrotherapy baths

Aerated baths are used as a hydrotherapy treatment in the majority of health spas, using a hose to direct air over the body. The hydrotherapy unit is shaped like a bath with grab handles to assist the client to get in and out. The inside of the hydrotherapy unit is fitted to the shape of the client's body more so than an ordinary household bath. The unit is filled with warm water, the selected essence is added and the compressor is switched on allowing air to aerate the bath gently through the duck board. The client is helped into the bath and the therapist switches on the hose which is worked methodically over the muscle groups. The treatment time is generally around 20 minutes.

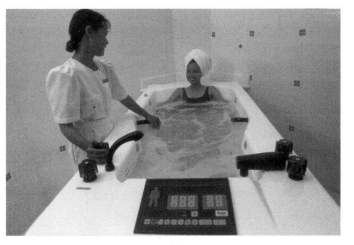

Fig. 8.7 *Hydrotherapy bath*

Contraindications

to hydrotherapy baths

- Heart conditions.
- Infections skin conditions.
- Circulatory conditions.
- After a heavy meal or after consuming alcohol.
- Athlete's foot.
- Verrucas.
- Pregnancy.
- Diabetes.*
- Epilepsy.*

* Only to be carried out with medical approval.

Effects of a hydrotherapy bath

- Body temperature is raised.
- Perspiration is induced.
- Circulation is increased.
- Muscle fibres are relaxed.
- Metabolism is increased.

Preparation of the hydrotherapy bath

1. Observe general safety precautions.
2. Fill bath with warm water.
3. Add essence required.

Hydrotherapy treatment

1 Client is greeted at reception and taken to changing facilities.
2 Consultation is carried out and the effects of the treatment are explained.
3 Client removes items such as contact lenses, spectacles and jewellery, etc., and showers to remove deodorant, fragrances, body lotions, etc.
4 Compressor is switched on for gentle aeration of the water.
5 The client is helped into the unit, where they rest in a semi-reclined position.
6 The hose is switched on and the therapist guides it over the client's body for approximately 15–20 minutes before the hose is switched off.
7 The compressor is switched off and after a few minutes the client is helped from the bath.
8 The client is taken to a relaxation area to rest.

Whirlpools

Whirlpools are sometimes called spa baths and are commonly known by the name of the American manufacturer who brought them to commercial success – Jacuzzi™. They are found in the majority of health spas, hydros, clubs and hotels and even in individual homes. They vary in size, shape and price. The larger ones can accommodate up to eight people at the same time. They are commonly found near the swimming pool in most health spas where the benefits of contrast baths can be achieved.

There are a number of factors to consider when fitting a whirlpool:

1 The floor must be:
   ◊ reinforced to take the large weight of the filled pool
   ◊ tanked and drained.

2 The plant room which houses the controls must:
   ◊ have a suitable power supply
   ◊ be within five metres of the pool
   ◊ be well ventilated.

3 The pool should have:
   ◊ a filtration system
   ◊ a heavy duty control panel to withstand constant wear and tear.

ACTIVITY

Research:

a the range of spa pools available
b the recommended chemical additives and how they are added, e.g. automatically or manually
c the manufacturers' procedures for checking the water quality and filters
d the manufacturers' procedures for maintaining the pH and ensuring hygienic practices.

Compare your findings to the SPATA (Swimming Pool and Allied Trades Association) code of practice.

Effects of the whirlpool

- Increases circulation.
- Stimulates the skin and aids desquamation.
- Increases metabolism.
- Relaxes muscles.
- Relieves aches and pains (whilst in pool).
- Produces a sense of wellbeing.

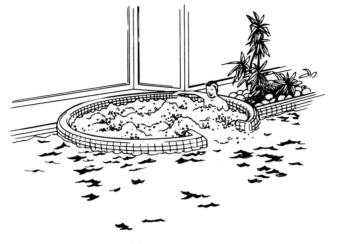

Fig. 8.8 *Whirlpool bath*

The whirlpool generally has two massage effects; a gentle effect and a strong one. The gentle massage effect is created by compressed air flowing through small holes at the base of the pool. The strong whirlpool massage effect is created by jets of air pummelling the skin along with the action of the fast moving water of the pool. When these two effects are combined they create a fast stream of bubbling water.

ACTIVITY

With a colleague, select three different spa treatments that would benefit each of you. Taking the roles of client and therapist undertake the treatments selected and evaluate their physiological and psychological effects on you. Discuss and compare your findings with your colleague.

Hydro-oxygen baths

This treatment involves the client reclining in a bath-type cabinet that contains jets which are used to blast the client's body with hot water and to diffuse oxygen into the cabinet. The treatment is extremely stimulating and makes the skin more sensitive. An infra-red treatment would not follow due to skin sensitivity.

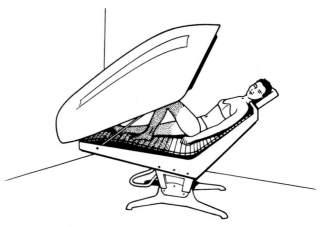

Fig. 8.9 *Hydro-oxygen bath*

Effects of hydrotherapy treatments

Hot baths:

- Relieve pain.
- Induce perspiration.
- Have a cleansing effect.
- Increase temperature.

Cold baths:

- Relieve pain.
- Have a stimulating effect.
- Have a diuretic effect.
- Reduce temperature.

Cold baths used to be very popular, particularly after a sauna. However clients today tend to prefer cool baths. Perhaps tolerance of different temperatures has altered with the advances in technology which brought about such development as central heating and air conditioning.

Thalassotherapy

Thalassotherapy is a salt water hydrojet massage used to ease aches and pains, and to trim and tone tissues. It is renowned for its healing properties. The treatment will also restore balance and energy to the body.

Thalassotherapy consists of a large pool which can hold up to fifteen people at a time and consists of different areas with pressure jets situated underneath. The treatment takes 30 minutes during which time a person progresses around the pool to the different areas. The treatment can also be combined with an algae wrap.

The pool contains one ton of salt which consists of three main elements:

- magnesium, a natural sedative to make the client feel relaxed and sleepy
- zinc, which has healing properties and is especially good for sufferers of eczema and psoriasis
- sodium, which has a firming and toning effect, particularly when used in conjunction with the side jets in the pool.

Main benefits of thalassotherapy treatment

- Relieves stress.
- Regulates blood pressure.
- Purifies the body of toxins.
- Regulates hormonal activities.
- Strengthens the cardio-vascular system.
- Increases body metabolism.
- Cleanses the sinuses and respiratory passages.
- Improves the quality of skin and hair.

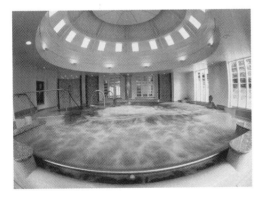

Fig. 8.10 *Thalassotherapy*

Contrast baths

Contrast baths describe the situation where two different temperature baths are found next to each other so that the client can move from one to the other. The treatment time may vary slightly dependent on the temperature of the baths, but generally the client would spend between 1–5 minutes in the hot bath and 15–60 seconds in the cool bath. The total treatment time would last approximately 10–30 minutes.

The Scotch douche treatment utilises hot and cold water which is alternatively run up and down the client's spine to stimulate the spinal nerves by sluicing blood in and out of the spinal area. This treatment is believed to help sufferers of migraines and other ailments such as aches and pains in the back.

The Sitz bath treatment from Germany also uses the effects of contrast bathing. Two baths are used, one containing hot water the other cold. For the first 5–10 minutes the client sits in the hot bath with their feet immersed in cold water. The client then changes and sits in the cold bath with their feet immersed in the hot water. The cold water causes the blood vessels to constrict which in turn will force the blood supply to the area of the body immersed in hot water. The overall effect of this treatment is to flush the blood into the pelvic area bringing nourishment to it then to flush it out taking away waste. This type of bath was recommended for any illness which effects the lower part of the body.

Another treatment using the effects of differing temperatures is the Spanish mantle treatment. Cold, damp, cotton sheets are wrapped around the client and hot water bottles are placed around the body or a radiant heat lamp is used to induce perspiration. The client would be left to perspire for up to three hours. It was claimed that when the sheets were finally removed the elimination of toxins from the body changed the colouring of the sheets.

ACTIVITY

Research the different spa treatments offered by three different health spas.

Progress Check

1   State the different treatments you might find in a spa area.
2   List four contraindications to each of the following treatments:
    a foam bath
    b hydrotherapy bath.
3   State two effects for each of the following treatments:
    a foam bath
    b hydrotherapy bath
    c whirlpool.
4   Explain the preparation of the foam bath.
5   State the effects of hydrotherapy treatments.
6   Briefly describe the following treatments:
    a hydro-oxygen baths
    b contrast baths.

Key Terms

You need to know what these words and phrases mean. Go back through the chapter to find out.

- ⬥ Aerated baths
- ⬥ Floatation treatments
- ⬥ Foam baths
- ⬥ Heat treatments
- ⬥ Hydro-oxygen baths
- ⬥ Hydrotherapy
- ⬥ Hydrotherapy baths
- ⬥ Sauna
- ⬥ Steam cabinets/rooms
- ⬥ Thalassotherapy
- ⬥ Whirlpool

After working through this chapter you will be able to:

- outline the key principles of the electromagnetic spectrum
- state the differences between ultra-violet and infra-red treatments
- list the three bands of ultra-violet rays and explain their main effects
- give the main benefits and uses of infra-red and ultra-violet treatments
- list the contraindications and safety precautions to both treatments.

There are two main forms of radiation that the therapist needs to be aware of, each forming part of the electromagnetic spectrum. *Ultra-violet* is used mainly for its skin tanning effects while *infra-red* is used as a method of warming the tissues for therapeutic purposes.

The electromagnetic spectrum

The electromagnetic spectrum consists of a continuous band of radiation given off from the sum in varying frequencies and wavelengths. The radiation given off can be divided into bands according to their wavelength:

- Gamma rays (shortest wavelength).
- X-rays.
- Ultra-violet rays.
- Visible light (red, orange, yellow, green, blue, indigo, violet).
- Infra-red rays.
- Radio waves (longest wavelength).

Wavelengths are typically measured in nanometres (nm). A nanometre is a millionth of a millimetre. The wavelengths of visible light are in the range between 400 and 770 nm with the lower (shorter) wavelengths being at the blue end of the visible spectrum and the higher (longer)

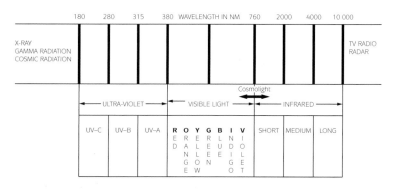

Fig. 9.1 *Spectrum of electromagnetic radiation*

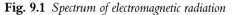

wavelengths being at the red end of the visible spectrum. Infra-red rays have wavelengths in the range of 770 to 4000 nm while ultra-violet rays have wavelengths between 200 to 400 nm.

Electromagnetic rays can be uniquely defined in terms of their wavelength. The wavelength is defined as the distance form the point on one wave to the same point on the next wave. Rays also have a frequency which is defined as the number of cycles or complete waves that pass a fixed point each second. Frequency is calculated and shown as a reading of hertz, i.e. the number of cycles per second. Shorter wavelengths such as ultra-violet will have a higher frequency than longer wavelengths such as infra-red because they require more cycles to cover the same distance.

The bands of radiation used in therapy treatments are ultra-violet and infra-red.

Infra-red radiation

As mentioned previously, infra-red rays have wavelengths of the order 770 to 4000 nm which means that they have longer wavelengths than visible light. This form of radiation can be divided into two bands:

- Infra-red rays which are longer wavelength rays of approximately 4000 nm
- radiant heat rays which are shorter wavelength rays of approximately 1000 nm.

In infra-red lamp or non-luminous lamp type emits a gentle warmth with a barely detectable glow. The lamp operates at a fairly low temperature so the intensity of the output is also low.

A radiant heat lamp or luminous lamp type emits a more intense heat with a very visible glow. The lamp operates at a much higher temperature with an output of heat radiation and visible light.

Infra-red and radiant heat lamps are used in therapy treatments to warm the tissues and the difference in the wavelengths produces varying effects. Traditionally, in beauty therapy, a warm source is used to produce the infra-red energy and the bulbs are then coated red to indicate a hot surface.

Infra-red rays penetrate the epidermal layer only irritating the cells to release histamine which results in the blood vessels dilating thus generating heat in the tissues. This redness is often termed *hyperaemia* and has a soothing effect as opposed to a stimulating one as the nerve endings are not greatly affected.

Radiant heat rays penetrate into the dermal layers causing immediate dilation of the blood and lymph vessels which forces the fluids away from the skin into the underlying structures producing a deep heat effect.

Types of infra-red equipment

Infra-red and radiant heat lamps normally come in the following forms:

- **Fireclay lamp** – this is basically a wire coil surrounding a clay support with a reflector shield.

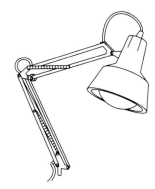

Fig. 9.2 *Infra-red heat lamp*

- **Filament lamp** – this is like a large light bulb that also contains a built-in reflector shield and is made from red coloured glass. Dimmer devices are added so the intensity of the lamp can be reduced to emit infra-red rays as opposed to radiant heat.
- **Quartz heat lamp** – this type normally contain quartz rods with a heating element inside. (Sometimes seen as old-fashioned bathroom heaters.)

There is a European recommendation that when using high wattage bulbs the cowl, the part that holds the bulb, should be double skinned to allow an outer and an inner space between the bulb and the cowl. This creates a cooling effect as air drawn into the lower ventilating holes or slits warms, rises, and flows out through the upper ventilation holes or slits.

General effects of infra-red and radiant heat on the body

Infra-red and radiant heat are used in the therapy clinic as a general heat treatment to help relax the client and to relieve pain and tension. These effects are achieved as:

- Metabolism is speeded up as a result of the increased heat which will ultimately increase the demand for oxygen and nutrients and speed up the excretion of waste and toxins.
- Vasodilation occurs due to the heat on the blood vessels increasing blood circulation.
- Sudoriferous gland activity is increased due to the vasodilation effect (this will bring about further elimination of waste products).
- There is a soothing effect on sensory nerve endings.

Contraindications
to infra-red and radiant heat treatments

- Heart and vascular conditions.
- Fever, heavy colds and influenza.
- Skin diseases and disorders.
- High or low blood pressure.
- Burns and sunburn.
- Metal pins and plates.
- Diabetes (due to impaired circulation).
- Oedema.
- Cuts, scars and skin abrasions.

Harmful effects of infra-red and radiant heat treatment

If the treatment is not carried out correctly any of the following may occur:

- Burning of the skin.
- Giddiness or fainting.
- Headaches.
- Permanent eye injury.

Safety precautions for infra-red and radiant heat treatment

1. Always carry out a detailed consultation before treatment checking for any contraindications.
2. Always follow manufacturer's instructions with regard to operating any equipment.
3. Accurately time and position the lamp according to the cosine and inverse square laws (see below and p. 258).
4. Protect the client's eyes.
5. Ensure skin is properly prepared and carry out a skin sensitivity test prior to treatment. (See Chapter 6.)
6. Ensure lamp is secure with no trailing wires, is dust free and is regularly serviced.
7. Preheat lamp before positioning over treatment area.
8. Do not leave the client unattended.

Progress Check

1. List the key principles of the electromagnetic spectrum.
2. Name the three types of infra-red equipment available.
3. What is the average wattage of an infra-red bulb?
4. List four effects of infra-red/radiant heat.
5. List five contraindications to infra-red and radiant heat treatments.

The cosine law

The cosine law shows the comparison between intensity of rays and the angle at which these rays make contact with the skin. The lamp should be placed perpendicular to the skin ensuring the rays fall at right angles to the body which will give maximum intensity.

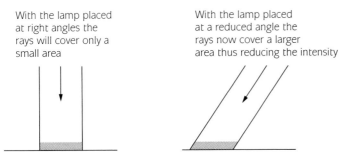

With the lamp placed at right angles the rays will cover only a small area

With the lamp placed at a reduced angle the rays now cover a larger area thus reducing the intensity

Fig. 9.3 *The cosine law*

The inverse square law

With any radiation treatment distance is extremely important and in particular it is important when using ultra-violet where very little heat is generated. It goes without saying that the closer a lamp is to the body the higher the intensity of radiation will be. The inverse square law states that *the intensity of radiation will differ inversely with the square of the distance from the lamp*. This means that if the distance from the lamp is doubled the intensity of the rays will be quartered. In practical terms the intensity of radiation at a distance of 30 cm is four times that at 60 cm, i.e. four minutes' treatment at 60 cm will give the same effect as one minute's at 30 cm.

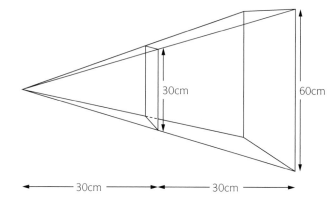

Fig. 9.4 *The inverse square law*

ACTIVITY
Research the uses of infra-red heat treatments within a health spa.

Ultra-violet radiation

Ultra-violet rays have wavelengths within the range of 200 to 400 nanometres, i.e. beyond the violet end of the visible light spectrum. They are invisible to the naked eye and are classified as follows:

- UVA rays.
- UVB rays.
- UVC rays.

UVA rays

UVA rays have wavelengths of 315–400 nm and penetrate deeply into the dermal layer of the skin. This damages the collagen and elastin fibres causing premature ageing together with increasing the risk of skin cancer. UVA rays expand melanin already present within the skin causing a short-term tanning effect.

UVB rays

UVB rays have wavelengths of 280–315 nm and will penetrate only to the basal layer of the epidermis. UVB stimulates melanocytes present in this layer to produce more melanin causing a much deeper, longer lasting colour than UVA alone. It is UVB which causes thickening of the epidermis and is also responsible for sunburn and for the development of skin cancers.

- If a client chooses or is recommended to have a UVB treatment, a pre-sensitisation and a skin sensitivity test (see Chapter 6) must be carried out in addition to the therapist observing contraindications and safety precautions.
- It is paramount that the cosine and inverse square laws are implemented.

Pre-sensitisation test

This should be carried out 24 hours before the client wishes to have the UVB treatment. One way to carry out such a test is to take a sheet of paper and cut four small holes in a line about 1 cm apart. Place the sheet over the forearm and mount the UV lamp at the standard distance. Expose the area to UV rays for one and a half minutes then cover over the first hole, continue UV exposure and after a further half a minute cover over the second hole, after another half a minute cover the third hole and the final hole after another half a minute. The arm should be inspected the following day to see which of the areas most closely resembles a first degree erythema so the appropriate exposure time can be worked out for the client.

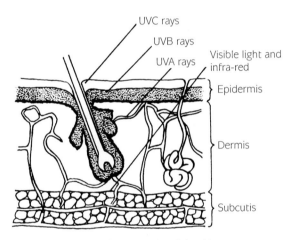

Fig. 9.5 *Ultra-violet and infra-red penetration of the skin*

UVC rays

UVC rays have a wavelength shorter than 280 nm and are harmful to living cells. UVC rays are absorbed by the Earth's atmosphere and therefore are not found in natural sunlight or used in salon tanning treatments.

The effects of ultra-violet radiation

Current research into the effects of ultra-violet radiation have proved that it is responsible for premature ageing of the skin together with being the primary cause of skin cancer. In extreme moderation however there are some beneficial effects:

- Stimulates the production of vitamin D needed for healthy bones and teeth.
- Has a slightly germicidal effect on the skin.
- Causes hyperkeratinisation which is thought to help with some skin conditions such as acne vulgaris and psoriasis.

- Gives a psychological feeling of wellbeing.
- Produces a tan.

Harmful effects of ultra-violet treatment

- May cause sunburn if exposure is too long.
- Is the primary cause of skin cancer.
- Thickens the epidermis giving a 'leathery' appearance.
- Irreversibly damages collagen and elastin fibres leading to premature ageing.
- Causes dehydration of the skin tissues.
- Can cause allergic reactions.
- Can produce dark pigmentation patches.

The tanning mechanism

Ultra-violet rays are absorbed by the skin where they stimulate an enzyme called *tyrosinase*, found within the epidermis, which converts into an amino-acid known as *tyrosin* which then changes into *melanin*. This is an immediate response to exposure to ultra-violet and is followed by the increased production of new skin cells which quickly migrate to the stratum corneum layer to develop in colour. Prolonged exposure to UVB in particular will stimulate greater melanocyte production causing a deep and lasting tan.

The way in which this tanning mechanism works will depend on the individual skin type and colouring. These skin types are normally categorised as follows:

- Group 1 – very sensitive, burns easily and never develops a tan.
- Group 2 – sensitive skin which burns easily and tans with difficulty.
- Group 3 – normal skin which tans fairly slowly and may burn slightly.
- Group 4 – tans very easily without burning.
- Group 5 – genetically pigmented skin which rarely burns.

Sunburn

Sunburn is the result of damage to the skin and is the body's way of protecting itself. Sunburn presents as erythema a few hours after exposure. Erythema is the result of histamine being released in the tissues which causes dilation of the blood capillaries. In extreme cases plasma exudes from the blood vessels into the tissues causing blisters.

There are four degrees of erythema which are as follows:

- First degree – presents as slight redness with no irritation and disappears after 24 hours.
- Second degree – presents as a more marked redness with irritation lasting for 2–3 days.
- Third degree – presents as very hot skin which is sore and swollen with pigmentation and lasts for up to one week; desquamation will occur.
- Fourth degree – this is similar to a third degree with the addition of blisters and peeling. This can be quite serious and require medical treatment.

1   Briefly explain the relevance of the cosine and inverse square laws.
2   Give the three bands of ultra-violet rays and explain their main effects.
3   State the purpose of the skin sensitivity and pre-sensitisation tests.
4   List the contraindications to ultra-violet treatments.
5   Give five harmful effects of ultra-violet radiation.
6   Briefly outline the stages of tanning.
7   Give a brief description of the four degrees of sunburn.

Types of ultra-violet equipment

Within the beauty salon ultra-violet radiation can be utilised in four ways:

- Mercury vapour lamps.
- Solarium.
- Sun-bed.
- Wood lamp.

Mercury vapour lamps

This type of equipment consists of a lamp surrounded by a layer of quartz which allows UV rays to pass through. The space between contains argon gas and a small amount of mercury. Two electrodes are encased at either end. When the unit is switched on ionisation of the argon gas occurs and electrons flow through the tube; this, together with the ionisation of the mercury, produces ultra-violet radiation. This type of equipment is rarely used in the therapy clinic but can be seen in hospitals for the treatment of certain skin conditions such as psoriasis.

Solarium

These normally consist of a lamp or a group of lamps suspended in an overhead fashion and often combining infra-red bulbs with UVB emitters. Traditionally these were used for either preparing the client's skin for exposure to sunlight by using UVB rays or for preparing the client for further salon treatments such as massage by using the infra-red lamps contained within the unit. Modern technology has seen the development of solarium-type units which encompass a padded bed area and air conditioning together with a small, high-pressure area for the face. Some also include music facilities. Those with infra-red as well as ultra-violet rays generate more heat and thus have a relaxing effect for the client. Individual manufacturer's instructions need to be followed closely to calculate treatment exposure and classify the type of UV rays emitted.

Sun-bed

These are the most popular form of UV equipment seen in the salon today and normally consist of a single or double sided plastic covered bed containing UV tubes. Modern beds are usually contoured to ensure even tanning treatment. The tubes are often made from a product called Vita-glass™ which allows the UV rays to pass through. Vita-glass™ has a phosphorous lining which absorbs UVC and most UVB rays thereby

> **USEFUL INFORMATION**
> * There is a large variety of sun-beds on the market today including the popular high-intensity type favoured by health spas.
> * The most recent development in suntanning is the sun cubicle or 'room'. Clients stand and are exposed for approximately 6–15 minutes only and as a result little perspiration occurs.

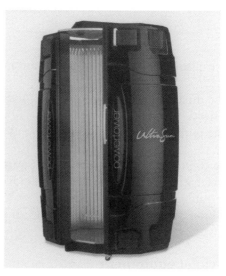

Fig. 9.6 *Ultrasun Powertower*™

emitting almost exclusively UVA. At the ends of the sun-bed tube the rating and specification will be stamped. Those with a built-in reflector will be marked R-UVA. Great care must be taken to ensure the correct type of replacement lamp is chosen for each sun-bed.

Note. R-UVA tubes should not be fitted into early models of sun-bed which have reflector panels between each lamp fitting position because a 'striped' tan will result! Check ratings of lamps carefully and consider the overall intensity per bed according to the number of lamps used.

POINTS TO NOTE

- Always ensure the plastic surfaces have been cleaned between clients using a specific product for the purpose as the wrong type of cleaner can damage them.
- Always use the manufacturer's recommended emission tubes and keep detailed records of tube use.
- Never leave a client unattended throughout the treatment.

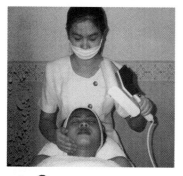

Fig. 9.7 *Wood lamp and skin scanner*

Wood lamp

Wood lamps can be used to assist the therapist in the analysis of their client's skin. 'Black' ultra-violet tubes illuminate skin conditions in degrees of reflected light, which gives a far clearer view than the naked eye sees in normal light. A variety of lamps is available; traditionally they are designed to be used in a darkened room. Some incorporate the use of a magnifying lamp and a black-out screen; the most consumer conscious enable the client to view their skin 'illuminated' at the same time as the therapist. An accurate and very visual analysis of their skin condition is very motivating and encourages a client to follow the treatment and home care schedule recommended by their therapist.

Ultra-violet treatment

As with any salon treatment, a detailed consultation should be carried out with the client before using UV equipment. Contraindications and a skin sensitivity and/or pre-sensitisation test should be checked thoroughly.

Contraindications

to ultra-violet treatments

- Any person who does not tan naturally in the sun.
- Any person prone to frequent bouts of cold sores (herpes simplex).
- Pigmentation disorders: vitiligo, chloasma.
- Vascular problems.
- Migraine and headache suffers.
- Any person prone to fainting.
- Pregnancy (as this may lead to increased pigmentation – chloasma).
- Previous history of skin cancer, problems with moles.
- Fever, colds and high temperature.
- Certain drugs may cause photosensitisation: antibiotics, tranquillisers, diuretics, contraceptive pills, anti-diabetic tablets, cold injections, quinine, blood pressure medications. (Consent from the client's GP will be required in these cases.)

Safety precautions for ultra-violet treatment

If it is considered safe to give treatment the client must:

- Remove all make-up and perfume and ensure that the skin is completely dry.
- Remove watches and jewellery and contact lenses.
- Shower with an unperfumed product.
- Cover hair, especially if treated with colours or permanent wave solutions.
- Avoid applying any suntan preparations except those recommended for UV treatments by specialist manufacturers.
- Wear protective goggles at all times.

Check the client's skin type and colouring. Explain all procedures clearly to the client and supervise the treatment at all times. Ensure that high standards of hygiene are maintained in the treatment area and that the manufacturer's instructions are clearly followed. Specialist clothing which has a UV protection factor of 40 can be purchased.

GOOD PRACTICE

- Treatment should be discontinued if the client has any adverse reaction to the treatment.
- Accurate records should be kept of all treatments given.
- Ideally, perspiration during a sun-bed treatment should be minimal. Most beds contain body-cooling fans to reduce sudoriferous gland activity.
- It is essential that the sun-bed room has sufficient ventilation.

ACTIVITY

Research the variety of suntanning equipment available. Compare their cost, size, facilities, durability and cost-effectiveness within a salon environment.

1 Explain the benefits of using a wood lamp in the salon.
2 State the differences between ultra-violet and infra-red treatments.
3 State the main benefits and uses of infra-red and ultra-violet treatments.
4 List the safety precautions to be observed when carrying out:
   a solarium treatment
   b infra-red treatment.
5 Explain why pressure marks from a sun-bed do not tan.

Key Terms

You need to know what these words and phrases mean. Go back through the chapter to find out.

- Cosine law
- Electromagnetic spectrum
- Infra-red
- Inverse square law
- Pre-sensitisation
- Radiant heat
- Solarium
- Sun-bed
- Sunburn
- Tanning mechanism
- Ultra-violet
- Wood lamp

REMEDIAL CAMOUFLAGE

After working through this chapter you will be able to:

- identify the different conditions that can be treated with camouflage make-up
- list the contraindications to camouflage techniques
- have knowledge of the basic principles required to carry out treatment
- carry out a basic camouflage make-up treatment.

In today's society great emphasis is placed on physical appearance. Whether we like it or not, we are all influenced by media pressure to look the very best that we can even if this is sometimes an unhealthy attitude to possess.

For some this can be made worse by unnatural disfigurement caused either at birth or through illness or accident. While surgery may be an option for some, it is not possible or necessary for others, yet they still feel embarrassment every time they face the outside world. This can have serious repercussions, in some cases making the individual loathe to face anything or anyone new. It can affect career prospects and even the forming of relationships.

The therapist who can provide and instruct on remedial camouflage can greatly enhance an individual's life and gain tremendous job satisfaction.

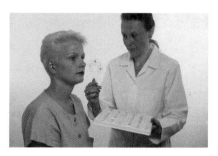

Fig. 10.1 *Remedial camouflage make-up*

Role of the cosmetic camouflage therapist

It goes without saying that the therapist working in cosmetic camouflage is entering into a field slightly different from the normal course of work, with the exception maybe of electrology. This area of work requires a very discreet approach and a sympathetic attitude so as to prevent the client suffering undue stress or discomfort. The therapist should have a good understanding of the different types of disfigurement possible and be able to identify the client's needs and anticipated outcomes. The experienced therapist should be able to expertly cover any blemishes or disfigurement and most importantly be able to instruct the client on how to do so. This should always be carried out in an atmosphere of peace and tranquillity.

Client consultation

The importance of a correct client consultation cannot be overstated if the treatment is ultimately going to be a success. The first objective is to establish a rapport with the client and instil confidence in the therapist's ability and willingness to help whilst at the same time being realistic in the treatment's outcomes.

It is wise to try and gather information about the scar/disfigurement at the time of booking the consultation so that a general practitioner's note can be provided ahead of time where necessary. This is preferable to referring the client to her/his GP at the time of consultation as it could possibly lead to lost custom through embarrassment or frustration.

It is also most important to allow the client to tell you what is troubling them rather than just presuming. A wrong assessment could cause untold harm to an already sensitive client and this could have serious long-term repercussions on the individual's self-image.

A detailed record card should be completed carefully with the client. An example of such a record card is shown in Fig. 10.2.

Name of client:	Name of doctor:
Address:	Address:
Telephone: Day	Telephone:
Evening:	
Source of referral:	
Type/age of scarring:	
Area(s) of scarring:	
Signature of client:	Signature of therapist:

Fig. 10.2 *Example of a remedial camouflage consultation card*

On the back of the card the following information should be recorded:

- Products used.
- Shades of creams.
- Number/method of application.
- Results.

A similar card should be given to the client after treatment detailing the products used and the method of application so that it can be used for reference. In some cases it may be necessary to also send a copy of the consultation card to the client's own doctor, especially if consent was required or if there is to be any follow-up medical treatment.

Types of client
Unlike in any other area, the therapist working in remedial camouflage will be dealing with a diverse range of clients: men, women and even children. Some will be new to the clinic, some existing and many will be extremely nervous.

Male approach
Men who come to the clinic for remedial camouflage may often be more inhibited than women. This is partly because they consider salons to be

the domain of women, especially if there is feminine-style décor and because they see cosmetics as a predominantly female medium. When dealing with a male client the main objective is to make the remedial camouflage as undetectable as possible and to ensure appropriate surroundings.

Female approach

The female client will often be more used to cosmetics and therefore less inhibited about using them. She may however be more concerned about her appearance than a male client so may need extra reassurance and even help and guidance with normal cosmetic application.

Child approach

When dealing with children for remedial camouflage it is important not to make them feel that their disfigurement is unacceptable. Often it is a parent who has instigated treatment and this can draw attention in the child's mind to a problem that never really bothered them before. Depending on the age of the child it may be a case of teaching the parent how to apply camouflage techniques. It should be suggested that in this case the child returns at a later date to be given expert advice as well.

Also it is worth mentioning that some childhood disfigurements disappear with age in some instances.

Progress Check

1 State the importance of the consultation procedure.
2 Explain how you would handle a child requiring cosmetic camouflage.

Remedial camouflage conditions

Pigmentation disorders

The most common pigmentation disorders are outlined here.

Chloasma

This is a smooth, irregularly shaped patch of brown pigmentation which occurs when there is increased production of the melanocyte stimulating hormone. It occurs most frequently in pregnancy or when taking the contraceptive pill. Exposure to ultra-violet radiation exacerbates the condition.

Vitiligo (leucoderma)

This is an absence of melanin in small patches on the skin caused by the destruction of melanocytes in the basal layer of the epidermis. Sometimes large areas can be affected and the small patches merge into one. The condition is obviously more noticeable on a darker skin. The other key feature of vitiligo is that as there is no protective melanin present, the areas affected are photosensitive and will burn if exposed to UV radiation.

Melanoderma

This is a general term for patchy pigmentation of the skin. There are many reasons for melanoderma but the main cause is allergic reaction to a product being applied to the skin and reacting with UV radiation, e.g. perfume.

Types of naevus

The medical definition of a naevus is a birthmark or circumscribed area of pigmentation due to dilated blood vessels. Many forms of naevus exist including;

- Strawberry naevus. These are normally present at birth or occur shortly afterwards and normally start as a small red spot which enlarges fairly quickly. They are normally raised above the surface of the skin and can become quite large. In most cases they fade with time and will have completely disappeared by the age of about seven when just a red patch remains.
- Angioma (Port wine stain). So named because it tends to be dark red or purplish in colour. Angioma can be extremely disfiguring. It is an area of profusely dilated capillaries and often affects the face and neck. The individual is born with this condition.
- Spider naevus (stellate haemangioma). These can appear at any age and are small, red central spots with superficial veins radiating from them. They can occur on any part of the body, but are usually seen on the face and upper cheek area.
- Epidermal benign naevus (moles). Moles can be found all over the body and vary in size and texture. They can be raised or flat, pigmented or normal skin colour, and some contain hairs. Most pigmented moles occur through overgrowth of melanocytes in the basal layer of the epidermis which is an indirect result of exposure to ultra-violet radiation.

Types of scar

A scar is a mark which is left on the skin after it has healed from some form of trauma. There are many different types of scarring, but the main categories are outlined here.

Hypertrophic scar

This is a large unsightly scar which is raised and shiny in appearance.

Ice-pick scar

As the name suggests, this type of scar is rough and pitted. It is a common post-acne blemish.

Keloid scar

This type of scar is fibrous and lumpy as the body continues to produce extra collagen after a wound has healed. Keloid scars are more prevalent on black skin types.

Quiescent scar tissue

This term describes scar tissue which is at rest or has healed. The rate at which a scar heals will vary from one person to another. There are general signs that indicate that a scar is healed:

- there is no evidence of inflammation
- it is not painful or sensitive to the touch
- it is not weeping or moist.

Skin disorders

Psoriasis

This is caused by an abnormally fast rate of cell renewal in the epidermis with cells sometimes reaching the stratum corneum in a few days instead of the normal 28–30. This results in clusters of cells forming characteristic oval, dull-red plaques together with silvery scales.

The cause of the condition is not clear but hereditary factors play an important part and it is thought to be exacerbated by stress.

Rosacea

This normally affects the over thirties age group and often women of menopausal age. It begins with a flushed appearance, particularly in response to stress, spicy foods and alcohol. The flushing then becomes permanent as the blood vessels in the area become dilated. This increases the temperature of the skin stimulating sebum production and this in turn leads to papules, pustules and open pores becoming present. It is a chronic disorder of the blood vessels of the face.

Skin conditions

Tattoos

It has long been fashionable for people to have tattoos. A tattoo is where a permanent pigment is put into the skin. Unfortunately many people live to regret having a tattoo and although removal is now possible it is both painful and expensive. Camouflage make-up is an alternative option to successfully hide such marks.

POINT TO NOTE

Camouflage make up will generally last longer on dry skin types.

Varicose veins

Varicose veins produce a characteristic bulging effect and can be quite disfiguring. They are the result of valves within the veins collapsing through an inherited weakness and/or poor circulation.

Contraindications

to camouflage make-up

As with any treatment there are some conditions that the therapist should not treat. Examples include:

- Infectious skin conditions.
- Warts.
- Cuts/Abrasions.
- Skin irritations.
- Swelling.

1   List four contraindications to camouflage make-up and explain why each is a contraindication.
2   Describe four types of scar tissue.
3   Name three remedial camouflage conditions which can be successfully camouflaged.

Equipment required for camouflage make-up

A camouflage make-up kit is needed by the therapist which should be kept in an immaculate and hygienic condition. Firstly it will be necessary to have a range of skin care products to prepare the skin for treatment. The client may already be wearing some form of make-up but if not it is still necessary to cleanse and remove any traces of sweat, sebum and general dirt. Toner must be used to remove any residue left by the cleansing medium otherwise the camouflage creams may 'slide' on application and also be unstable. Moisturiser should also be applied, but avoid the blemished area for the same reasons.

Secondly it will be essential to have a good range of cover creams, there are many different types available and it is up to the individual therapist to decide which range is best for them. Great improvements have been made over recent years in the production of camouflage make-up. Many manufacturers produce sample kits of all the colours in their range with replacements available for the colours that are used the most. It will also be important to carry a range of stock for the client to purchase for immediate use.

Within the kit it will be necessary to have a setting or fixing powder. Some manufacturers supply these powders whilst others recommend the use of translucent powder. Retail powder should also be available for the client to purchase. Finally, a range of sponges and good quality sable brushes together with some form of mixing palette will be needed for professional application. Some of the palettes available today are made from clear Perspex with a central magnifier which allows the therapist to blend the creams and hold it up to the skin to check the colour compatibility. (An example of this type of palette is the one produced by Rita Roberts™.)

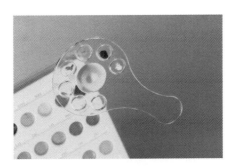
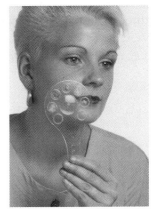

Fig. 10.3 *'Blend-in' palette*

Lighting

The source and type of lighting is very important when carrying out a camouflage make-up treatment as it will affect the colour of the cosmetics.

The colour of the pigment within the skin will vary depending on the type of light that is illuminating it. Natural daylight is composed of all the colours of the spectrum and will therefore define the face clearly. Artificial (white) light may consist of many hues (colours) some of which may be stronger than others, therefore if the coloured hue falls on a pigment that is able to reflect it, the colour of the lighting is seen, however if it falls onto pigment and the rays are absorbed then the pigment colour will be distorted.

Example. If white light falls on a red lipstick, the pigment within the product reflects the red light and absorbs the other six colours of the spectrum making the lipstick appear red. However if pure blue light falls on the lipstick, it will be absorbed and as there is no red light for it to reflect it will appear black.

ACTIVITY

Research the effects of lighting on make-up.

Camouflage make-up creams

When choosing a range of camouflage make-up it is important to consider the following points:

- Colour range. There should be a wide range of colours available to cater from the palest to the darkest skin colouring.
- Even consistency. The products should blend easily on contact with the skin, they should not drag or feel unduly tacky.
- Waterproof. The products should be waterproof to allow the user to participate in normal activities, e.g. swimming.
- UV filters. As scar tissue can be sensitive, cover creams should have in-built UV filters.

Blending techniques

If the therapist is to become skilled in the blending of camouflage make-up it is essential to have a good understanding of the principles of colour and to practise.

The colour wheel

There are three primary colours; red, blue and yellow. To make a colour you more around the wheel, e.g. red + yellow = orange.

POINT TO NOTE

Opposite colours neutralise, e.g. green neutralises red.

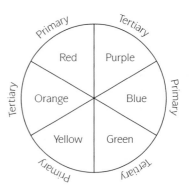

Fig. 10.4 *The colour wheel*

Colourings

The colour of skin can alter through life as it is affected by different factors such as climate, illness and certain products.

Skin contains varying amounts of the pigment melanin which is genetically passed from parent to child. Skin colour can be divided into four basic categories.

1   **Caucasian skin**. This is the most fragile of all skin types, prone to sun damage, broken capillaries and pigmentation irregularities. Scarring tends to leave pink pigmentation marks that can be quite noticeable. It has blue and pink tones present from the blood capillaries behind which is a basic tone normally of either yellow or pink. It can vary from being very pale to quite a deep tan depending on UV exposure and hereditary factors.

2   **Oriental skin**. This type is more resilient than Caucasian skin and most often is of even tone. However it can develop pigmentation discoloration if exposed to ultra-violet radiation. This skin type will have more melanin present and be mainly of one colour tone. It has a basic yellow undertone.

3   **Asian skin**. This type is normally strong and adaptable. It can have a tendency towards uneven colouring and in particular dark shadows around the eye area. Scarring tends to leave dark pigmentation marks which are slow to fade. It can vary in tone from being quite olive to very dark, but always has a yellow undertone.

4   **Black skin**. This skin type has the greatest amount of protective melanin pigment and therefore is the slowest to show signs of ageing. As with Asian skin types scarring tends to leave dark pigmentation marks that are slow to fade. There are many varying colour tones from light brown to deep ebony.

ACTIVITY

Complete a detailed case study on a client with a disfigurement, keeping photographic evidence where possible. Evaluate your findings including client feedback.

Matching skin colour (basic application techniques)

As mentioned previously, when purchasing a camouflage make-up kit it is essential to choose one with a good variety of depths and tones of shades to meet the diverse range of skin colours.

1   It will be necessary to establish the depth and tone of the client's skin and to choose the nearest colour to match the client's skin accordingly.
2   Neutralise any irregularities present, e.g. green will neutralise red, but it must be remembered that the principle of camouflage make-up is to disguise the abnormality by blending it to the client's skin colour.
3   Mix the depths and tones so that when applied to the treatment area it will blend and match the client's skin colour.
4   When choosing the correct colour, if the client's skin is midway between two shades, blending equal quantities of both should produce the exact match.
5   If a client's skin is closer to one of the shades, blending two parts of the closer to one part of the other should produce a good match.
6   Another important point is to write down exactly what has been blended as it is easy to forget.

Once you have mixed the correct shade it will be necessary to test the cream near the treatment area. If the match is perfect it can be applied to the disfigurement. However if it is deeply pigmented it may not be sufficient to adequately cover, in which case it will be necessary to apply a thin coat then set it with powder and then apply a second coat and set that.

POINT TO NOTE

A dampened cosmetic sponge is used when a light coverage is required. For example a camouflage treatment for rosacea to give a natural look will allow some of the skin's natural colouring to show through.

There are many methods for applying camouflage make-up and whichever method is chosen it will require a lot of practice to become proficient. There are a few basic principles which the therapist should observe:

- Always thoroughly prepare the area before treatment with cleansing, toning and moisturising procedures but avoid putting moisturiser directly over the scar.
- Always study the skin colour and type of disfigurement carefully.
- Always apply camouflage creams sparingly as this will achieve a more natural effect and is less likely to come off on clothing.
- Apply the creams in layers, setting between applications (except where an additional cream is to be added to the basic shade as in the case of toning-in with a surrounding area, in which case the powder is applied at the end).
- Always allow a few minutes for the products to set properly and then brush off the powder in a downward action.

The finger can be used in
several ways: in a rubbing
action, a pressing action or
in a stippling action. This
means that you can
control the amount of
surface stimulation of the
blood capillaries which is
very important in certain
conditions.

- Blot the area gently with damp cotton wool to remove any detectable traces of powder.
- Use either a brush, dampened cosmetic sponge or even a finger to apply cosmetic camouflage depending on the size and area of the treatment, and always work in a hygienic fashion.
- Use feathering strokes to fade-in the edges around the camouflage area.
- Always explain procedures to the client and give home care advice on general skin care, removal, application at home, etc.
- Ask the client to book in for a further consultation so that any queries can be dealt with and you can see how they are progressing with their application techniques.

GOOD PRACTICE

- Remember to try to contain the cosmetics to the area requiring camouflage for the most natural effect.
- The appearance of stubble will sometimes need to be added to men and this can be achieved by carefully stippling a grey coloured cream.

ACTIVITY

With a colleague, practise camouflaging disfigurements such as freckles, scars, birthmarks, etc. Take the role of the client and therapist and carry out a detailed consultation. Evaluate your findings.

Home care advice

1 Camouflage make-up should be removed thoroughly with an appropriate product.
2 Be careful with soap or soap-based products as these can sometimes dislodge the creams.
3 When drying with a towel after bathing or swimming always pat dry and do not rub the camouflaged area.
4 Climate can have an effect on the durability of the products as heat tends to loosen the creams more readily. For this reason a client will need to take great care whilst in any hot environment.

POINT TO NOTE

Artificial freckles sometimes need to be added to restore balance to the face.

Prosthetics

This is the term used to describe any manufactured appendage used to enhance or complete the human body. Obvious examples include artificial limbs, but false nails and eyelashes also fall into the category and an understanding of the filament prostheses available will be of benefit to the camouflage therapist.

1 State the main conditions you may encounter in the field of camouflage make-up.
2 Give three important points to consider when selecting camouflage creams.
3 Explain the importance of lighting when carrying out a camouflage make-up treatment.
4 Give four classifications of skin colour and explain two characteristics of each.

Key Terms

You need to know what these words and phrases mean. Go back through the chapter to find out.

- Blending techniques
- Cosmetic camouflage
- Client consultation
- Equipment required for camouflage
- Matching skin colour
- Prosthetics
- Remedial camouflage conditions

AROMATHERAPY

After working through this chapter you will be able to:

- define an essential oil
- outline the factors governing the quality of essential oils
- describe the effects of the main chemical categories of essential oils
- describe the main qualities of a selected number of essential oils
- describe the qualities of a number of carrier oils
- select the amounts of carrier and essential oil for massage
- carry out a consultation for an aromatherapy massage
- prepare a plan for an aromatherapy massage
- select oils which blend together well for aromatherapy massage
- prepare a client for aromatherapy massage
- adapt the principles of body massage to aromatherapy massage
- outline the basic principles of shiatsu pressures
- apply these principles to body massage
- apply these principles to face and scalp massage
- apply these principles to massage of selected parts of the body
- give home advice to clients following aromatherapy massage
- describe other therapeutic ways of using essential oils
- recognise how aromatherapy is being used in medical settings.

Aromatherapy is the name given to treatments that use essential oils – the pure, volatile portions of aromatic plant products. There has been a huge surge of interest in such treatments as part of the growing regard for holistic therapies and complementary medicine. There are many books and courses now for anyone interested in becoming an aromatherapist; beauty therapists, massage therapists and medical personnel such as nurses, occupational therapists and chartered physiotherapists are all becoming involved. It is a subject which can be studied to many levels, so that some people will call themselves aromatherapists who have only a limited knowledge of oils and others will have studied and practised for many years. As more people become aware of the benefits of aromatherapy, training standards will be raised and the levels standardised with a full qualification necessary to practise.

This chapter is meant to provide a starting point for the beginner and to provide a basis for future development. As with other therapies, learning must start somewhere but should never stop. Aromatherapy becomes more fascinating the more you learn.

Skin absorption

There are many factors which determine how much of a chemical penetrates the skin. Some of these factors are:

- the amount and concentration of the chemical applied
- the length of time the chemical is in contact with the skin
- the skin's temperature and moisture content
- the concentration of hair follicles and sweat ducts in the skin in the area where the chemical is applied
- whether the skin is damaged in any way.

All of these are likely to affect the absorption of substances such as aromatherapy oils.

Although there is little information on the absorption of essential oils as such, there has been research on the skin penetration of fragrance chemicals. This research shows that absorption is greater over areas of thinner, more delicate skin, such as that on the face and eyelids, and less on the thicker skin on the palms of the hands and soles of the feet. Children's skin is more permeable than adults'.

The two major factors governing the level of absorption of such chemicals by the skin appear to be the strength of the dose applied and the size of the area to which it is applied. Massage and heat may also encourage absorption as will covering the area with clothes or towels.

Allergy

Substances applied to the skin may cause the skin to react allergically against the substance. The reaction of some of the cells of the dermis is to release histamine, causing the tissue to become red, warm and swollen. The first contact with the substance may leave the tissue sensitised so that later contact can cause a more severe and generalised reaction. Once a person has become sensitised to a substance it must be completely avoided.

GOOD PRACTICE

- Clients should always be asked if they are allergic to any substances used in products being applied to the skin. If there is any doubt, perform a patch test. Apply some of the substance to a small patch of skin and check for any reaction after 24 hours.
- Aromatherapy products which contain the essential oils of plants are often considered safe because they are pure and natural. However they are potent, concentrated, natural chemicals and some can be toxic. For example, the oil from the pennyroyal plant contains a liver toxin and cinnamon bark oil can cause allergic skin reactions. The contraindications of individual oils must be checked before use on the skin.
- The commonest way of applying these essential oils is by massage which increases the flow of blood to the area and this may enhance absorption of the substances into the body.

Photosensitivity

Certain chemicals cause the skin to react more strongly than usual when exposed to sunlight. The best known of these used in perfumery and aromatherapy is oil of bergamot. The result can be 'sunburn' or a rash after a very short exposure to ultra-violet light. It follows that any product containing a photosensitiser should not be applied to the skin before exposure to natural or artificial sunlight (e.g. a sun-bed).

Because essential oils are said to be good for physical and mental conditions there is a temptation for the practitioner to regard aromatherapy as a form of medicine. If that were so, then beauty therapists and those without some medical training would not be using it. Aromatherapy is the use of essential oils to help maintain people in good health and to improve their wellbeing. Clients with medical conditions should always be referred to their doctor.

Essential oils

Essential oils are aromatic substances present at very low concentrations in different parts of plants: in leaves, flower petals, berries and even twigs. When they are extracted from plants and bottled as pure essential oils, their concentration is 100%. They are available for purchase in this form by the general public as well as aromatherapists and should always be adequately diluted for safe use.

Extraction
Oils are extracted from plants by several different methods.

Expression
A few essential oils, such as the citrus oils where the oil is contained in the outer part of the skin, can be obtained by simple pressure. (Examples: lemon, orange, bergamot.)

Distillation
Some essential oils are obtained by distillation. The plant parts are heated in water or steam and the vapour given off is cooled to produce a liquid which is a mixture of essential oil and water. The essential oil can then be easily separated and drawn off to leave perfumed water behind as a by-product.

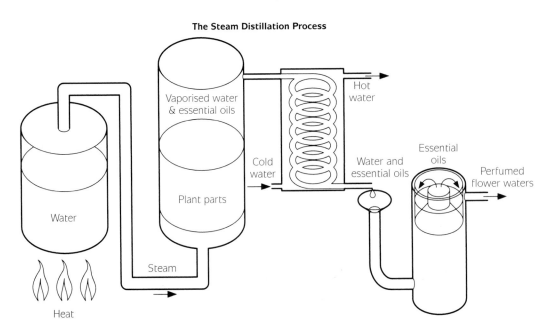

The Steam Distillation Process

Fig. 11.1 *Distillation of essential oils*

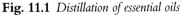

Solvent extraction

Solvent extraction is a method used to obtain some floral oils. The plants are immersed in hydrocarbon solvents to dissolve the essential oils. The solution is then distilled to leave behind a mixture of wax and oil known as a 'concrete'. The wax can then be dissolved in alcohol which in turn can be evaporated off leaving an 'absolute'. Absolutes differ from true essential oils in that they are generally thicker and more viscous. They are more often used in perfumery than in aromatherapy.

More recently carbon dioxide has been used as a solvent to extract essential oils successfully. By using carbon dioxide in a state known as 'hypercritical' at high pressure, it becomes a very effective solvent which does not contaminate the oils. This method requires bulky and expensive equipment but the number of essential oils extracted by this method that are commercially available is increasing.

Enfleurage

Enfleurage is a traditional method of extraction that is only used today for some very expensive oils such as rose and jasmine. It involves spreading the petals of the plant on fat or oil which absorbs the essence and then extracting it from the fat by using solvents to separate them. However even rose and jasmine these days are mostly extracted by the more commercial solvent or distillation methods.

Quality

The quality of essential oils is most important and care must be taken to use only oils which are pure and unadulterated. The best advice when starting is to deal only with a reputable supplier who is known to stock oils of the highest quality. Good suppliers are also the best source of advice on which oils to order, for example there are a number of different oils called lavender each with its own qualities and a good supplier will be able to advise you of the differences.

All plants have a common English name and a recognised scientific Latin name which identifies it more accurately and it is wise to become familiar with the Latin name to avoid mistakes when ordering and using the oils.

Factors which can affect the quality of oils include:

- choice of the best possible member of the plant species
- where the plant was grown
- whether it was grown organically

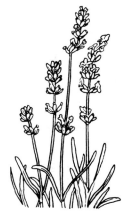 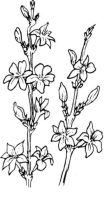

Fig. 11.2 *Lavender and jasmine*

- how it was harvested and at what time of day
- what method of extraction was used
- how the oils have been stored.

Categories of oils

There are a number of ways of classifying oils

1 By their volatility rate – that is how quickly they evaporate into the air.

   Top notes evaporate the fastest, act quickly and tend to be stimulating. Examples: lemon and other citrus oils.

   Middle notes evaporate more slowly and are most often used to help the general metabolism. Examples: geranium and other floral and fruity oils.

   Base notes evaporate slowly and are relaxed and sedating. Example: sandalwood.

   Some therapists will take this into account when mixing a blend of oils, using a base note oil to hold and 'fix' a top note oil. If you smell a mixture of oils containing different 'notes', you will smell the top notes first followed by the middle and base notes.

2 By the eastern yin and yang philosophy. The terms yin and yang are descriptions of opposite 'energies' or qualities. Yin describes cool, moist, calming, feminine qualities (e.g. rose, geranium), whereas yang describes hot, dry, stimulating, masculine qualities (e.g. juniper). Many oils fall between these extremes and the nearer they are to the middle the more 'balancing' they will (e.g. sandalwood). Some therapists take this into account when selecting oils for a particular client and when deciding what effects they need to produce – calming, balancing or stimulating.

3 By the chemical constituents of the oils. This is a much more complex matter as each essential oil will consist of many chemical components which may even vary in oils of the same name depending on where the plant was grown and under what conditions.

Oils contain chemicals in varying proportions and tend to be classified according to which of the chemicals is predominant. These chemicals can be put in place on a chart according to their general yin or yang qualities. The chemicals also have general effects which can be described. Fig. 11.3 summarises the effects of certain chemicals and shows their relation to the yin and yang qualities.

Selection of oils for use

Selection of oils for use with a particular client is the most important part of aromatherapy and can be very daunting for the beginner.

When starting, select from the limited list, 8–10 oils should be enough, growing to 15–20 as experience increases. In the selection you choose include more calming and balancing oils than stimulating oils, select the more commonly used oils and be guided by a good supplier. Make sure you know if any of the oils have any contraindications or can have harmful effects.

A possible list might include the following oils. The oils are listed alphabetically along with their Latin names, predominant chemical category, their best known effects and some of the oils that can be used with them to make a good blend.

YIN (calming)

Aldehydes – anti-inflammatory, antiseptic, anti-rheumatic, very calming and soothing.

Ketones – healing, good for skin and scars, sedative, loosens mucous and softens fat, so often used for people with bronchitis and cellulite. **(Ketones should not be used for too long or in high concentrations when they may be toxic.)**

Esters – the most widespread group of chemicals found in essential oils; anti-spasmodic, anti-inflammatory, anti-parasitic, cooling and soothing.

Ethers – anti-inflammatory, anti-spasmodic and anti-stress.

Sesquiterpenes – anti-inflammatory, anti-allergic, anti-parasitic; good for people with heart conditions and asthma.

——— Balancing line ———

Sesquialcohols – act as a general tonic.

Alcohols – germicidal; some are very stimulating, but others are much less so.

Terpenes – antiseptic and anti-inflammatory; they can help to improve the blood and lymphatic circulation.

Oxides – expectorant and decongestant, helping people to cough. Some are anti-parasitic, anti-viral and antiseptic.

Phenols – anti-bacterial, anti-viral, antifungal and anti-parasitic. **(Oils in the phenol category are very stimulating and are never used in aromatherapy massage.)**

YANG (stimulating)

Fig. 11.3 *The properties of essential oils*

Yin oils

Basil (*Ocimum basilicum*) – top note, ether.

- Steadying, good for nervous clients, good for muscle aches and pains and for coughs and colds.
- Blends well with bergamot, geranium.

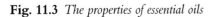

GOOD PRACTICE

Basil should not be used during pregnancy.

Bergamot (*Citrus aurantium bergamia*) – top note, ester.

- Uplifting; good for people who are anxious or depressed and having difficulty sleeping.
- Blends well with lavender, neroli, basil.

GOOD PRACTICE

- Bergamot has been shown to sensitise skin to ultra-violet so do not use within three hours of going out into the sun or using a sun-bed.
- Bergamot should not be used on children.

Clary sage (*Salvia sclarea*) – middle to base note, ester.

- Good for exhaustion and overwork, a good muscle relaxant, anti-depressant.
- Blends well with citrus oils, frankincense, geranium, juniper.

Chamomile (*Matricaria chamomilla*) – middle note, sesquiterpene.

- Soothing; a very gentle oil, good on the skin, very calming and good for people suffering from tension, anxiety and related conditions.
- Blends well with lavender, patchouli, geranium, benzoin.

Lavender (*Lavandula angustifolia*) – middle note, ester.

- Boosts the immune system, calming, balancing, healing (especially burns), muscular pain, problem skins. The most versatile and useful oil.
- Blends well with other oils especially floral and citrus oils.

Lemon grass (*Cymbopogon citratus*) – top note, aldehyde.

- Strengthening; good for muscle aches and pains, stomach upsets.
- Blends well with geranium, lavender.

Peppermint (*Mentha piperita*) – top to middle note, ketone.

- Cooling; traditionally used for stomach upsets, also for clearing the head and for coughs and colds. Very good for tired feet.
- Blends well with benzoin, rosemary.

Petitgrain (*Citrus aurantium*) – top note, ester

- Anti-stress, good for oily skins and stomach upsets.
- Blends well with rosemary, lavender, geranium, bergamot, clary sage.

Rose geranium (*Pelargonium graveolens*) – middle note, alcohol/ester.

- Balancing; good for dry and red skins, it stimulates the lymphatic system and can be used for cellulite.
- Blends well with most oils, especially citrus oils, lavender, bergamot and basil.

Rosemary (*Rosemarinus officianalis*) – middle note, ketone.

- Uplifting – after lavender, the most commonly used oil. It is useful for people with colds or other respiratory problems. Good for stiffness and discomfort in the muscles.
- Blends well with basil, citrus oils, frankincense, peppermint.

Yang oils

Black pepper (*Piper nigrum*) – middle note, terpene.

- Stimulating, good for the circulation and conditions related to poor circulation. Can stimulate the appetite.
- Blends well with frankincense, sandalwood.

Eucalyptus (*Eucalyptus globulus* or *radiata*) – top note, oxide.

- Decongestant helping people with colds or bronchitis to cough. Also relieves muscular or rheumatic pain.
- Blends well with benzoin, lavender, pine.

Frankincense (*Boswellia carteri*) – base note, terpene.

- Rejuvenating, very good on older skins, good for chest conditions – especially stress-related ones.
- Blends well with basil, black pepper, citrus oils, lavender, sandalwood.

Juniper (*Juniperus communis*) – middle note, terpene

- Diuretic, good for people with fluid retention or cellulite and can be helpful in cases of cystitis. Good on some problem skins, e.g. acne. Can be used as a disinfectant.
- Blends well with benzoin, lavender, sandalwood.

Lemon (*Citrus limon*) – top note, terpene

- Useful for clients recovering from viral-type illnesses. Also stimulates the circulation, so useful over areas of fat and cellulite and in rheumatic conditions. Refreshing.
- Blends well with lavender, neroli, ylang ylang.

Rosewood (*Aniba roseadora*) – middle note, alcohol.

- Gentle, very good for skin and stress-related conditions.
- Blends well with most oils, especially citrus and floral oils.

Sandalwood (*Santalum album*) – base note, sesquialcohol.

- Balancing; good on the skin and for stress-related conditions and nervous tension.
- Blends well with lavender, black pepper, bergamot, geranium.

Tea tree (*Melaleuca alternifolia*) – top note, alcohol.

- One of the best known of the essential oils and now being incorporated into creams and soaps for its anti-fungal, anti-bacterial and anti-viral qualities. Particularly useful in helping fungal conditions such as thrush and athlete's foot. It seems to stimulate the immune system and is particularly valuable if a cold or flu might be developing.
- Blends well with lavender, rosemary, clary sage.

Ylang ylang (*Cananga odorata*) – base note, sesquialcohol.

- Warming; soothes and boosts confidence, traditionally known as an aphrodisiac.
- Blends well with rosewood, bergamot.

Oils such as rose, melissa and jasmine are much too expensive to include in a starting list.

GOOD PRACTICE

Note that some of these oils are contraindicated during pregnancy. Until fully qualified it is wise to avoid using essential oils to treat children and women who are pregnant or breast feeding.

Progress Check

Check that you remember the main effects of each of the chemical categories.

Aldehydes	Sesquialcohols	Alcohols
Ketones	Sesquiterpenes	Terpenes
Esters	Oxides	Phenols
Ethers		

Carrier oils

Essential oils are very concentrated and should never be used undiluted on the skin. For an aromatherapy massage they must be mixed with a carrier oil which will provide lubrication for the massage as well as carrying the therapeutic essential oils being used.

Although mineral oils such as baby oil are sometimes used for massage they are not suitable as carrier oils as they are not easily absorbed by the skin. You can use any vegetable oil so long as it is fairly light and does not have a strong smell which would overpower the essential oils. Just as a good cook will insist that the olive oil they use should be of the finest quality, so an aromatherapist will use only carrier oils that are organically grown, unrefined and cold pressed. Again, the advice of a reputable supplier is invaluable.

The carrier oil chosen can be used on its own with the essential oils or can have small amounts of other oils mixed with them. When beginning to mix oils, grapeseed oil is probably best used as a carrier oil as it is easily available and not expensive. Sweet almond oil is also an excellent choice. Other oils may be mixed with the carrier oils in small amounts before blending in the essential oils.

Examples are:

- Apricot/peach kernel oil contains vitamins A and minerals. It is beneficial to mature, dry skins but can be used on all skin types.
- Calendula oil has anti-inflammatory properties and is beneficial for cracked dry skin and as a base for treating dry eczema.
- Grapeseed oil contains a high percentage of linoleic acid and a small amount of vitamin E. It is light in texture and non-greasy, making it a very popular carrier oil.
- Jojoba oil contains vitamin E and has anti-inflammatory properties. It is beneficial for psoriasis, eczema, arthritis, rheumatism and dry skins. It is also an anti-oxidant useful for clients with wheat allergy.
- Sunflower oil contains vitamins A, B, D and E and is high in fatty acids. It is a light, non-greasy texture and is suitable for all skin types.
- Sweet almond oil is rich in protein, containing vitamins A, B1, B2 and B6 and a small amount of vitamin E. It nourishes and protects all skin types and has a calming effect on skin irritations.

POINT TO NOTE

All of the above carrier oils can be used on their own to make up 100% of the carrier oil mix or with other oils.

- Avocado oil contains vitamins A, B and D and is also rich in lecithin. It is rich and nourishing and is especially good for dry, dehydrated or ageing skins.
- Carrot oil contains vitamins A, B, C, D and E and fatty acids. It is beneficial for dry skins, psoriasis and eczema.
- Evening primrose oil is a rich source of gamma linoleic acid and vitamins. It is beneficial for dry scaly skins, psoriasis and eczema and mature skins.
- Wheatgerm oil contains vitamins, minerals and proteins and, in particular, it has a very high content of vitamin E and is beneficial for scarred or dry and mature skin. It is an anti-oxidant and so acts to prevent other oils going rancid.

POINTS TO NOTE

- If any of these oils are to be used, they are usually added to the carrier oil in the proportion 10% to 90% main carrier.
- All vegetable carrier oils will go off and become rancid eventually and will become unfit for use. They should be kept cool and not mixed with essential oils until ready for use.
- Carrier oils have a limited life shelf of approximately six months as they all oxidise with exposure to air.
- Carrier oils should be carefully selected to complement the essential oils and the condition of the client's skin.

To prepare a blend for massage you will need:

- A glass measuring bottle that is marked in millilitres.
- A glass rod for stirring.

The amount of carrier oil needed for the massage is measured into the bottle and the drops of essential oils added. It is then stirred with the glass rod or shaken if there is a stopper, and then it is ready for use.

Amounts of oil needed for massage will vary but a useful 'rule of thumb' is: for a full body massage allow 10 ml for a small person, 14 ml for a medium size and up to 20 ml for a large person. In women, the dress size is a good indicator.

Try not to mix too much oil as it will be wasted.

For body massage the essential oils should form 2% of the blend. It is not practical to measure the essential oils in millilitres as 2% of essential oil in 10 ml of carrier oil would be 0.2 ml. The essential oils are therefore measured in drops. 1% of essential oils in 10 ml of carrier is 2.5 drops and 2% in 10 ml of carrier is 5 drops. So if you divide the millilitres of carrier oil by two the answer gives you the same number of drops of essential oils to give a 2% solution, i.e. up to 5 drops of essential oils can be added to 10 ml of carrier, up to 7 drops in 14 ml and up to 10 drops in 20 ml.

For facial massage the essential oils should form 1% of the blend, half the strength of that used for the body.

The scalp can be treated with a 2% blend and will need at least 5 ml of carrier oil as the hair tends to absorb some. Or, if face and scalp are being treated at the same time, a 1% blend can be used for both.

The oils selected for use are always the result of a careful consultation process which will take into account client preference. One, two or three essential oils may be used to make up a blend.

Factors to be considered in making up a blend

- Appropriate choice of essential and carrier oils for condition of client.
- Fragrance of individual oils acceptable to client.
- Fragrance of mix of oils acceptable to client.
- Oils with very strong fragrance used in small amounts so that they do not dominate, e.g. eucalyptus.
- Oils that complement each other.

The selection and blending of oils for use with a particular client is the most important part of the aromatherapy treatment. Some oils blend together well and are said to be acting synergistically as they seem to help each other's effects. Other oils may inhibit each other's effects and do not blend so well together. If a start is made by using the oils that the client is attracted to and which fit into the category that will help the main problems the client presents, then that is an excellent start.

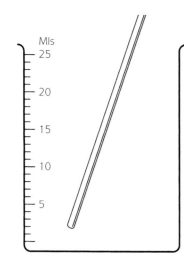

Fig. 11.4 *Mixing equipment*

Examples of oils that work well together are given in the lists of essential oils.

An example of selecting a blend may be for a client who has worries at work and gets constant cold-like symptoms:

● Select the general categories that suit the problems, i.e. an ester for the cooling, soothing qualities, an oxide to help the cold symptoms and maybe a ketone to loosen mucus if the cold is a chesty one.

● From the available oils, choose the ones that the client likes and that you think will go well together, e.g. lavender, eucalyptus and rosemary.

Experience will lead you to an instinctive blend of oils.

Consultation

ACTIVITY
Re-read Chapter 3 on consultation procedures.

The consultation process is especially important in clients attending for aromatherapy massage. This is because the effects of massage and the effects of the essential oils have to be considered.

The purpose of the consultation is to find out firstly that it is safe to treat the client and secondly how best to help the client.

Consultation should take into account:

1 The medical background: contraindications, problem areas.
2 Lifestyle.
3 Personality: temperament, emotional state.

POINT TO NOTE

Check for contraindications to specific oils as well as to the massage itself.

The consultation procedure to establish the medical background is fully covered in Chapter 3.

Lifestyle and personality

Information about lifestyle and personality helps to give an overall picture of the person and indicates how you may best help them. Questions should not be too direct or probing but should be open questions allowing the client to express themselves fully.

Examples of open questions are:

- What do you feel the problem is?
- How do you think aromatherapy can help you?
- What makes you feel good/bad?

Most questions beginning with 'how', 'why', 'where', 'what', 'when' will be open questions that will give the client the opportunity to talk. Any question that can elicit the answer yes or no is a closed question. Listen to what the client wants and how they perceive their problem.

One useful way of asking how a client feels emotionally is to ask them to consider how they feel on a scale of 1–10 on a bad day, a good day and at the present time.

POINT TO NOTE

Consultation is an ongoing process which should continue throughout treatment.

Any counselling skills that you can acquire will be of real use here in dealing with clients who have problems.

Contraindications

to treatment with essential oils

- Any condition requiring medical attention.
- Broken skin.
- Skin infections/diseases.
- Swellings.
- Severe bruising.
- Recent scar tissue.
- Fractured bones.
- Varicose veins.
- Alcohol in bloodstream.
- Fever/unwell.
- Thrombosis.
- Diabetes.
- Severe circulatory disease.
- Recent inoculations.
- Hepatitis/liver problems.
- Pregnancy (treatment should not be given in the early stages of pregnancy and care in latter stages should be taken on selection of oils as some are contraindicated during pregnancy).
- Young children (treatment of babies and young children is a very specialised area and should be given only by those qualified in advanced aromatherapy).
- Clients with nut or wheat allergies.
- Sunburn.

**AROMATHERAPY
CLIENT RECORD CARD I**

Name of client: First .... Last .... Name of therapist ....

Address of client ....

Telephone .... Date .... Date of birth: Month .... Day ....

☐ Under 21
☐ 21–30
☐ 31–40
☐ 41–50
☐ over 50

The following profile should be completed for all clients. This is to correctly evaluate the client's special needs in both salon treatment and home maintenance. This is completely confidential and to be used only for this analysis.

1.	MEDICATION: Are you taking any tablets or pills prescribed by a doctor? if YES, please give details. If NO, please indicate if you have had a need to visit a doctor in the last 6 months, or visit a dentist in the last 3 weeks.
2.	FEMALE: When is your period due? If your periods have stopped, please indicate whether naturally or surgically.
3.	CHILDREN: Please give ages.
4.	ALLERGIES: Any known allergies in your family (asthma, hayfever, etc.)? Do you smoke – or have you smoked in the past?
5.	OCCUPATION: Please give details/type of occupation (sitting, standing, driving).
6.	SLEEP: Please give details of your sleep pattern
7.	EATING: Please give details of your eating pattern, times, etc., also amount of fluid intake daily.
8.	HEADACHES: Do you get headaches? Do you experience motion sickness or fear of falling? Do you wear contact lenses or glasses?
9.	EXERCISE: Do you take regular exercise?
10.	HABITS: Are there any habits you might be aware of (biting nails, biting lip etc.)?

The above information will help us to recommend the correct essential oil blend and treatment for your personal needs

PLEASE INDICATE THAT THE ABOVE INFORMATION IS CORRECT BY SIGNING HERE

Signature .... Date ....

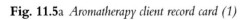

Fig. 11.5a *Aromatherapy client record card (1)*

**AROMATHERAPY
CLIENT RECORD CARD II**

Client: ....

Therapist: ....

TREATMENT OBSERVATIONS

POSTURE   Standing
                Sitting
                Walking
                Lying on couch

Hands/Arms
Legs
Feet
Back
Face
Neck

BLEND/FORMULATION RECOMMENDED

COMPARATIVE ANALYSIS

Foot chart

Right foot   Left foot

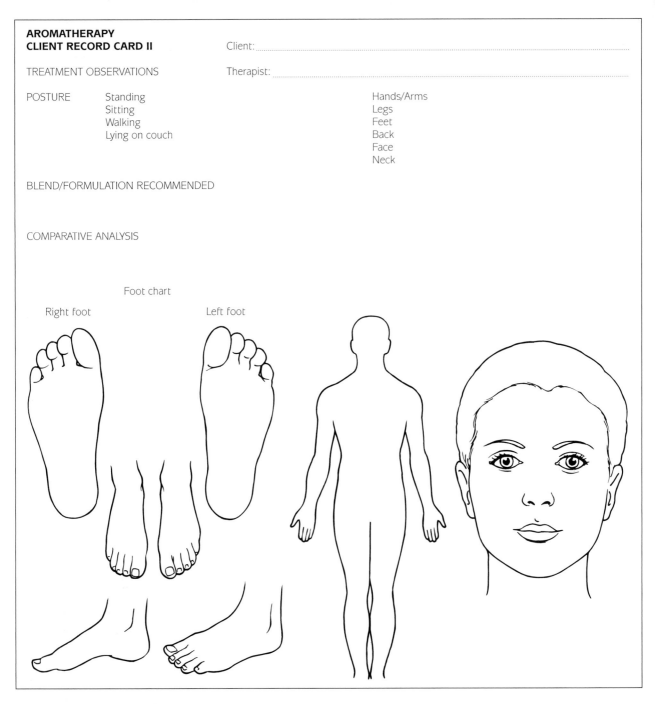

Fig. 11.5b *Aromatherapy client record card (2)*

AROMATHERAPY CLIENT RECORD CARD III   Client: ....

Date:			
Treatment given:			
Advice given to client after treatment:			
Essential oils recommended for use at home:			
Directions given on their use at home:			
Bathtime blends recommended:			
Complementary treatments recommended:			
Products purchased:			
Return treatment recommended:			
Therapist:			

Fig. 11.5c *Aromatherapy client record card (3)*

Progress Check

With a colleague acting as a client, carry out a consultation with the aim of selecting suitable oils for the client. Ask the colleague to explain how effective the questions were in eliciting relevant information.

Treatment plan following full consultation

- Decide on the aims of treatment, focusing on the client's main and secondary problems.
- List the essential oils suitable for use with these problems.
- Select two or three compatible oils from this list.
- Ask the client to smell and approve each individual oil.
- Ask the client to smell and approve the oils together.

Decide treatment method:

- Full body massage.
- Full body massage with facial massage.
- Part body massage.

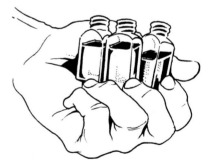

Fig. 11.6 *Letting the client smell the selection*

Agree time scale and charges with client
Many clients may feel uncomfortable if the therapist assumes that there will be a series of treatments. Always ask if a client wants to book a series or individual treatments.

POINT TO NOTE

It is important to consider the client's availability when discussing the length and number of treatments.

Once the treatment method and time scale have been decided the treatment plan is carried out.

Complementary home care advice should be given with the opportunity to purchase aromatherapy products. Advice might include the use of a bath oil that will complement the treatment or the use of an aromatic burner with appropriate oils.

Example

Following full consultation with a middle-aged, female client you decide the aims of treatment are:

1 General relaxation (very busy, tense lifestyle).
2 Improve sluggish circulation (cold hands and feet).

Time scale/financial constraints

- Ideally over a period of six weeks.
- Full body aromatherapy massage every other week alternating with an aromatherapy facial treatment.
- Costs will be as per clinic price list.

POINT TO NOTE

Courses of treatments paid for in advance act as an incentive to the client and help the therapist.

Suitable oils to use for relaxation are:
- Lavender.
- Rose geranium.
- Bergamot.

Suitable oils to use to stimulate the circulation are:
- Rosemary.
- Juniper.
- Black pepper.

Ask the client to smell each oil briefly and reject any not liked.

Select two oils the client has approved, one from each group, say lavender and rosemary, and let client smell them together. If the combination is approved by the client the oils can be mixed.

- For the full body massage, in 15 ml carrier oil mix five drops of lavender and two of rosemary.
- For the facial massage, in 6 ml of carrier oil mix two drops of lavender and one of rosemary.

More than two essential oils can be used but not more than four. If three oils are preferred for the body massage the blend may be: four drops lavender, two drops rosemary, one drop bergamot.

POINT TO NOTE

Bergamot must not be used on skin to be exposed to natural or artificial sunlight.

Offer to mix oils or products for home use or take the opportunity to sell aromatherapy products. When the client returns for the next treatment always discuss the effects of the previous treatment and be ready to adjust the oils and method of application to suit the client's needs.

Other useful essential oils

Less common essential oils are listed here in alphabetical order along with their Latin names, predominant chemical category and the effects they are best known for.

Aniseed (*Pimpinella anisum*) – middle note, ester.

- Warming, antiseptic, expectorant.

Benzoin (*Styrax bensoin*) – base note, ester.
- Anti-inflammatory, warming, good for joint conditions, colds and the skin.
- Blends well with sandalwood.

Cedarwood (*Cedrus atlantica*) – base note, terpene.
- Antiseptic, astringent, expectorant, bronchial and urinary infections, catarrh.
- Blends well with rosewood, bergamot, ylang ylang.

Cinnamon (*Cinamomum zeylanicum*) – middle note, aldehyde.
- Astringent, stimulant (circulatory, cardiac and respiratory), poor circulation, rheumatism.
- Blends well with ylang ylang, mandarin, benzoin.

Clove (*Syzygium aromaticum*) – middle note, ketone.
- Anti-histamine, anti-oxidant, antiseptic, nausea, rheumatism.
- Blends well with rose, clary sage, bergamot.

Cypress (*Cupressus sempervirens*) – middle to base note, terpene.
- Anti-rheumatic, vasoconstrictor, diuretic.
- Blends well with juniper, lavender, pine.

Fennel (*Feniculum vulgare*) – middle note, ether.
- Eases wind and stomach upsets, traditionally used for obesity.
- Blends well with geranium, lavender, sandalwood.

Fennel, sweet (*Foeniculum vulgare*) – top note, terpene
- Diuretic, detoxifying, cellulite, nausea, odema, amenorrhoea.
- Blends well with geranium, rose, lavender.

Geranium (*Pelargonium graveolens*) – middle note, ester.
- Anti-depressant, antiseptic, acne and oily skin, pre-menstrual tension, eczema.
- Blends well with lavender, patchouli, neroli.

Immortelle (*Helichrysum angustifolium*) – middle note, ketone.

- Expectorant, good for aches and pains, skin conditions and breaks in the skin.
- Blends well with chamomile, clary sage, geranium and lavender.

Jasmine (*Jasminium grandiflorum*) – middle note, ester.

- Relaxant, anti-depressant, sedative, coughs, muscular spasm.
- Blends well with rose, sandalwood, citrus.

Mandarin (*Citrus reticulata*) – top note, ether.

- Antiseptic, sedative.
- Blends well with other citrus oils such as neroli.

Marjoram (*Origanum majorana*) – middle note, alcohol.

- Warming, sedative, soothing, good for joint conditions.
- Blends well with lavender, rosemary, cypress and eucalyptus.

GOOD PRACTICE

Marjoram and cinnamon should not be used during pregnancy.

Melissa (*Melissa officinalis*) – middle note, terpene.

- Asthma, coughs, menstrual problems, eczema and skin problems.
- Blends well with lavender, geranium, citrus.

Myrrh (*Commiphora myrrha*) – base note, sesquiterpene.

- Healing, good for the chest, sedative.
- Blends well with frankincense, sandalwood, benzoin, juniper.

GOOD PRACTICE

Myrrh should not be used during pregnancy.

Myrtle (*Myrtis communis*) – middle note, oxide.

- Good for catarrh, slightly sedative, soothing.
- Blends well with begamot, lavender, rosemary and clary sage.

Neroli or orange blossom (*Citrus aurantium*) – base note, alcohol.

- Calming, anti-stress, good for shock and depression.
- Blends well with most oils.

Niaouli (*Melaleuca viridiflora*) – top note, terpene.

- Antiseptic acne, respiratory problems, poor circulation.
- Blends well with lavender, rosemary, clove.

Orange, sweet (*Citrus sinensis*) – top note, terpene.

- Anti-depressant, digestive problems, oily skins, cold, flu.
- Blends well with lavender, geranium.

Patchouli (*Pogostemon cablin*) – base note, sesquialcohol.

- Good for depression, anxiety, healing skin.
- Blends well with vetiver, sandalwood, geranium, neroli.

Pine (*Pinus sylvestris*) – middle note, terpene.

- Good for colds and chest infections, stimulating.
- Blends well with tea tree, rosemary, lavender, juniper.

Rose otto (*Rosa damascena*) – middle note, ester.

- Astringent, thrush, labour pains, period pains, menopause, anxiety, insomnia.
- Blends well with jasmine, bergamot, lavender, clary sage.

Sandalwood (*Santalum album*) – base note, terpene.

- Astringent, expectorant, catarrah, coughs.
- Blends well with black pepper, clove, jasmine.

Thyme (*Thymus vulgaris*) top note, terpene.

- Coughs, sinusitis, poor circulation, bruise cellulite.
- Blends well with lemon, rosemary, melissa.

Valerian (*Valeriana fauriei*) – top note, ester.

- Anti-spasmodic, bactericidal, sedative, insomnia, nervous indigestion.
- Blends well with pine, lavender, rosemary.

Vetiver (*Vetiveria zizanoides*) – middle note, sesquialcohol.

- Calming, stimulates the circulatory system.
- Blends well with sandalwood, patchouili, lavender and clary sage.

Progress Check

1. What is an essential oil?
2. Give five factors governing the quality of an essential oil.
3. Select pairs of oils that would be suitable for use with clients who:
   a have a very stressed lifestyle
   b have problems sleeping
   c have weight and cellulite problems
   d tend to get stiff and sore after an activity such as gardening.

Aromatherapy massage

Although essential oils can be used in many ways, massage is the most important and commonly used method of applying them in aromatherapy. This is because massage combines the therapeutic power of touch with the properties of the oils. Massage provides a very effective way of introducing the oils into the body. As the skin absorbs the oils, a useful amount will be taken into the bloodstream in the relatively short time that a body massage takes.

In general the conditions and legislation that cover the practice of aromatherapy will be the same as those covering the practice of massage.

The effects of aromatherapy massage will consist of:

- the effects of the massage
- the effects of the oils used.

Aromatherapy oils can be administered to the body using a typical body massage routine and different aromatherapists will have quite different techniques depending on their training and experience. However, in general the massage used in aromatherapy treatments is a relaxing massage using mainly effleurage and stroking movements and omitting the percussion and more vigorous petrissage movements. Instead of these more vigorous movements many therapists integrate finger pressures into their massage which may be called acupressure, shiatsu pressures or neuro-muscular techniques.

> **Contraindications**
>
> to aromatherapy massage will consist of:
>
> ♦ contraindications to massage
> ♦ contraindications to the oils to be used
> ♦ contraindications to acupressure.

Acupressure

Acupressure refers to many treatment systems that manipulate the acupuncture points on the body by pressure rather than by needles as is the case with acupuncture. The acu points are found along twelve pairs of meridians or channels which pass down the body. It is said that energies flow along these meridians which govern the body's systems.

When pressure is applied to a point on a meridian it stimulates local nerves and tissues and also influences the flow of energy through that and other meridians. The basic philosophy of acu points comes from

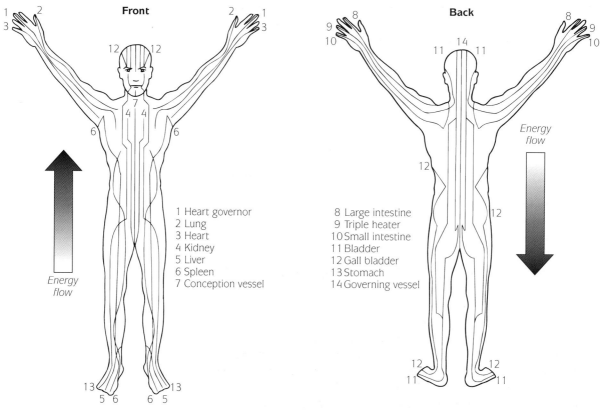

Front

Back

Energy flow

Energy flow

Energy flow

1 Heart governor
2 Lung
3 Heart
4 Kidney
5 Liver
6 Spleen
7 Conception vessel

8 Large intestine
9 Triple heater
10 Small intestine
11 Bladder
12 Gall bladder
13 Stomach
14 Governing vessel

Fig. 11.7 *The meridian system*

traditional Chinese systems of healing, however most Eastern societies will have pressures in their massage therapies.

Shiatsu

The Japanese word shiatsu (*shi* – finger, *atsu* – pressure) describes pressures on the acu points which may be applied with the fingers, other parts of the hand and even the elbows or feet. The massage itself is just one part of a whole philosophy of treatment attempting to return the energy, or chi, of the body to a state where yin (negative) and yang (positive) qualities are in balance.

A shiatsu treatment is very different from the usual Swedish-style massage. No oil is used and there are no smooth, flowing strokes; just pressure and stretching are used. However some shiatsu-type pressures applied with the fingers or the thumb can be integrated into a Western-style massage very successfully and more can be used as a knowledge of the meridian lines is gained. Sliding pressures applied with the thumb or the hand along meridians are particularly useful as oil is being used.

Pressures

The thumbs are the usual tools used for applying pressures as the acu points are mostly placed in thumb-sized hollows. In some areas a finger may be used, often supported by the adjacent finger. The heel of the hand may be used over larger areas such as the side of the buttocks.

Pressure should be applied in a firm, controlled manner with body weight controlling the amount of pressure. No poking or roughness should be used and pressure should be moderate to light. When sliding pressure is applied it should be even and the sliding movement steady with care being taken not to cause discomfort by pulling on hair or skin.

The client should breath out when pressure is applied to the back or chest and breath in between pressures.

Pressures are usually performed only once over the area whereas the traditional massage movements will be repeated a number of times depending on the time available and the speed of the strokes.

GOOD PRACTICE

Contraindications to pressures are the same as those for massage; don't press over any tender or fragile areas and if pain occurs, use very light pressure. Take care that nails do not dig in.

POINT TO NOTE

Use your eyes to check the client's responses to the pressure applied.

Routine for an aromatherapy treatment

- Consultation – which should take at least half an hour in the first instance.
- Complete consultation card.
- Obtain the client's signature.
- Check for contraindications to massage and oils.
- Select appropriate oils and check acceptability with the client.
- Mix oils and check acceptability with the client – mix enough 5% mixture for the body and 1% mixture for the face.
- Check that all necessary oils, creams, towels, cotton wool and tissues are close to hand.

- Suggest the client empties the bladder.
- An infra-red treatment may be given to warm the client, but saunas and steam baths are not suitable.
- The client should be lying supine, warm and well covered by towels.
- Cover the hair with a light, loose cloth or towel unless the scalp is to be included.
- If the scalp is to be included ask the client if oil may be used on the hair.
- Deep cleanse the face if facial massage is to be included.
- Place a little of the 1% oil mixture on the client's hands and ask them to inhale and lightly stroke the cheeks with the oil mixture. If there is only 2% mixture available apply a little to the client's upper lip.

The following aromatherapy routine is reproduced courtesy of the Eve Taylor Institute of Clinical Aromatherapy. Note the diagrams are for guidance only.

Back of legs movements

1 Start with the left leg. Using the base of your hands and commencing with your left hand, stroke up the back of the whole leg and follow through with your right hand to the popliteal area only. Repeat 3–6 times.

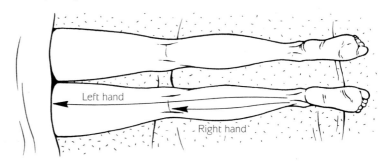

Fig. 11.8 *Movement 1*

2 Lift (about 15 cm/6 in) and support the client's ankle and using the palma pad of your hand, slide up the centre of the calf to the popliteal area. Repeat 3–6 times.

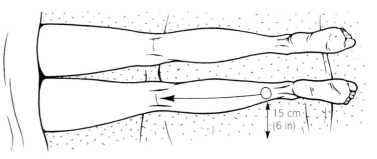

Fig. 11.9 *Movement 2*

3   Tilt your thumbs upwards and thumb slide from the ankle to the knee. Repeat 3–6 times.

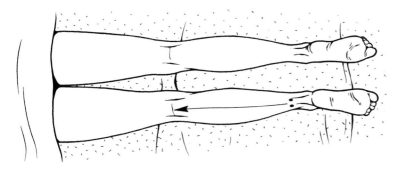

Fig. 11.10 *Movement 3*

4   Slide your fingers up and finger slide over the calf to the popliteal area.

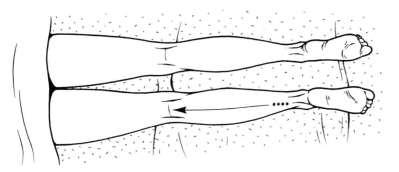

Fig. 11.11 *Movement 4*

5   Repeat movement 2 (Fig. 11.9).
6   Repeat movement 1 (Fig. 11.8).

Repeat movements 1–6 on the client's right leg.

Back movements
Group one: searching and finding

1   Using cushioned fingers, perform a figure-of-eight movement up and out over the client's back using both hands. Repeat 3–6 times.

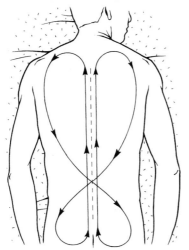

Fig. 11.12 *1 Figure-of-eight*

2   Using your thumbs, work down each side of the spine separately using a press and release movement. Repeat 3–4 times.

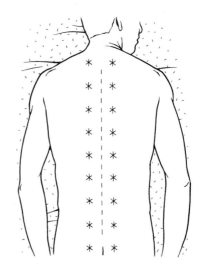

Fig. 11.13 *2 Thumb press, release and move*

3   Using your thumbs, work down each side of the spine separately using a press and slide movement. Repeat 3–4 times.

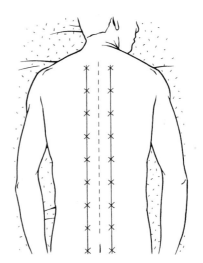

Fig. 11.14 *3 Thumb press and move*

Group two: heat movements

1   Using cushioned fingers and working both hands simultaneously on either side of the back, work up the upper back area. Repeat 3–4 times.
2   Using cushioned fingers, work one hand followed by the other up over one side of the upper back then repeat on the other side. Repeat 3–4 times.
3   Place one hand cupped like a pyramid over the base of the elimination area of the back whilst the other hand operates like a corkscrew twisting up and out over the upper back and shoulder area. Repeat on the other side. Repeat 3–4 times.

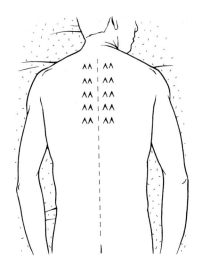

Fig. 11.15 *1 Double heat with cushioned fingers*

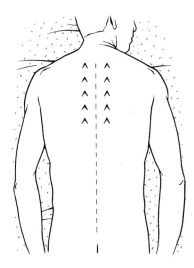

Fig. 11.16 *2 Single heat with cushioned fingers*

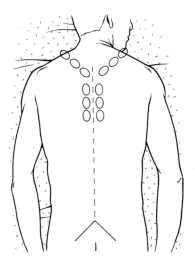

Fig. 11.17 *3 Pyramid and corkscrew movements*

Group three: erase, loosen and drain

1 Using the sides and base of your hands, loosen the connective tissue working by pumping from the spine out to the side of the body then repeat on the other side. Repeat 3–4 times.

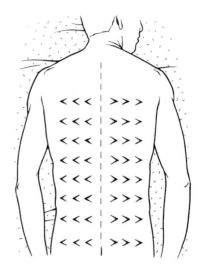

Fig. 11.18 *1 Loosen connective tissue*

2 Using cushioned fingers, drain from the spine out to the outside of the body, then repeat on the other side. Repeat 3–4 times.

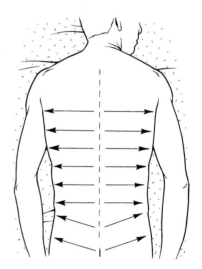

Fig. 11.19 *2 Slide out with cushioned fingers*

3 Spread your hand to make a fan shape and use your fingers to stroke up and out over one side of the lower back, quickly followed with alternate hands. Repeat this over the other side of the lower back. Repeat 3–4 times.

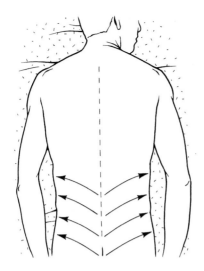

Fig. 11.20 *3 Repeated fan movements*

Movements on the neck

Support the client's head and check the five points on the base of the skull for sensitivity using the fingertips in a gentle pumping action. If there is any sensitivity, work the area gently.

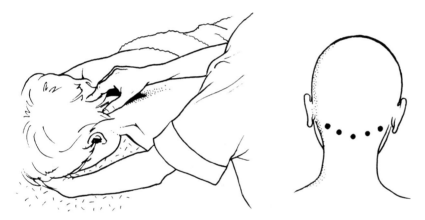

Fig. 11.21 *Movements on the neck*

Foot movements

Part one: wake up routine

1   Using your knuckle on the solar plexus point, press in and up on both feet simultaneously. Then start work on the client's right foot (see Fig. 11.22).
2   Work the pituitary area using your thumb and a pumping technique (see Fig. 11.23).
3   Work the neck area using your thumb and a pumping technique (see Fig. 11.24).

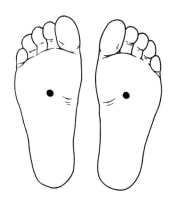

Fig. 11.22 *Movement 1*

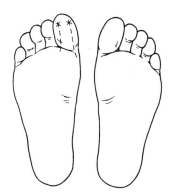

Fig. 11.23 *Movement 2*

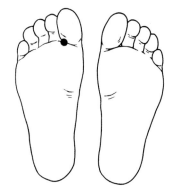

Fig. 11.24 *Movement 3*

4 Work the reproductive area using your thumb and a pumping technique.
5 Massage the spinal reflex area from the inner foot to the reflex area followed by massaging the heel to the kidney area using your thumb and a pumping technique.
6 Using the thumb pumping technique, massage from the kidney reflex to the bladder reflex.

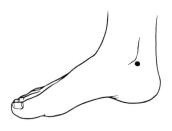

Fig. 11.25 *Movement 4*

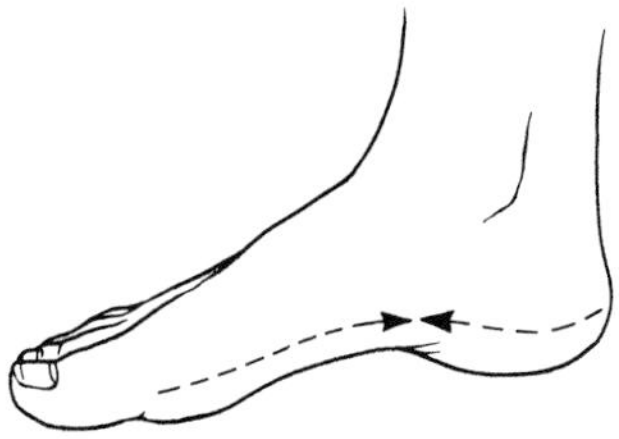

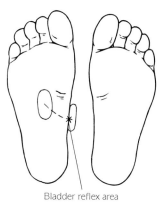

Bladder reflex area

Fig. 11.26 *Movement 5*

Fig. 11.27 *Movement 6*

Repeat movements 2–6 on the left foot.

Part two: wake up technique

1 Using your left hand to hold the sole of the right foot, your right thumb massages the solar plexus area whilst your fingers rotate the toes three times. Repeat on the left foot.
2 Placing your thumbs on the solar plexus points and your fingertips on top of the feet, push up on the plexus and drain out with your fingers. Repeat by moving your fingertips out slightly.
3 Rotate the client's foot outwards with your left hand gently gripping the foot, then grind out over the sole of the foot with the thumb of your right hand. Repeat on the other foot.
4 Using your thumbs, apply pressure to both solar plexus points. Close your eyes and as your client breathes in push up gently. Release as the client breathes out.

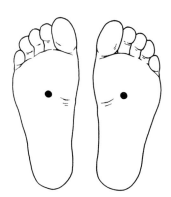

Fig. 11.28 *Movement 1*

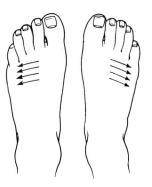

Fig. 11.29 *Movement 2*

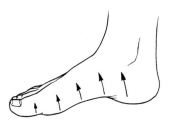

Fig. 11.30 *Movement 3*

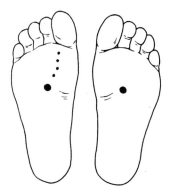

Fig. 11.31 *Movement 4*

Face and décolleté movements

Wash your hands and apply appropriate oil for this area.

NB All the following movements are repeated 3–4 times.

1   Place your fingers just above the client's ears and your thumbs between the eyebrows. Using your thumbs press, release and repeat gliding back to the hairline.
2   Keeping your fingertips in the same position, use your thumbs to press and slide using a gentle pumping action until you reach the hairline.

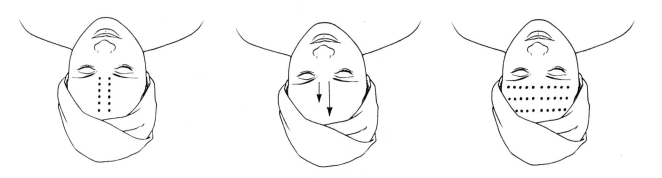

Fig. 11.32 *Movement 1*   Fig. 11.33 *Movement 2*   Fig. 11.34 *Movement 3*

3 With your fingers still resting over the ears use your thumbs to press and slide out from eyebrows to temples.
4 Using the palma pad of your hands slide out over the forehead and drain down towards the ears.
5 Place your thumbs between the eyebrows and use cushioned fingers to drain out from the nose towards the ear, first above the bone, then below the bone.
6 Using two fingers, drain with both hands simultaneously from the centre of the jawline out towards the ear.

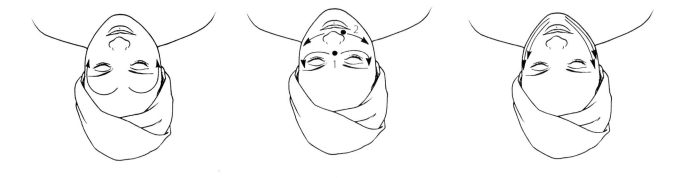

Fig. 11.35 *Movement 4*   **Fig. 11.36** *Movement 5*   **Fig. 11.37** *Movement 6*

7 Drain with your fingertips with both hands simultaneously up the jawline to the face and use the palma pad of your hands to drain out over the forehead back down the face.
8 Using your fingers of both hands simultaneously drain down to the clavicle, release the pressure in your fingers, press down and back on the shoulders three times, and push down on the shoulders towards the client's feet three times.

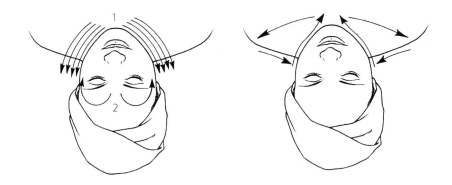

Fig. 11.38 *Movement 7*   **Fig. 11.39** *Movement 8*

9 Slide your fingers from the shoulders to the neck along the trapezius until they meet at the spine and flow up into the neck, and release.
10 Place one hand under the client's neck on the occipetal area, the other gently cupping the jaw (mandible) area on the front of the face. Very gently, move the head from side to side. This slightly stretches the spine. Bend your knees to gain the correct posture and support the client's head and neck by resting their neck on

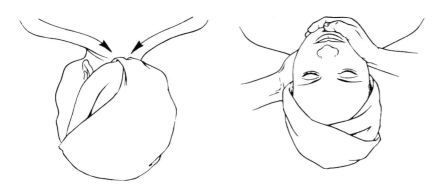

Fig. 11.40 *Movement 9*   **Fig. 11.41** *Movement 10*

your hands and head on your wrist and arms. Tell the client which way you are going to move and slowly move your leg rather than your body from side to side.

Arm movements

1   Support the client's arm by gently resting their fingers on your wrist and your fingers on their wrist. Using the side of your hand slide and glide using a pumping action working up the arm. Repeat 3–4 times.

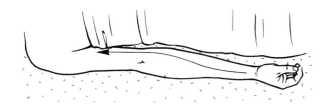

Fig. 11.42 *Movement 1*

2   Using the same supportive technique and action, work up the inner fore arm, then the outer upper arm, then the inner arm. Repeat 3–4 times.

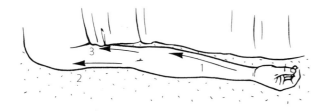

Fig. 11.43 *Movement 2*

Repeat movements 1–2 on the client's left arm.

Clavicle and abdominal movements

1   Using three fingers above the bone, drain out over the clavicle and slide your thumbs down into the axillary groove. Repeat 3–4 times (see Fig. 11.44).

2 Using the fingers of your left hand, make a large circle moving up the ascending colon, across the transverse and down the descending colon, immediately following through using your right hand to make a small circular movement over the intestines. Repeat 3–4 times.

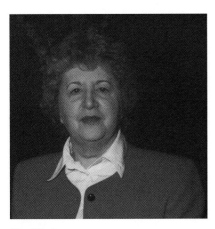

Fig. 11.44 *Movement 1*

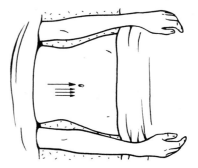

Fig. 11.45 *Movement 2*

3 If the client's abdomen is distended with air, place your hands over the abdomen and ask the client to breathe in and push their stomach up, hold for 7 seconds and then breathe out. As the client breathes out, gently press down. Repeat 3–4 times.

USEFUL INFORMATION

Eve Taylor's routine is available on video through Eve Taylor Institute of Clinical Aromatherapy, 9 Papyrus Road, Werrington Business Park, Werrington, Peterborough, Cambridgeshire PE4 5BH.

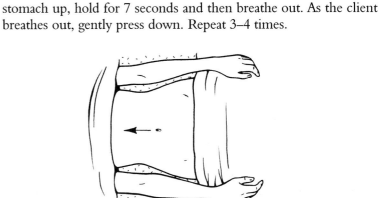

Fig. 11.46 *Movement 3*

4 Resting your fingers gently on either side of the rib cage, use your thumbs at the base of the sternum to drain lightly down over the transversus to the umbilicus. Then repeat using finger and thumb sliding. Repeat 3–4 times.

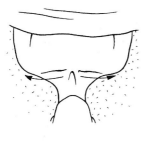

Eve Taylor

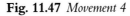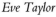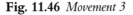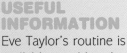

Fig. 11.47 *Movement 4*

5   With overlapping hands, drain out around the diaphragm in light
    pumping movements then repeat on the other side. Repeat 3–4
    times.
6   From the waistline, use strong draining movements over to the
    pubic zone using alternate hands. Repeat on the other side.

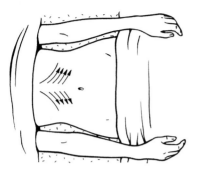

Fig. 11.48 *Movement 5*

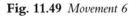
Middle finger of left hand

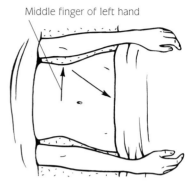

Fig. 11.49 *Movement 6*

POINT TO NOTE

As the massage comes to an end, make the movements slower and lighter.

Progress Check

Practise the back routine until you are able to perform
it fluently.

A whole body massage may not be required or appropriate. Individual
parts of the body may be treated by aromatherapy massage taking less
time and costing a proportional amount, for example:

- back massage – 30 minutes
- feet and lower legs – 15 minutes each leg
- face and scalp – 30 minutes
- face, chest and shoulders – 30 minutes.

If only a small part of the body is to be treated the essential oils used may
be used in slightly stronger concentrations. 3% to 5% mixes may be used
on the body, but not the face, and only if the safety of the oil has been
checked.

ACTIVITY

Consider what types of client would benefit most from an
aromatherapy massage consisting of:

a   full body
b   feet and lower legs
c   face and scalp
d   face, chest and shoulders.

After care and home care advice

Following a body massage a client should be advised to leave the oils on the body for a few hours in order to maximise the effects. It is also wise to tell the client whether the oils used could have a sedative or stimulating effect, especially if the client is driving.

The following advice should be given to the client.

1 Drink 6–8 glasses of water.
2 Do not sunbathe or use sun-beds for 24 hours.
3 Avoid heat treatments such as sauna or steam.
4 Where possible avoid using machinery or driving for 12–24 hours.

Further uses for essential oils

Essential oils can be used effectively in ways other than massage. They can be used in skin care by mixing them with a bland cream or adding them to a basic facial mask, in compresses, baths and diffused into the atmosphere.

Compresses
Compresses can be hot or cold. For a hot compress, a few drops of oil can be added to a bowl of hot water and a cloth or flannel dipped in and wrung out. This can then be placed on the affected area. They are useful to place on the back, for instance, while the rest of the body is being massaged.

A cold compress is prepared in the same way using ice cold water and is suitable for the forehead if the client has a headache.

POINT TO NOTE

Take care that the temperature of the compress is not too hot or cold before applying it to the skin.

Baths
Essential oils can be added directly to bath water just before getting in or can be mixed with a little carrier oil first. If added directly to the water, mix the oil well in to the water before sitting in the bath to avoid them coming into direct contact with the skin. If used with a carrier oil, be careful not to slip.

Suggested oil for the bath:

- **Relaxing** – 6 drops lavender with 4 drops of geranium or 7 drops chamomile with 3 of basil.
- **Colds** – 6 drops of pine with 6 of eucalyptus.
- **Aches and pains** – 4 drops of rosemary with 3 of chamomile.

Diffusion
Oils can be diffused into the atmosphere in a number of ways. The commonest way is to use a pottery burner which contains a night light candle. A few drops of oil are placed in warm water in a saucer shaped bowl above the candle. The heat from the night light speeds the evaporation of the oil into the atmosphere.

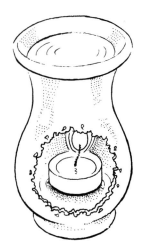

Fig. 11.50 *Pottery oil burner*

Specific oils can be chosen for their effects, e.g. frankincense and lavender for a relaxed atmosphere and eucalyptus or sweet myrtle when people have colds.

A more effective way of spreading oils into the atmosphere is to use an electrically operated nebulizer which propels the oil into the air in a very fine mist.

All these methods can be used to enhance and complement aromatherapy massage.

Massage and aromatherapy in a medical setting

The recent growth in popularity of complementary therapies is reflected in the number of health care professionals who are showing an interest in training and in using these therapies in the treatment of patients. There is a real desire among nurses, physiotherapists and occupational therapists to return to their caring role rather than the medical model that has been the trend for many years. The term 'holistic approach' is being used more and more where all aspects of the individual being treated are considered rather than just the physical.

Some recent examples of massage and aromatherapy being used in such a way follow.

Labour ward
Midwives at the John Radcliffe Maternity Hospital in Oxford wanting to find a way of relieving pain and calming women in labour set out to evaluate the use of essential oils for the purpose. The project lasted six months and the oils used were lavender, clary sage, peppermint, eucalyptus, chamomile, frankincense, jasmine, rose, lemon and mandarin.

The oils were used in baths, footbaths, inhaled or massaged. The most effective oil used was lavender. Peppermint and clary sage also showed good results. There was a high degree of satisfaction from the women and the midwives and the use of essential oils has been retained in the labour ward.

Intensive care
Research in the intensive and coronary care unit of the Royal Sussex County Hospital showed that massage and the use of essential oils reduced the heart rate and breathing rate in most of the patients tested and seemed to be more effective than massage alone.

The feet were massaged with lavender in a carrier oil and comparison was made with patients who were massaged with carrier oil alone. The drop in the heart rate was significantly greater in the lavender group.

Occupational therapy

Aromatherapy and massage are currently being used by many occupational therapists in a variety of settings to develop relationships, relieve anxiety and to help physical function. One example is where the occupational therapist massages the hands of children using lavender oil to relax and mobilise the hands before exercise. Other uses may be to diffuse into the atmosphere to promote concentration or relaxation.

Sleep patterns

A trial to evaluate the effects of lavender diffusion on the sleep patterns of patients with dementia was carried out in 1993 at Newholme Hospital, Bakewell. The trial ran over a seven week period using an electric diffuser. The results showed a significant improvement in the sleep patterns of the patients.

ACTIVITY

Try to carry out a literature search in professional journals and collect references to the use of massage and aromatherapy in a variety of medical settings.

Key Terms

You need to know what these words mean. Go back through the chapter to find out.

- Acupressure
- Anti-inflammatory
- Anti-oxidant
- Antiseptic
- Base note
- Compress
- Diffusion
- Distillation
- Expression
- Middle note
- Sedative
- Shiatsu
- Solvent
- Synergistically
- Therapeutic
- Top note
- Volatile

ARTIFICIAL NAILS

After working through this chapter you will be able to:

- appreciate the range of nail technology services
- advise on the suitability of different artificial nail systems
- apply and maintain sculptured and pre-formed nails
- apply and maintain nail extensions using tips and overlays
- describe contraindications to treatment
- carry out appropriate health and safety procedures
- Provide advice on after care.

Nails have become important fashion accessories and professional nail treatments now make a major contribution to the continuing growth and success of the beauty industry. Almost every high street has at least one specialist nail clinic and many hairdressing and beauty salons employ qualified nail technicians. Artificial nails are big business. They are very profitable and there is considerable scope for associated retail sales.

Artificial nail systems

There are many different artificial nail systems and technology is advancing at such a rate that new, improved methods seem to be appearing all the time. Fortunately, the companies who distribute nail systems in the UK provide very good training which ensures that technicians keep up-to-date. The main aim of research and development in the nail industry is to produce an artificial nail which not only looks natural, but feels and reacts like a strong, healthy natural nail: comfortable, lightweight, resilient and not prone to cracking or splitting.

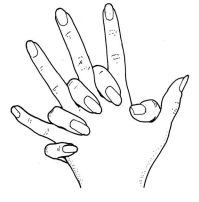

Fig. 12.1 *Artificial nails*

GOOD PRACTICE

Make sure you keep up-to-date with new nail systems as they come on the market. Clients will want the latest treatments. Keeping up with changing fashion trends and new systems will keep you one step ahead of your competitors.

ACTIVITIES

1. Conduct a survey of the salons in your area and discover which ones offer artificial nail treatments. Find out which nail systems they use and the range of services they offer. Compare the prices of artificial nail treatments offered by different salons.
2. Keep up-to-date with advancements in nail technology. Read professional journals and visit trade exhibitions. Gather product information and take any opportunity you can of seeing new nail systems being demonstrated.

Products and equipment

The following are specialist items used for nail technology treatments. Some of these are basic requirements of all artificial nail systems. Others are used only with certain treatments. These are identified in the relevant treatment sections.

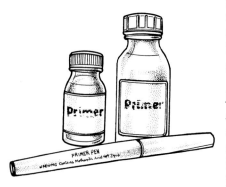

Fig. 12.2 *Primer*

Nail sanitisers

These are alcohol based and are usually applied from a spray pump to prevent bacterial or fungal growth occurring between the client's natural nails and the artificial ones. The sanitiser should have a 'chalky' white appearance when it has dried, indicating that all grease and moisture has been removed from the nail surface. This is important for preventing the artificial nail from lifting after it has been applied.

Primer

A primer is used to 'etch' the natural nail chemically. This removes surface oil and bacteria and provides a more adherent surface for the acrylic to stick. If primer is not used, the acrylic lifts more easily, increasing the risk of infection. When used for infills, primer must not be allowed to run over the surface of previously applied acrylic as it can weaken and discolour the remaining 'nails'.

Acrylic liquid

This is used to bond with acrylic powder to create an acrylic nail. Acrylic liquid has a very strong odour which can cause dizziness, sickness and headaches if there is inadequate ventilation. Once the acrylic nail has set, the fumes disappear.

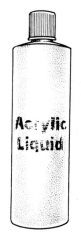

Fig. 12.3 *Acrylic liquid*

Acrylic powder

When liquid and powder acrylic are mixed, a chemical reaction takes place creating a structure which is strong and durable. Acrylic powders come in a range of colours which produce very natural effects:

- pink and white for a French manicure look
- ivory and peach which are especially attractive for clients with black skin
- overlay (slightly opaque) for applying over nail tips.

Some powders have smaller particles which allow the acrylic mixture to set more quickly. These are used by more experienced nail technicians.

GOOD PRACTICE

Always use acrylic liquids and powders according to the manufacturer's instructions as they vary for different systems.

UV gel

The gel hardens on exposure to ultra-violet light leaving a sticky residue which must be removed with a finishing wipe or cotton wool soaked in sterilising fluid before buffing to finish.

POINT TO NOTE

Gel will go hard in the pot if exposed to direct sunlight. The nails will also turn yellow with persistent exposure to sunlight or sunbeds.

UV lamp

This is used for 'curing' (setting) UV gel and UV acrylics.

Fibreglass/silk mesh

Available in either strips or pre-cut in various sizes. The mesh usually has a sticky backing to aid application. Good quality meshes should not fray or show through after the application of resin. When resin has been applied, a hard, resilient structure is formed which either strengthens the natural nail or provides extra support for a nail extension.

Resin glue

This product may be used with a fabric mesh for applying overlays or nail extensions. It sets hard and glossy. Although resin glue will set without using a curing product, it will not be as hard and will take longer to set. The finish will not be as durable.

Resin activator

This contains setting agents which dry and harden the resin so that it becomes non-porous and stronger. The room must be well ventilated when using this product. If you prefer not to use a spray, brush-on activators are available.

Nail forms

Nail forms are used to help create a nail extension if a tip is not being applied. The false nail is built up over the nail form. Care must be taken to ensure a good fit or the acrylic will run underneath and build up the nail incorrectly, resulting in a thick, lumpy edge. Nail forms are available as:

- re-usable: soft metal forms which can be shaped to fit any size of nail and finger. They can be sanitised and used again.
- disposable: paper forms with a sticky undersurface which come in various sizes and shapes to fit a range of clients.

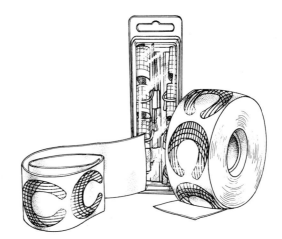

Fig. 12.4 *Disposable nail forms*

Brushes

These are usually sable, wooden handled brushes which come in various sizes. Slender, shorter brushes give the nail technician more control. Using the wrong brush with the right product makes application difficult.

Brush cleaner

This must be used with caution as it contains very harsh chemicals which can damage the skin. The bristles are immersed in the cleaner immediately after use to avoid the acrylic setting and hardening on the brush. The brush must be suspended in the cleaner so that the bristles maintain their shape.

Files (boards) and buffers

There are various shapes and sizes of cushioned boards and block buffers which are graded according to their 'grit' size. The coarser the surface, the lower its grit number; 60–200 grit are classed as coarse grade and are used mainly for etching the nail plate, first stage acrylics and shaping the natural nails. There are different combinations:

- 80 / 80: a heavy duty buffer used for the first stage of acrylics
- 100 / 100: for shaping natural and artificial nails
- 100 / 180: for second stage buffing of acrylics, fibreglass and brush-on gel systems.

180–280 grit are classed as medium grade and are used mainly for smoothing and finishing natural nails and shaping and blending. The combinations found are:

- 100 / 240: buffer for use on strong natural nails and artificial nail extensions
- 180 / 240: for shaping natural nails.
- 280–900 grit are classed as fine grade and are used mainly for blending and smoothing.
- 1000–2500 grit are classed as micro-abrasive and are used to buff and shape natural and artificial nails.

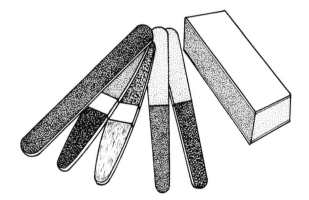

Fig. 12.5 *A selection of files and buffers*

Cuticle oil

Cuticle oil is used to:

- soften and nourish the skin around the nails
- avoid damage to skin during the removal of false nails
- help produce a high shine during the final buffing process
- improve the look (and smell) of the finished 'nail'
- help hide any tiny imperfections.

Nail tips

Nail tips are applied to extend the natural nail. Products are then overlaid to give extra strength to the nail extension. Nail tips come in a wide range of shapes, sizes and shades. The size and shape of the client's natural nails must be assessed accurately to ensure a perfect fit. If the nail tip does not fit well, this may cause discomfort or the tip will not adhere well to the natural nail.

Nail glue

Nail glue is used with care for applying a nail tip to the natural nail. The glue is applied sparingly to the 'well' on the underside of the nail tip. It can also be used in an emergency to apply a false nail which has 'lifted'.

Cuticle pusher

A plastic hoof stick is used to push back the cuticles gently.

Tip cutters

These are specially formulated to cut cleanly through the artificial nail structures without damaging the natural nails.

Dappen dish

This small glass or plastic dish is used to hold small amounts of product during the treatment. This avoids contaminating products by using them straight from their container.

Terminology

Some frequently used terms have a specific meaning in relation to artificial nail treatments.

Porosity

This refers to the ability of the nail or artificial nail structure to absorb substances. The natural nail is porous and absorbs oils and moisture. Some products applied as overlays are porous which is why they can be removed with solvents.

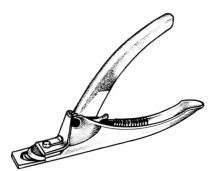

Fig. 12.6 *Tip cutters*

Friction heat

This is caused by filing and buffing too vigorously or too hard and is very uncomfortable for the client.

Product curing heat

When curing or setting a product, a chemical reaction occurs which creates the hardened finish. Curing products are *exothermal*. This means they give out heat while curing. This can sometimes be uncomfortable for the client.

Dehydrating

It is important to dehydrate the natural nails before applying nail extensions. Any moisture, oils or bacteria left on the nail plate will become trapped under the product and may cause the artificial nail to lift, the nail plate to soften and even mould or fungal growth to appear.

Lifting

If an overlay is applied too thickly or has been applied on to the surrounding skin, it will lift. Lifting can occur for various reasons. Glue may be used to repair the lift. This is best done by a technician in the salon. It is important to ensure that the nail is clean and dry before applying the glue as water or bacteria left under the overlay will cause problems.

Consultation

A consultation is essential. The receptionist should allow time for this when the appointment is booked. Your client needs to agree the treatment plan and understand what is involved. They need to be fully aware of the necessary aftercare and maintenance procedures and their costs.

It is important to choose the system which will best meet the needs of your client. Make sure that you explain what can be achieved so that they have realistic expectations before the treatment begins.

POINT TO NOTE

Always fill in the client's record card during and on completion of treatment.

Use open and closed questions to find out:

◊ why the client wants nail extensions: are they for a one-off occasion, for example a holiday, or are they required for permanent wear?

◊ has the client any previous experience of nail extensions? Was it a good or bad experience? Has it made the client sceptical?

◊ the client's lifestyle: how much time does she have available for looking after her nails? Will she be able to return every fortnight for maintenance? Does she have small children? If she does, she may frequently have 'fiddly' jobs to attend to like fastening buttons, which make long nails impractical.

◊ her occupation: the job she has may influence which system and products are used.

◊ has the client got pre-conceived ideas about what can be achieved? Can the desired shape and length really be achieved?

POINT TO NOTE

The nail extension should be no longer than half the length of the nail bed. Any longer than this weakens the structure.

Contraindications

to artificial nails

◊ Severely bitten nails.
◊ Thin, flaking nails.
◊ Any signs of bacterial or fungal infection.
◊ Allergy to nail products.
◊ Inflammation or swelling in the area.
◊ Open wounds, cuts and abrasions.

Preparing the nails for treatment

The methods described here are typical of most nail systems currently available. Before starting treatment, always:

◊ remove all traces of nail enamel and wipe over the hands and nails with sanitiser

◊ check that there are no contraindications

◊ file the nails to an even length and tidy up the cuticles if necessary.

POINT TO NOTE

If there is a lot of work required on the cuticles, this is best done during a full manicure the day before.

Acrylic nails

This method of nail extension involves building up an artificial nail over a nail form or plastic nail tip, using a liquid and powder acrylic mixture. Some systems use a drill with an abrasive head to smooth down the hardened compound to the correct thickness and shape. Considerable skill is required to apply and blend in tips and produce a natural shape. Maintenance work is required every 2–3 weeks following initial application to compensate for the effects of natural nail growth. Acrylic nails look natural and are very strong and resilient. They will withstand normal wear and tear.

Selling points

- Very strong.
- Natural appearance.
- Need only a small area of natural nail to ensure a firm attachment.
- Flexible.
- Resilient.
- Can be used to disguise bitten nails so long as the nail bed is not exposed and there are no signs of infection.
- Can be adapted to any size or shape of natural nail.
- Effects last up to 2–3 months if regular infill treatments are provided.
- A full set application of acrylic nails takes approximately 1 hour 15 minutes.

POINT TO NOTE

Acrylic nail products can also be applied as an overlay to strengthen the natural nails as they grow.

Disadvantages

- More expensive than temporary methods due to the treatment time, products used and costs of maintenance.
- Weakens the natural nails.
- 'Infill' treatments required every 2–3 weeks after initial application.
- The treatment products have a pungent smell which can be unpleasant for the client and the technician.
- Too 'heavy' for use on weak nails and could cause nail trauma.
- Are porous, therefore natural moisture can escape but moisture can penetrate the artificial nail causing a fungal infection.
- Acrylic nails may discolour with prolonged exposure to UV, going a yellowy colour.

POINT TO NOTE

The primer which is used during acrylic nail treatments is caustic and can have an adverse effect on the natural nails. This only becomes apparent when the acrylic nails are removed.

Products and equipment

You will need:

- bactericidal hand and nail cleanser
- nail sanitiser
- selection of graded files and buffers
- nail forms

- nail primer
- acrylic powder(s)
- acrylic liquid
- cuticle oil
- tip clippers
- brush sable brushes
- dappen dishes
- brush cleaner.

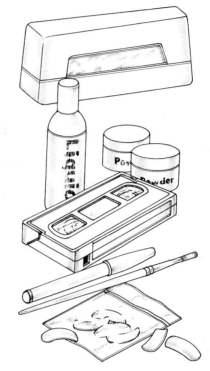

Fig. 12.7 *Products and equipment for acrylic nails*

POINT TO NOTE

Depending on the system being used, you may also need a (UV) light box and an abrasive drill.

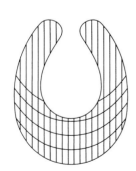

Fig. 12.8 *Disposable nail form*

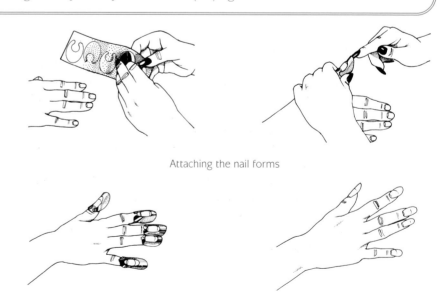

Attaching the nail forms

Sculptured products applied over nail forms

Fig. 12.9 *Using nail forms for sculptured nails*

Procedure

1 Wash your own hands and cleanse the hands of your client.
2 Remove nail enamel and check for contraindications.
3 Push back the cuticles on both hands.
4 Score over all the nails with a fine grit file, from cuticle to free edge.
5 Sanitise the nails to remove any surface bacteria.

POINT TO NOTE

The nails should dry to a cloudy finish. This shows that all oil has been removed which would otherwise cause the artificial nail structure to lift.

6 Fit the nail forms 'snugly' or apply tips.
7 Prime the natural nails ensuring that the product does not run into the cuticle or under the free edge.
8 Dip brush in liquid acrylic, removing excess product by stroking the brush on the edge of the dappen dish.
9 Dip the tip of the brush into the powder acrylic to produce a small ball. Apply this to the nail form or tip extension in a rolling motion (roll the brush between your own fingers and pull back).

POINT TO NOTE

Any kinks in the nail form will result in an uneven nail and cause problems during filing.

10 Wipe the brush on paper towel to absorb excess liquid and any stray acrylic powder.
11 Allow the product to flow gently over the nail form.

POINT TO NOTE

Too much liquid will result in a weak free edge. The drier the free edge, the stronger it is.

12 Pat the product into shape, following the guidelines on the nail form, to ensure the correct length and width of the artificial nail structure. The acrylic will be setting while you are doing this.
13 Apply a second ball of product to the main body of the nail, gently patting it with the brush towards the nail grooves.
14 When the product is 3mm away from the nail grooves, brush forwards over the product to flatten it, ensuring that it does not overlap the grooves.
15 Next, using a slightly wetter brush, apply a smaller ball of product and taper it off towards the cuticle with the brush.
16 Finally, a ball of product, using natural powder, can be applied over the stress area (just below the flesh line) for added strength, as this can be the weakest point.

POINT TO NOTE

The extension must adhere to the nail plate, otherwise lifting may occur.

17 Continue this procedure on all ten nails, checking the length and shape of each new nail.

GOOD PRACTICE

Throughout the procedure you must check the shape, profile and barrel view of the artificial nail structure to ensure that natural looking nails are developing.

18 As soon as you have finished forming the artificial nail structure, clean your brush. Suspend it is a bottle of brush cleaner, making sure that the bristles do not become distorted.
19 Check that the acrylic has set by tapping it lightly with an orange stick. If there is a clear 'tap' sound, the acrylic has set. If a 'thud' sound is heard, the acrylic has not yet set.

POINT TO NOTE

Acrylic does not stick to the skin but it can irritate it.

20 When you are sure the acrylic has set, remove the nail forms and begin to shape the sides of the nail, removing any product which may have strayed into the grooves.
21 Supporting the nail firmly with your free hand, file on top of the nail. You will need a coarse grit file where the acrylic is thick or slightly lumpy. Use a medium grit file for more refined work.
22 When filing near the cuticle, use your thumb to cover the cuticle and nail walls so that the file does not cut the skin. Because you are working on an artificial structure, you can use a see-saw action with the file but always support the nail from above with your thumb to avoid vibrations.
23 Use a medium grit board to file the free edge. For a square nail, hold the file at a 90° angle to the free edge. If a more curved shape is required, tilt the file slightly.
24 Change to a fine grit file and, once the desired shape is achieved, use a 3-sided buffer to eliminate scratches and produce a shine.

GOOD PRACTICE

When creating a French manicure effect you must ensure that the white acrylic powder does not stray beyond the flesh line. Try to avoid having to apply coloured nail enamel as the look of the nails will help sell your work.

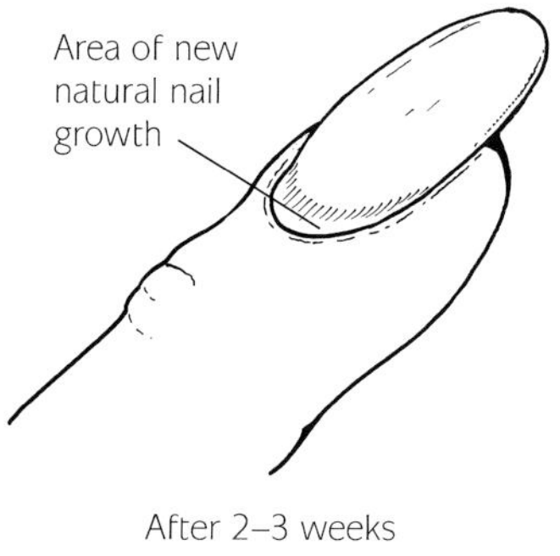

Area of new natural nail growth

After 2–3 weeks

Fig. 12.10 *Infills*

25 Always give the client home care advice and book her maintenance appointment two weeks ahead. If the appointment has to be made later than two weeks, advise the client to purchase a maintenance kit for emergencies.

After care
Approximately two weeks after the nail extensions have been applied, some new natural growth will show at the base of the nail, close to the cuticle. You may also see some lifting of the product in this area. This will look a slightly different colour and will become loose. Check for any

cracks or lifting and signs of infection, especially if the client has used 'emergency' glue.

Infills and maintenance

1. Cleanse the hands and nails thoroughly using a bactericidal cleanser.
2. Dehydrate the nails and tidy cuticles.
3. Using a suitable file, buff away any product which has lifted. Continue until you have created a smooth surface and removed any shine.

4. If there are any cracks or chips in the acrylic, these can now be treated so the nails look like new. New acrylic will adhere to old acrylic. If cracks appear lower than the flesh line, they can be buffed and filled as long as the natural nail is not cracked.

5. Prime the nail growth area (it is not necessary to prime the existing acrylic).
6. While the primer is still wet, apply a ball of the product to the growth area and level it out to the existing acrylic.

7. Buff until you have achieved a smooth surface.
8. Apply cuticle oil and polish to a shine with a 3-way buffer.

Maintaining a French manicure

If a French look was created originally, this will need a 'back' fill. Smooth the surface of the white acrylic and file a well between the white and pink, indicating the natural flesh line. Fill in with white acrylic. No primer is necessary at this stage (primer applied on top of acrylic causes yellowing).

Gel nails

These are quite strong, non-permeable and have an attractive, high gloss finish. Acetone does not break down gel nails, therefore they have to be removed by buffing. Minimum lifting occurs. Gel nails require setting by either ultra-violet light emitted in a light box, or by brushing or spraying with setting gels.

Gel nails are recommended for clients with brittle nails to help keep them protected as they grow. The gel coating hardens on the nails so that the client has to return every 3–4 weeks to have the small ridge created by new growth buffed away and new gel applied.

Nail extensions can be produced by applying the gel over artificial nail tips or nail forms. This system produces longer, natural looking nails but re-gelling is required every 2–3 weeks. The appearance and consistency of the nail produced depends upon the manufacturer and the gel product used for each stage of treatment. Some gel systems involve the use of an ultra-violet light to 'cure' (set) the gel.

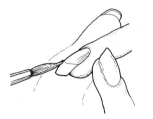

1 Applying gel over artificial nail tip

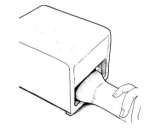

2 Curing the gel in a UV light box

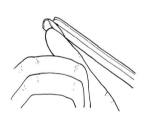

3 Buffing the hardened gel

4 The finished natural effect

Fig. 12.11 *Gel nails*

Selling points
- Very natural appearance.
- Do not require nail enamel.
- Quite strong.
- Effects last up to 2–3 months if regular infill treatments are provided.
- A full set application of sculptured gel nails takes approximately 1 hour.

Disadvantages
- Not as strong as acrylic or fibreglass systems.
- More expensive than temporary methods due to treatment time, products used and costs of maintenance.
- Can weaken the natural nails if primer used.

POINT TO NOTE

The gel is non-porous and prevents natural moisture from escaping. This can be a problem for fragile nails. It can be used as a top coat for other nail systems to prevent water from penetrating the artificial nail. Because it is non-porous, gel is very difficult to remove.

Products and equipment
You will need:

- bactericidal hand and nail cleanser
- nail sanitiser
- selection of graded files and buffers
- gel products: different colours are available to create a French manicure effect
- sable brushes with flat, square shaped bristles
- nail primer (some systems do not use primer)
- lint free wipes and acetone to clean any sticky residue in between the different stages of the treatment
- tip clippers
- a UV lamp or light box to 'cure' the nails (this may not be required for some gel systems).

POINT TO NOTE

Gel nails are not always cured in a light box. Sometimes a brush or spray activator is used. The brush should be cleaned before each layer is applied. Activator must be sprayed from 25 cm (10 in) away to prevent the gel nails from curing too quickly. If this happens, the client experiences a severe heat reaction.

Procedure
Prepare the hands and nails exactly as for the procedure for acrylic nails up to and including step 6 (page 323).

7   Brush the base product (product 1) over the surface of the nail in circular / dabbing movements working from the base to the free edge. Ensure that the product does not overlap into the nail grooves. Complete this procedure on all the fingernails of the one hand and cure for 2 minutes. While these nails are curing, repeat the procedure on the fingernails of the other hand. When all the fingernails have been cured, treat both the thumbs and cure them together.

8   If applying a 'French' look, apply white gel to the free edge. This product is thicker and should be applied to a nail form or nail tip extension in circular movements. This product can shrink slightly during curing so apply it to just beyond the flesh line. Cure for 2 minutes and then remove any sticky residue.

9   Apply pink gel to the main body of the nail checking the profile and barrel view of the developing nail shape.

10 The pink gel must meet the white free edge. Cure the pink gel for 2 minutes and remove any residue.

11 It may be necessary to apply a coat of clear gel to bond the pink and white together and to achieve the desired shape. This should be done before proceeding to the next stage.

12 Finally, apply a top coat in the same way as you would a nail enamel, from the base of the nail to the tip. This will create a permanent shine. Cure for 2 minutes and remover any residue.

13 Apply cuticle oil.

After care
Recommend the client to return fortnightly for a gentle buffing and manicure. Monthly appointments should be made to re-shape and file

away ragged edges, buff and re-apply the gel. It is not usual to remove the false tip. This is normally allowed to grow out with the natural nail, being eventually filed away.

Infills and maintenance

Infills may be required every 2–4 weeks depending on the rate of nail growth.

1 Clean and sanitise the nails.
2 Dehydrate the nail and tidy cuticles.
3 Using a suitable file, gently buff away any ridges to blend in the remaining gel with the area of new natural nail growth.
4 Prime the area of new nail growth (not the existing gel) and allow this to dry.
5 Apply the gel to the area of new nail growth and sweep it over the nail with the brush. Press down firmly to avoid building up on existing gel.
6 Cure under the lamp as usual and repeat if necessary.
7 Wipe off any sticky residue and buff to a smooth finish.
8 Apply cuticle oil and polish with a 3-way buffer.

POINT TO NOTE

To maintain a French manicure look, a backfill may be necessary.

Fabric overlays and nail extensions

Different types of fabric can be used with a special glue to reinforce the natural nails or create nail extensions by securing false tips to the natural nails. Pieces of fabric are cut to the size of the nail and then eased into position over a layer of glue, taking care to avoid the cuticle. Extra layers are built up and the resulting 'nail' is buffed smooth until it is transparent.

Fabric products

Materials such as fibreglass and silk are used with a resin glue to produce a strong overlay over natural nails or nail extensions. The thickness and openness of the fabric mesh used determines the strength and resilience of the resulting nail structure. A thick, coarser open mesh material will hold more resin and will therefore set harder and stronger:

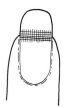

- Fibreglass: this is the thickest, strongest material which produces the most natural looking nails. The resin breaks down the fibreglass so that the detail of the mesh can not be seen when the product has hardened.
- Silk: the thinnest material which may be seen through the resin so the effect is not as natural. Silk is used mainly for repairing natural nails.

Fig. 12.12
A fibreglass stress strip

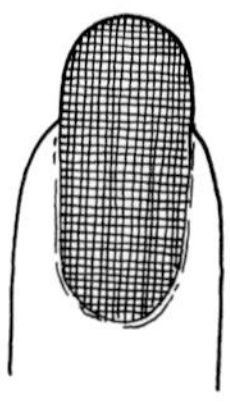

Fig. 12.13
Fibreglass mesh over whole nail

POINT TO NOTE

It is not possible to free form a nail using these products, they are used to provide strength and rigidity, not length. A narrow fibreglass stress strip can be applied across the nail to strengthen the area of weakness. This will help the nail to grow longer without breaking.

Fibreglass nail extensions provide the most natural effect. They are also the least harmful to the natural nails. This is because fewer chemical substances are used during the process.

Selling points

- Very natural appearance.
- Very strong and flexible.
- Extremely light and thin.
- Can be used effectively for matching odd broken nails.
- Suitable for clients with weak and brittle nails.
- There is less trauma to the natural nail so can be worn for longer periods of time.
- A full set of fibreglass nail extensions takes approximately 1 hour 15 minutes.

Disadvantages

- Quite expensive due to the time involved and the cost of materials.
- Cannot be used on clients who bite their nails due to the relatively small area of natural nail plate available.

Products and equipment

You will need:

- bactericidal hand and nail cleanser
- nail sanitiser
- resin glue
- resin activator
- fibreglass / silk mesh
- selection of graded files and buffers
- cuticle oil.

Procedure

1 Prepare the natural nails using the standard cleansing and sanitising procedures.

POINT TO NOTE

Some companies recommend applying resin to the natural nail first to avoid damaging it when blending in the tip.

2 Apply tips to all 10 nails and blend in to the natural nails.
3 Apply resin to the natural nail and extension.
4 Apply the previously cut fabric to the whole surface of the nail, leaving a 1–5 mm gap around the cuticle and nail groove area. It does not matter if there is an overlap beyond the free edge as this can be buffed away later.
5 If too much glue has been applied remove it now or it may cause lifting. If not enough glue has been applied, add more or use a clean plastic sheet to spread the resin down the nail and flatten the material used.
6 Set the product using activator.
7 Apply another coat of resin until three layers have been applied. Activate each application.
8 Buff to a shine and apply cuticle oil.

After care

This will be required every 2–3 weeks as the nail grows. Buff the area closest to the cuticle to blend in with the natural nail. It may only be necessary to apply resin to the area of new growth. Do not use extra mesh fabric for the first infill as this may cause bulk in the cuticle area.

Infills and maintenance

1. Clean and sterilise the nails.
2. Dehydrate the nails and tidy cuticles.
3. Using a suitable file, buff down the existing product until it is level with the area of new nail growth.
4. Gently buff the whole nail to take off the shine.
5. Apply resin to the growth area and spread it, avoiding build up of the product over existing resin.
6. Activate the resin and allow it to dry. If necessary, re-apply resin (or mesh and resin if second or subsequent infill treatment).
7. Buff with a suitable file to create a smooth surface.
8. Apply cuticle oil and polish to a shine with a 3-way buffer.

Semi-permanent nails (nail tips)

Tips are applied to the natural nails to provide extra length for just a short time. The tips are made of plastic. The most popular shades are clear, opaque and white. There are different shapes and sizes. It is very important that the nail tips fit snugly without causing discomfort or lifting off. Artificial nail tips appear very natural but, because they are applied only to the tips of the natural nails, they are not very strong. A seamless join has to be created where the false tip is attached to the natural nail. This is the weakest part of the nail extension which can be strengthened with an overlay of gel, fibreglass, acrylic or silk.

GOOD PRACTICE

Look closely at the shape of the client's natural nails. Look at their profile and barrel view. The nails will not all be the same shape. Select the tip which will be the most suitable shape and then identify the correct size. Press the tips against the nails to check for fit. Write the number of each top on the client's record card for future reference.

POINT TO NOTE

If the client's nails are badly bitten, a tip with a small well will be necessary as the tip should cover only one third of the client's natural nails. If you only have a limited supply of tips, they must be customised to fit by cutting and filing the well.

Selling points

- Very natural effects.
- Ideal for special occasions when the hands are on show.
- Can temporarily disguise a broken nail.
- Good, short term solution for people who are not normally able to have long nails.

- Easy to remove.
- Full set application takes approximately 45 minutes.
- With overlays, treatment takes approximately 1–1½ hrs.

Disadvantages

- Weakest type of nail extension.
- Temporary effects (7–10 days).
- Easily damaged.
- Great care needed when doing manual jobs and when hands are near sources of heat.

Products and equipment

You will need:

- bactericidal hand and nail cleanser
- nail sanitiser
- selection of graded files and buffers
- quick-setting glue
- nail tips
- tip clippers
- overlay product
- lint-free pads.

Procedure

1. Before applying the tips, the natural nails must be prepared to ensure good adhesion. If an overlay of strengthening product is to be used, for example acrylic, gel, resin, then the whole of the natural nail must be prepared otherwise lifting of the products may occur.
2. A quick-setting glue is used to attach the tips to the client's natural nails. This is applied to the well of the tip and then spread over the final one third of the natural nail while the tip is held in place, ensuring a close fit.

POINT TO NOTE

If the natural nail and the nail tip do not fit well, the tip may lift or dirt get trapped underneath.

3. After 5 seconds the glue has set. Cut and file the free edge to the desired shape and blend the tip into the natural nail.
4. Apply the required overlay.
5. If too much glue has been applied, spray with sanitiser and remove excess with a lint free pad.

Make sure the client understands that her new nails are not indestructible! In the event of a heavy blow, they will break. This is much better than the possible damage to the nail bed which could occur if they did not break.

Temporary nails (pre-formed)

For some clients, nail extensions are not practical for everyday wear. Temporary, pre-formed nails are effective for special occasions or one-off

USEFUL INFORMATION

There are many products on the market which help to blend the tip into the natural nail. Acetone is effective but must be used with care as it dissolves the plastic tip quickly and can dehydrate the natural nail. Files and buffers can be used on their own without the aid of products but great care must be taken to avoid mechanical damage to the natural nail.

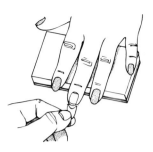

1 Matching the nail tip to the natural nail

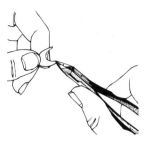

2 Trimming with clippers for perfect fit

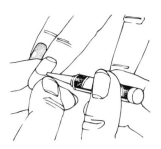

3 Holding the tip in place while adhesive is applied

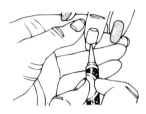

4 Extra adhesive applied to the seam

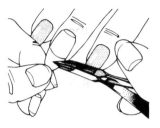

5 Clipping the new artificial nail before shaping

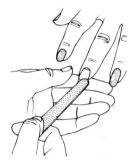

6 Smoothing over the seam with a buffer

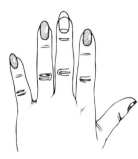

7 Nail tips in place

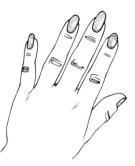

8 Nail enamel applied

Fig. 12.14 *Applying nail tips*

events. They can be worn for up to 7–10 days if applied well and looked after carefully by the client. The nails are made from plastic and come in many shapes and sizes. Some of them are already coloured so that nail enamel does not have to be applied. After two weeks, the natural nail has grown sufficiently to create a noticeable gap between the false nail and the cuticle.

Selling points
- Ideal for special occasions when the hands are on show.
- Relatively inexpensive.
- Can disguise a broken nail if nail enamel is being applied.
- Do not weaken the natural nails.
- Quick results: a full-set application takes approximately 30 minutes.

Disadvantages
- The least natural looking of all the artificial nail systems.
- Must be worn with nail enamel.
- Temporary effects (maximum 7–10 days).

USEFUL INFORMATION
Temporary pre-formed nails are not bonded as closely to the natural nails as with other systems and if water and other substances become lodged behind the false nail, the natural nail plate may weaken and become spongey.

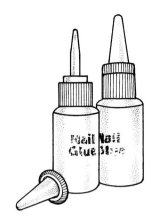

Fig. 12.15 *Nail glue*

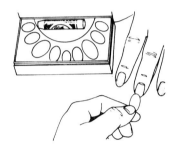

Fig. 12.16 *Pre-formed nails*

♦ Not very strong.

♦ Great care needed when doing manual jobs and when hands are near sources of heat.

Products and equipment

You will need:

♦ bactericidal hand cleanser
♦ nail sanitiser
♦ orange stick
♦ selection of graded files and buffers
♦ pre-formed nails
♦ nail glue.

Procedure

1 Wash your own hands and cleanse the client's hands.
2 Remove old nail enamel and check for contraindications.
3 Sanitise the nails, ensuring that no moisture or grease is left on the nail plate.
4 Choose the appropriate style and shape of false nails and measure them against the natural nails, matching up their width at the base. If the exact size and shape required is not available, choose a larger nail and file it down to fit, using a fine grit.
5 Lay out the nails on a clean tissue in the order they are going to be applied.
6 Starting with the thumbs, apply glue with the nozzle of the applicator to the underside of the false nail or directly to the centre of the natural nail, allowing space for the glue to spread. This will happen when the false nail is applied.

POINT TO NOTE

Any glue which strays on to the skin can be wiped off with a little of the special remover on a tipped orange stick.

7 Holding the pre-formed nail by the free edge, gently slide it up towards the cuticle then hold it in place with your thumb for a few seconds while the glue sets.
8 Repeat the procedure on all the nails.
9 Test that the false nails are secure before applying base coat and nail enamel in the normal way.

After care

The nails can be stored in their container and re-used so long as all traces of glue are removed from the contact surface. Never try prising the nails off without first loosening them with a special glue solvent:

♦ hold the hand up vertically and apply a drop of solvent behind the tip of each false nail: wait a couple of minutes for the solvent to penetrate and then gently rock the nails from side to side, gradually loosening them and lifting them from the nail plate
♦ any remaining glue can be cleaned from the natural nails and false nails using the special solvent.

Removing artificial nail structures

Clients should be advised to return the salon to have their false nails removed. This will ensure minimal damage to the natural nails.

You will need:

- tip remover (acetone)
- cuticle oil
- manicure lotion
- non-plastic bowl
- orange stick
- coarse file
- strong tissues or cotton pads
- 3-way buffer.

POINT TO NOTE

Gel nails are non-porous so you will have to spend much more time buffing the nails to remove extensions with gel overlays.

Procedures

1 Place tip remover in the bowl and add one teaspoon of cuticle oil.
2 Wipe a small amount of manicure lotion over the client's hands.
3 Buff the nail extensions to create a rough surface. This encourages absorption of the solvent by the nail.
4 Place the client's fingertips in the bowl and allow to soak for 5 minutes.
5 Remove from the bowl and wipe the surface of the nails with tissues or pads. Buff if necessary.
6 Use an orange stick to gently 'tease off' the product, taking care not to scrape the nail.
7 Repeat the soaking and wiping until the product is completely removed.
8 Ask the client to scrub their hands thoroughly.
9 Reshape the natural nail and massage cuticle oil into the nails and cuticles.
10 Re-apply a new set of extensions if required, otherwise buff with a 3-way buffer.

General home care advice

Make sure your client understands how to care for her new nails at home. This will ensure she gets the best value from her treatment:

- wear gloves for manual jobs such as gardening and washing up
- try to use the pads of the fingers or the knuckles for performing certain tasks such as turning on light switches
- use a pen or similar item for dialling a telephone number
- use a non-acetone nail enamel remover as acetone damages the surface of artificial nail structures
- if the nail 'snags' or chips, use a suitable file (purchased from the salon) to smooth the nail.

POINT TO NOTE

Nail enamel will last longer on artificial nails as there are no natural oils or moisture to lift them off.

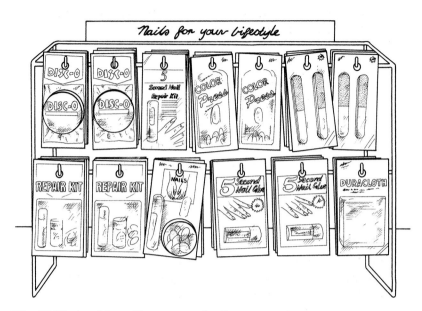

Fig. 12.17 *A nail bar selling a range of nail care accessories*

◊ any slight lifting can be resealed with a little glue purchased from the salon. Ensure the nail is clean and dry before repairing and inform the technician at the next maintenance visit so that the repair can be checked

◊ do not pull the extensions off. They must be removed properly with acetone, preferably followed by a manicure

◊ when on holiday, make sure the hands and nails are dried thoroughly after swimming and any oil or sun cream washed off the hands

◊ when bathing, try not to soak the hands for too long in the water and wash of any cream-based bath products

◊ use a nail brush very gently to remove any dirt or creams from under the free edge. Dirt is trapped very easily between the nail extension and the natural nail

◊ have regular manicures to maintain the cuticles and enhance the general appearance of the hands

◊ always apply a base coat under nail enamel to prevent 'yellowing' of the artificial nail.

POINT TO NOTE

Some artificial nail products are sensitive to UV light and turn yellow. This should be considered when having a sun-bed treatment.

Contra-actions

The following adverse reactions may appear following application of an artificial nail structure:

- Thinning of the natural nail plate, caused by excessive filing and buffing when preparing the nails and blending in a nail tip.
- Allergy to one of the many chemical products used during the process.
- Bacterial or fungal infection caused by inadequate hygiene procedures or incorrect home care.
- Softening of the natural nail plate as a result of prolonged exposure to harsh products such as nail primer.
- Physical damage to the nail plate, nail bed or cuticle showing as bruising, ridges in the nail plate and skin damage to the cuticles and nail walls.

ACTIVITIES

1. Explain, in detail, the appearance and specific causes of each of the contra-actions to artificial nails.
2. Explain the advice which should be given and the immediate action which should be taken for each contra-action.

Key Terms

You need to know what these words and phrases mean. Go back through the chapter to find out.

- 3-way buffer
- Curing
- Dappen dish
- Fibreglass
- Gel nails
- Grit
- Light box
- Liquid acrylic
- Nail extension
- Nail tips
- Overlay
- Porosity
- Powder acrylic
- Pre-formed nails
- Primer
- Resin activator

> After working through this chapter you will:
>
> ◊ have a greater awareness of what is involved in setting up a business
>
> ◊ recognise the roles and responsibilities of the employment hierarchy
>
> ◊ be able to identify the important legislative requirements necessary to conduct a successful business.

Beauty therapy is a diverse and exciting career offering many opportunities and working arrangements. There are few professions where so much choice is available. It is essential that the therapist has a good working knowledge of salon administration and related legislation whether they are a junior therapist, manager or self-employed as the success of the salon ultimately depends on efficient working practices.

Different countries have different legislation governing business practices. This chapter focuses on those business practices in England and Wales and is not intended to be a definitive one, but more of a guide and source of reference.

Forms of business arrangements

Legally all businesses fall into one of the following categories:

◊ Sole trader.
◊ Partnership.
◊ Limited Company.
◊ Franchise.
◊ Co-operative.

Sole trader
This is the simplest form of business organisation. One person controls finance and decisions. From a legal point of view there is nothing that needs to be done to set up in business as a sole trader.

Advantages
◊ Easy to set up – no lengthy legal formalities.
◊ Total control of the business.
◊ Immediate decision making.
◊ Taxed as an individual.
◊ Should benefit from close relations with suppliers.
◊ Easy to wind up.

Disadvantages
◊ Liable for any business losses.
◊ No legal distinction between the business and personal assets.
◊ Possible lack of continuity in management if the owner is ill.

- Does not have status.
- Possible lack of finances for expansion.

Partnership

By definition a partnership is when two or more people go into business together without registering as a limited company or a co-operative.

Again this form of business can be set up without legal formalities, but it is not to be recommended as severe disagreements could jeopardise the business. It is much safer to have a formal partnership agreement drawn up detailing the roles and responsibilities of all partners.

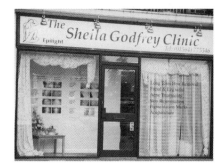

Fig. 13.1 *The salon*

Advantages

- A good way to start up a business that requires more capital than one person alone may have.
- Wider range of complementary skills and knowledge.
- Sharing of workload and general pressures of running a business.
- Sharing of any business losses.

Disadvantages

- All partners are responsible for any business debts even if they are caused by the actions of the other(s).
- Legal costs involved in drawing up a partnership agreement.
- Death or bankruptcy of one partner will automatically dissolve the partnership (unless previous arrangements have been made).
- Possible personality clashes can cause problems.

Limited company

A limited company is formed with a minimum of two shareholders, one of whom must be a director. A company secretary must also be appointed but he/she can be an outsider.

This is a company whereby any business debts are limited to the amount put in. Therefore if the business does go bankrupt, personal possessions cannot be taken to pay the company's debts.

A limited company prior to registration must produce and adhere to two legal documents:

- Memorandum of Association – this sets out the objectives of the company, as well as the company's share capital.
- Articles of Association – sets out additional rules by which the company will be governed.

Advantages

- Limited liability.
- Capital may be increased by selling shares.
- Better definition of management structures.
- Business not affected by death or bankruptcy of any of its shareholders.
- Higher level of status.
- Shareholders are employees of the company and therefore entitled to DSS benefits should the need arise.

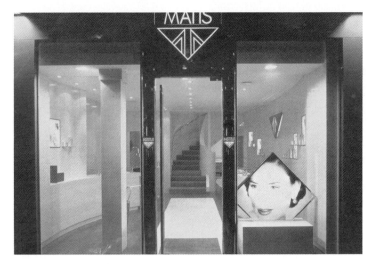

Fig. 13.2 *Matis' Paris salon*

Disadvantages

- Costly to set up with time-consuming legal formalities.
- The business will have to make public its accounts.
- As an employee of the company you will be subject to PAYE (see p. 374).

Franchise

A franchise is a business relationship between a franchiser (the owner of a name or method of business) and a franchisee (an operator of that business). The franchisee agrees to pay the franchiser a sum of money for the use of the business name, method of doing business, etc. Often there is an initial fee and an agreed percentage of sales afterwards is paid to the franchiser by the franchisee.

Advantages

- A tried and tested formula.
- A corporate image, instantly recognisable.
- Normally there is a wealth of knowledge available concerning most aspects of the business.
- Back-up services normally provided.
- Sharing of advertising costs.

Disadvantages

- Normally very expensive to set up.
- Business never truly your own.
- Franchiser may lay down certain requirements.
- May not be a flexible enough system to cater for changing needs of a local market.
- Profits normally have to be shared with the franchiser.

Co-operative

A co-operative is a business that is owned and controlled by the people working in it, therefore membership is usually open to all employees. The profits are not shared on the amount of capital put into the business by each individual but are distributed in proportion to the amount of work done by each person.

Choice and type of premises

When setting up in business one of the first things you will need to think about is the premises. The type and location of the premises are extremely important and it will be essential to thoroughly research this. Firstly you will need to establish that there is going to be a suitable potential market where you are looking. Local competitors will also need to be taken into account as will parking facilities and neighbouring businesses (you hardly want to be situated next door to a betting office!). If the premises you are interested in are not already occupied as a salon you will need to apply to the local council for a change of use.

POINT TO NOTE

Never agree to take on premises until you have been granted a change of use.

You then need to decide whether you are going to buy or rent premises. It will probably be the case that finances dictate your ultimate choice, but remember that sometimes large shopping complexes are owned by large companies or councils so the choice may be taken further from you.

Buying

If you decide that you are going to buy your premises you will need to contact a solicitor immediately to deal with the contracts involved and also to organise a land search. This is to check the ownership of the property and any plans in the future for redevelopment, etc. You will also need to establish if the property is freehold which means that the land and building would be yours if you purchased it, or whether it is leasehold which would mean that the building would be yours but the land that it is built on belongs to a third party and you would need to pay a ground rent.

Renting

Renting, or leasing as it is correctly known, is when you agree to occupy a building in return for an agreed sum of money. If you decide to rent a property you will again need the services of a solicitor to draw up a lease agreement which should include the following:

- How much rent is to be paid and how often (monthly, quarterly, etc.).
- When the amount of rent paid will be reviewed.
- How long the lease will run for.
- Who will be responsible for repairs, upkeep and decoration of the premises both internally and externally.
- What the rules are regarding subletting.
- Awareness of the Landlord and Tenant Act 1954.

Altering premises

Whether you are the owner of the property or just leasing, if you wish to alter the premises you will need to check the following:

- Planning permission.
- Building and fire regulations.
- Offices, Shops and Railway Premises Act 1963.

Progress Check

1 **a** List four forms of business arrangement.
   b Give two advantages and two disadvantages of each form of business arrangement.
2 State four important points to consider when looking for business premises.
3 Compare and contrast buying and renting as an option when deciding on business premises.

Basic business legislation

The Landlord and Tenant Act 1954

This piece of legislation gives the tenant security of tenure which means that you cannot be removed from the premises you are leasing unless the landlord can show a justified reason (not paying the rent, etc.). If the landlord wishes to remove you to sell the premises you will be entitled to compensation.

Offices, Shops and Railway Premises Act 1963

This piece of legislation relates in particular to hygiene, health and safety of the premises and covers such things as:

- Washing facilities.
- Toilets for both sexes and for client use.
- Sanitation.
- Safety on stairways.
- Eating and drinking facilities for staff required to stay on the premises at break-times.
- Adequate space for each employee (at least 400 cubic feet if the ceiling is 10 ft high).
- Fire exits and adequate fire fighting equipment.

Health and Safety at Work Act (HASAWA) 1974

This piece of legislation gives rights to both employers and employees.

Employers must provide:

- a safe and healthy workplace including maintenance of a reasonable working temperature of not less than 16 °C after the first opening hour, effective ventilation, suitable lighting and humidity levels and adequate toilets and washing facilities
- proper safety procedures – fire exits, notices, drills, handling and recording of accidents etc.
- safe equipment which is regularly serviced
- adequate training for all staff in safety procedures
- access to a written local health and safety policy.

Employees must:

- follow health and safety procedures
- act to protect themselves and others
- treat all equipment properly and report any faults.

Electricity at Work Regulations Act 1990

This piece of legislation states that all pieces of electrical equipment in the workplace should be checked annually by a qualified electrician. In particular, discontinue using any equipment that is broken or damaged, displays exposed wires or worn flexes or has a cracked or broken plug.

Also, you should take care never to overload sockets. Within a health and beauty and hairdressing business there is likely to be a great deal of portable equipment, e.g. hair dryers, epilation units, etc. which it is essential to have tested annually.

Fire Precautions Act 1971

This piece of legislation states that all employees should be trained and aware of emergency fire evacuation procedures. This should include such things as:

- the nearest fire exit (this should remain unlocked with clear access during working hours)
- the appropriate assembly point that everyone should meet at once the building has been evacuated
- in the event of a fire lifts must not be used

- where possible all windows and doors should be closed on leaving the premises
- all personal belongings should be left behind when evacuating the premises
- an awareness of the location and type of fire fighting equipment available on the premises.

Extinguisher	Type of fire
Blue band (dry powder)	Multi-purpose
Red band (water)	Solid material
Black band (carbon dioxide (CO_2) gas)	Electrical
Green band (halon gas)	Electrical
Cream band (foam)	Liquids
Red band (blanket)	Liquids and cloth

Fig. 13.3 *Fire-fighting equipment checklist*

GOOD PRACTICE

Each business should hold regular fire drills to ensure that their employees are fully prepared for their own safety and that of the clients in the event of a fire.

The Control of Substances Hazardous to Health Regulations (COSHH) 1988

These regulations lay down the ways in which substances which can be deemed hazardous to health (e.g. hydrogen peroxide) should be used and stored. Employers are responsible for assessing risks from hazardous substances and deciding upon action to reduce them. The majority of manufacturers issue clear instructions on the handling of products that fall within these regulations. It is essential that all employees should be made aware of the risks of such substances and where necessary be given training in such areas. Employees should always follow safety guidelines and take the precautions identified by their employer.

GOOD PRACTICE

In case a client becomes ill whilst waiting for or having treatment, it would be useful if the practitioner noted an emergency contact number on each of their clients' record cards.

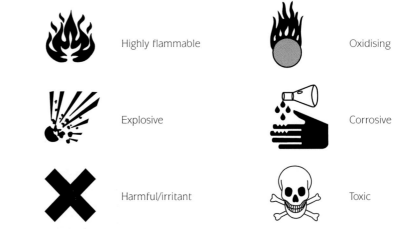

Fig. 13.4 *Common symbols used for substances hazardous to health*

Examples of hazardous substances that may be found within a health, beauty or hairdressing environment

Highly flammable

Highly flammable substances, e.g. acetone and solvents are deemed hazardous to health because if their vapours are exposed to naked flames or other means of extreme heat they can ignite.

Recommended storage

These products much be kept sealed and stored in a cool place. It is important not to store large quantities together as in the event of a fire they would cause a large explosion.

You should also be aware that some products are more flammable than others, e.g. ethanol-based products such as witch-hazel are far less flammable than acetone-based products such as nail varnish remover.

Recommended handling and usage

It is important to use flammable products in an area that is well ventilated and not to dispense them in an area where there is a risk of fire, e.g. whilst someone is smoking, near a naked flame or near an area of extreme heat. Extreme care must be taken when transferring products into dispensing containers to ensure that the labels are clear and correct. Care must be taken when using the product to avoid excessive inhalation, or contact with eyes and skin.

In the event that the product comes into contact with the eyes or skin emergency first aid of rinsing with water should be given immediately. If the casualty continues to have any sign of irritation they must be referred for medical advice. Medical advice must be sought if the product has been in contact with the eye or ingested. In the case of inhalation the person must be moved into fresh air.

Recommended disposal

These types of products must not be disposed of via sanitary systems as this leads to pollution. Advice on disposal should be sought from the practitioner's local environment health and trading standards department.

Recommended action

In the event of a fire evacuate the premises and notify the fire brigade of the location of stored flammables.

POINTS TO NOTE

- Acetone is used as a solvent in nail enamel removers. It can cause splitting and peeling of the nails and skin rashes on the fingers and hands. Inhalation of acetone can irritate the lungs.
- Alkyl sodium sulphates are used in shampoos for their cleaning ability and ease of rinsing from the hair. They may cause irritation to the skin.
- Ethanol is a colourless, clear and very flammable cosmetic ingredient. It is used as an antibacterial agent in mouth washes, liquid lip rouge, nail enamel, astringents etc. It is also used medicinally as a topical antiseptic, blood vessel dilator and sedative.
- Ethanolamide of lauric acid is used in soapless shampoos and is a mild skin irritant.
- Ether is used as a solvent in nail polishes. It is a mild skin irritant.
- Ethoxyethanol is used as a solvent and plasticiser for nail enamels. It is toxic when applied direct to the skin.

- Hydrogen peroxide is an ingredient used in lash and brow tinting, skin bleaches, hair bleaches, permanent colours and cold permanent waves for its oxidising and bleaching ability. If used undiluted it can cause burns to the skin.
- Salicylic acid is obtained from sweet birch, wintergreen leaves and other plants. It is used in small percentages as an antimicrobial and preservative in cosmetics such as face masks, hair tonics, hair dye removers, deodorants, suntan lotions etc. In medicines it is used in higher quantities in ointments, plasters, powders and lotions. Absorption via the skin may cause irritation such as skin rashes, vomiting, increased respiration and abdominal pain.

ACTIVITY

1   Select ten cosmetics from a bathroom, list their ingredients and research the effect of each.
2   List the products that due to their ingredients should be stored out of direct sunlight.

Explosive

Aerosols, e.g. hairspray, nail dry sprays, deodorants and air fresheners, are deemed hazardous to health as they are flammable and are explosive under certain heat-induced conditions.

Recommended storage

These products must be stored in a dry, cool place and away from direct sunlight.

Recommended handling and usage

Any product considered to be flammable should only be used within an area that is well ventilated. Care must be taken when handling such products to avoid contact with the eyes.

It is important when using aerosol/spray containers not to heat the canister or to tamper with the actuator. Care must be taken when using the product to avoid excessive inhalation and not to dispense it on to or near a naked flame or a very hot surface, which might cause combustion and fire.

Recommended disposal

In the event of a spillage, ventilate the area then, wearing disposable gloves and using a cloth or tissue, wipe up the spillage immediately.

Unless stated by the manufacturer dispose of small quantities in the normal manner ensuring that the canister can not be pierced or placed in extreme heat.

Recommended action

In the event of a fire evacuate the premises and notify the fire brigade of the location of stored aerosols.

POINTS TO NOTE

- Aerosol products under pressure when exposed to excessive heat e.g. in direct strong sunlight can explode and burst into flames
- Ensure canisters are not pierced and do not burn them.

Harmful/irritant products

Products such as hydrogen peroxide are deemed hazardous to health as they may cause irritation whether through direct contact, inhalation or absorption.

Recommended storage

These products should be stored carefully in a cool place within the business premises to avoid unnecessary exposure and possible irritation. The products must retain their lids and labels.

Recommended handling and usage

Care must be taken when handling harmful products including the wearing of gloves to protect the hands. Spillages must be removed immediately.

Recommended disposal

The majority of these products used within the health, beauty and hairdressing environment can be disposed of in the normal manner. It is important to observe manufacturers' instructions and if necessary seek the advice of the environmental health and trading standards department within the local authority.

Recommended action

Observe standard first aid procedures if ingredients come into contact with the eyes or skin or if inhaled or ingested.

POINT TO NOTE

It is important to remember that current legislation must be observed, in particular the Local Government (miscellaneous provisions) Act of 1982 which advises on the use and disposal of equipment such as needles used by practitioners for treatments such as acupuncture, electrolysis and ear piercing.

Health and safety legislation – the 'six pack' 1992

The new health and safety at work legislation is commonly referred to as the 'six pack' and was introduced to fulfil European Union directives. It is composed of the following six regulations (1–6).

1 The Management of Health and Safety at Work Regulations 1992

This is to ensure that the correct systems are in place to co-ordinate, control and monitor health and safety management. This regulation requires the employer to:

- assess the health and safety risks to employees, clients and other visitors to the business premises
- plan, implement, monitor and review preventative measures
- maintain accurate health and safety records, e.g. servicing and repair of equipment
- select and appoint appropriate people to implement fire evacuation procedures and first aid
- ensure that all employees are provided with detailed information on the company's health and safety procedures and are adequately trained and updated in these.

2 Provision and Use of Work Equipment Regulations 1992

The aim of this legislation is to clarify and join together the many regulations relating to equipment. This legislation ensures that all equipment, whether new or second hand, must be properly maintained and all employees must be correctly trained in how to use and maintain it. It also ensures that written records regarding its maintenance are accurately kept.

3 Manual Handling Operations Regulations 1992

This is to ensure that proper procedures are laid down by the employer for the manual handling of goods etc. within the workplace, e.g. lifting heavy loads which often results in industrial injury.

4 Workplace (Health, Safety and Welfare) Regulations 1992

These are to clarify and link together previous legislation relating to the working environment, safety facilities and 'housekeeping'.

5 Personal Protective Equipment at Work (PPE) Regulations 1992

These are to clarify and join together previous legislation including the use, type and storage of personal protective equipment. It is the employer's responsibility to ensure that all employees who may be at risk of being exposed to health risks or injury are provided, free of charge, with appropriate protective equipment. They must also ensure that such equipment is maintained in good working order and that all employees are trained in its use.

6 Health and Safety (Display Screen Equipment) Regulations 1992

These are to clearly identify rules and regulations to protect the health and safety of employees who use display screen equipment. As the use of computers in businesses has rapidly expanded these regulations were needed to ensure employees are protected from eye strain, muscular pain, etc. These regulations apply to both new and second-hand equipment and require employers to assess the work area and equipment to prevent risk of strain or injury to employees and to provide suitable desks, chairs and, if needed, spectacles along with the appropriate training.

The Management of Health and Safety at Work Regulations Act 1999

This is principally involved with risk assessment, which is covered in Chapter 3 in this book.

POINTS TO NOTE

- Inspectors of the Health and Safety Executive (HSE) are at liberty to enter any business at a reasonable time and investigate claims of unsafe practice with regard to health and safety. The inspectors have the power to serve an improvement notice if they find fault and the time limit given to rectify the fault, which is usually twenty one days. If the inspectors find that the fault may endanger personal safety they will serve a prohibition notice which requires the employer to cease activity immediately or face criminal prosecution.
- Statistics on health and safety are issued from time to time by the HSE.

The Safety Representative and Safety Committees Regulations 1977

This legislation ensures that safety representatives are appointed from the membership of a trade union recognised by the employer. It is their remit to liaise with the employers on all matters relating to health and safety. The number of representatives will obviously be dependent on a number of points, including the quantity of employees, the variety of occupations housed within the organisational structure and the varying types of work activities undertaken. It is the responsibility of the union to put forward their nominee in writing. This person must have been employed by the organisation for at least two years or have 'similar' employment experience in the previous two years. Once officially appointed to the role of health and safety representative the employee is entitled to time off for relevant training for the role, e.g. to attend seminars and meetings. The employer must give the representative sufficient consultation time on any new issues concerning health and safety.

The Health and Safety (First Aid) Regulations 1981

These regulations lay down the minimum requirements for the provision of first aid in the workplace. The requirements will obviously vary according to the number of employees and the type of work performed within the business. There should be at least one employee who has received training in first aid and continues to keep their skills current, e.g. a St. John's Ambulance First Aid certificate has to be renewed every three years.

First aid box

A standard first aid kit in the workplace should contain the following:

- guidance card
- sterile dressings of various sizes
- individually wrapped adhesive dressings
- eye pads
- triangular bandages
- safety pins.

The quantity of each of the above items will be dependent on the workplace. The contents should all be kept in a damp and dust-proof container which is exclusively used for first aid purposes. It is important to note that from time to time regulations may change or be updated. The container must be clearly labelled in accordance with current regulations.

GOOD PRACTICE

Always check the current regulations regarding the contents of a workplace first aid box.

POINTS TO NOTE

The first aid requirements of a workplace will vary according to:

- the number of employees
- the nature of the work undertaken within the business
- the size and layout of the business premises
- the employer's first aid policy.

Problem	Priority	Action
Minor cuts	To stop the bleeding	Apply pressure over cotton wool taking care to avoid contact with the blood.
Severe cuts	To stop the bleeding	Keep applying pressure over a clean towel until qualified help arrives. Put on disposable gloves as soon as possible.
Electric shock	To remove from source of electricity	Do not touch the person until they are disconnected from the electricity supply. If breathing has stopped, artificial respiration will need to be given by a qualified person. Ring for an ambulance.
Dizziness	To restore the flow of blood to the head	Position the person with their head between their knees and loosen their clothing.
Fainting	To restore the flow of blood to the head	Lie the person down with their feet raised on a cushion.
Nose bleed	To constrict the flow of blood	Sit the client up with their head bent forward. Loosen the clothing around their neck. Pinch the soft part of their nose firmly until bleeding has stopped. Make sure breathing continues through the mouth during this period. If bleeding has not stopped after half an hour, medical attention must be sought.
Burns	To cool the skin and prevent it from breaking	Hold the affected area under cool, running water until the pain is relieved. Serious burns should be covered loosely with a sterile dressing and medical attention sought.
Epilepsy	To prevent self-injury and relieve embarrassment	Do not interfere forcibly with a person during an attack. Gently prevent them from injuring themselves. Ensure the person's airways are clear and wipe away any froth which forms at the mouth. After the attack, cover with a blanket, comfort and give reassurance until recovery is complete.
Objects in the eye	To remove the object without damaging the eye	Expose the invaded area and try stroking the object towards the inside corner of the eye with a dampened twist of cotton wool. If this is not successful, help the person to use an eye bath containing clean warm water.
Falls	To determine if there is spine damage. To treat minor injuries if the fall is not serious	If the person complains of pains in the back or neck, then do not move them; cover them with a warm blanket and get medical aid immediately. For less serious falls, treat the bruises, cuts, sprains or grazes as appropriate.

Fig. 13.5 *First aid situations the practitioner may have to deal with*

The Reporting of Injuries, Diseases and Dangerous Occurrences Regulations 1985

These regulations cover all employees and members of the public who as a result of work-based activity suffer a condition or an injury.

Trade Descriptions Act 1968 and 1972

This act makes it a criminal offence to describe goods falsely, and to sell or offer for sale goods which have been so described. It covers many things including advertisements, display cards, oral descriptions and applies to quality, quantity, fitness for purpose and price. The part of the act passed in 1972 deals with labelling of the country of origin; a product must be clearly labelled so that the consumer can see where it was made.

The Sex Discrimination Acts 1975 and 1986 and The Race Relations Act 1976

The aims or these acts are to prevent direct or indirect discrimination against candidates when applying for work on the grounds of race, sex, or martial status. The Equal Opportunities Commission will investigate complaints made on any of the above grounds and it monitors job advertisements as well.

An employee can seek unfair dismissal on grounds of sex discrimination through an industrial tribunal irrespective of length of service.

Contract of employment

This is a legally binding document drawn up by the employer when a new member of staff is appointed. The reason for such a document is to give both the employer and the employee a certain degree of protection and security and to formalise specific points. By law any person working 16 hours or more a week must be given a contract of employment within 13 weeks of the starting date.

The contract should cover the following points:

- Name of the company and the employee.
- Date when employment began.
- Job description.
- Hours of work.
- Pay scale, how payment will be made and at what intervals (weekly, monthly, etc.).
- Holiday entitlement.
- Pension arrangements.
- Sickness and sick pay conditions.
- Length of notice which an employee is entitled to give and receive.
- Disciplinary procedures.

There are other conditions which may be added such as working at different locations, confidentiality, medical examination, etc. and these are sometimes presented in a separate staff handbook.

Equal Pay Act 1970

The aim of this Act was to ensure that people who undertake the same work must be employed on the same terms and pay.

ACTIVITY

Although there are laws relating to offences for equal opportunities the employer is not obliged by law to be an equal opportunities employer.

(a) Look through the classified section in your trade journal and local newspaper, and make a list of the number of advertisements which state that the employer is an equal opportunities employer.

(b) Classify the type of organisations which state that they are equal opportunities employers.

The National Minimum Wage Act 1998

This Act took effect from 1 April 1999 and it enforces the following pay rates:

- a minimum level of £3.70 an hour (at the time of going to press, an increase to £4.10 was to be implemented in October 2001, with a further 10p in October 2002)
- a minimum level of £3.20 for 18–21 year olds

- a minimum level of £3.20 an hour for workers of 22 and over for six months after starting a new job with a new employer if they are receiving accredited training.

Exemptions from the national minimum wage include:

- self-employed
- anyone under 18
- prisoners
- the armed forces
- share fishermen.

Working Time Regulations (1998)

On 1 October 1998 regulations to implement the European working time directive came into force. The regulations provide the following new rights.

- A limit on the hours which a worker can be required to work from an average of 48 hours per week though some may choose to work longer.
- A right to four weeks paid leave per year.
- A right to 11 consecutive hours rest in any 24-hour period.
- A right to an in-work rest break if their working day is longer than six hours.
- A right to one day off each week.
- A limit on normal working hours of night workers to an average of 8 hours in any 24-hour period and entitlement for night workers to receive regular health checks.

The Disability Discrimination Act 1995

This Act covers people who have had a disability in the past as well as those who are currently registered disabled. The disability of a person is defined in the Act as either a physical or mental impairment which has a substantial long-term effect on an individual's ability to carry out what are considered to be normal day-to-day activities. This Act has several clauses and one of these relates to employment making it unlawful for employers who have twenty or more staff to discriminate against any current or prospective employee because of a reason relating to their disability. Responsibilities of employers include such things as making reasonable changes to the working environment and general employment arrangements so that the disabled employee is not disadvantaged compared to their able-bodied colleagues.

There are exemptions under this Act including:

- police officers
- people serving in the armed services
- fire officers
- prison officers.

The Employment Rights Act 1996

This Act supersedes some of the points in The Trade Union and Employment Rights Act 1993 which was designed to improve the employment rights of part-time workers. It entitled all female employees to take up to fourteen weeks maternity leave irrespective of their length of service with the organisation. It also gave all employees, after a period of time, the right to be given written terms and conditions of employment and it enabled all employees to appeal against unfair dismissal.

The Employment Rights Act of 1996 states that an employee is entitled to ask for a written statement of their terms and conditions of employment after one month's employment, and have the right to receive this after the expiry of two months from the date of commencement of employment. This Act does not refer to a contract of employment but does give an employer a legal obligation to supply a written statement which should contain details of the salary or wages, hours of work, notice entitlements and obligations, holiday entitlement, date of commencement of employment, job description and workplace location. This Act does not require the employer to title the document as a contract, although in employment law the employee is deemed to have a contract of employment when the offer by the employer of the job and the acceptance by the employee indicates an intention to enter into a legally binding relationship.

If the employer does not provide the written statement then the employee has the right to make an application to an industrial tribunal who can order the employer to produce the written statement.

POINTS TO NOTE

- An employee who is dismissed whilst pursuing their right to a written statement of their terms and conditions of employment will have unfair dismissal protection irrespective of their length of employment.
- The Part-time Workers (prevention of less favourable treatment) Regulations 2000 came into force on 1 July 2000 to ensure part-time workers are treated no less favourably than comparable full-timers.

GOOD PRACTICE

A contract of employment can be used to the employer's advantage if probationary periods and performance targets have been included, agreed upon and are not fulfilled.

Misrepresentation Act 1967

This legislation protects a person who enters into a contract and allows them the opportunity to make a claim based on misrepresentation of terms which causes them to suffer damage.

GOOD PRACTICE

It is essential for the manager to keep abreast of any changes in the employment law. It may be in the case of a small business due to restricted legal knowledge that they decide to take advice from a legal business advisor.

Statutory sick pay (SSP)

All employees over the age of sixteen years of age are entitled to the payment of statutory sick pay (SSP) after they have been off work through illness for four consecutive days from their employer. The employer by law must pay this minimum amount to the employee and they must maintain records of SSP and the employee sickness for inspection by the Department of Social Security (DSS). These records must include details of the dates of absenteeism due to sickness and the days that the employee would normally be at work, i.e. the qualifying days which are generally Monday–Friday, but in the health, beauty and hairdressing industries are highly likely to be different.

Maternity and Parental Leave Regulations 1999
Maternity rights

In England and Wales women employees who satisfy the relevant qualifying conditions are entitled to the following statutory rights:

- paid time off to receive antenatal care. A woman who is advised by a properly qualified person to attend an antenatal clinic has the right not to be unreasonably refused time off during her working hours to enable her to keep an appointment.
- maternity pay, which is currently payable for eighteen weeks to a woman absent from work because of her pregnancy. There are certain qualifying requirements, however.

♦ the right to return to work after confinement. A woman can currently return to work at any time before the end of the period of twenty-nine weeks beginning with the week in which the date of confinement falls.

Parental leave

From 15 December 1999, employees who have completed one year of service with their employer will be entitled to 13 weeks parental leave for each child born or adopted after this date. They will be able to take this leave up until the child's fifth birthday or until five years have elapsed following placement in the case of adoption. Parents of disabled children will be able to use their leave over a longer period up until the child's eighteenth birthday.

POINTS TO NOTE

♦ A woman is automatically held to be unfairly dismissed if the sole reason or principal reason for the dismissal is either that she is pregnant or any other reason connected with the pregnancy.
♦ An employer should carry out a risk assessment on a pregnant employee.

Disciplinary procedures

All employees should receive a copy of the company's disciplinary procedure within their contract of employment. This will detail the company's policy for dealing with what it considers to be misconduct. The employee should be given a breakdown of the areas of misconduct. There should also be a description of the disciplinary action taken, i.e. verbal warning, written warning etc., the level of management to be involved in such a scenario together with an appeals procedure.

The majority of employers will stipulate that an employee will be given one verbal warning of misconduct followed by a formal (verbal and written) warning and a final written (verbal and written) warning followed by dismissal. Immediate suspension may take place if gross misconduct occurs, e.g. theft.

GOOD PRACTICE

The employer should:

♦ always investigate alleged misconduct
♦ involve all parties concerned
♦ allow time for improved conduct before taking further steps
♦ ensure that apart from an extremely serious offence no employee should be dismissed on the first occasion
♦ ensure that dismissal is fair before taking action.

POINTS TO NOTE

♦ Large companies tend to have their own clearly defined grievance and disciplinary procedures.
♦ The Department of Trade and Industry (DTI) publishes a booklet entitled *Individual Rights of Employees* and is available at Job Centres.

ACTIVITY

Design a grievance/disciplinary procedure suitable for a large hair and beauty chain ensuring that the following points are taken into consideration:

- protection of and respect for the physical and human resources of the company
- accurate, truthful completion of records, e.g. bookings, time keeping, stock taking, etc.
- employee's attendance, e.g. time keeping, illness, etc.
- confidentiality
- rules and regulations relating to food, drink, etc.

Termination of employment and redundancy

The manager at some time during their career may have to consider action or even possible termination of an employee's employment. It is paramount that they must consider carefully the legal implications such as unfair dismissal and ensure that they observe fully the employer's and employee's rights. It is wise to contact the local Advisory, Conciliation and Arbitration Service (ACAS) office for current legislation and advice.

Unfair dismissal – The Employment Protection (Consolidation) Act 1978

Under the Employment Protection Act 1978 an employee may claim unfair dismissal if they can prove that the employer has acted in an unlawful manner. The employee must have worked for the organisation for at least one year.

Grounds for unfair dismissal are:

- the joining of a trade union or choosing not to join a trade union.
- alleged redundancy due to the business changing ownership
- any other area where an employer does not adhere to stipulated procedures.

Unfair dismissal can also be sought, irrespective of the employee's length of service, on the grounds of:

- pregnancy

- discrimination due to the sex, race or marital status of an individual.

All of these rights are not affected by the signing of a contract of employment, which usually states 'this contract does not affect your statutory rights'.

Treatment and consumer legislation

This legislation relates to services offered within the business and its environment.

Local bye-laws concerning body massage treatments

In England and Wales licensing is controlled by the local authorities. Anyone wishing to set up a clinic offering body massage treatments may need a license to practise, depending upon the area of the country in which their business is located. This license is obtained from the local authority through the Environmental and Trading Standards Department. To qualify for such a license the applicant normally submits information concerning their premises, staff and qualifications. Inspection of the premises is then carried out and once approved by the authority an annual fee, which varies from authority to authority, is paid.

Local Government (Miscellaneous Provisions) Act 1982

This Act is monitored through the local Environmental Health and Trading Standards Department (EHTS). Any practitioner using needles for treatments, such as acupuncture, epilation, sclerotherapy, collagen injections, semi-permanent make up or ear piercing, must apply for a license to practise under the above Act. This is to ensure that correct hygienic practices are used for storage, use and disposable of 'sharp' implements.

The Sale and Supply of Goods Act 1994

This Act replaces the Supply of Goods and Services Act 1982 and the Sale of Goods Act 1979. It relates to all goods including food regardless of where they are purchased. Terms under the Act state that the seller has to ensure that the goods are:

- of satisfactory quality: this is defined as the standard that would be regarded by a reasonable person as satisfactory having taken into account the description of the goods, the price and any other relevant circumstances

- reasonably fit: the goods must be able to meet whatever the seller claims they do, e.g. a car must reach 0–60 miles per hour in the number of minutes stated.

Once the contract has been made between the seller and the buyer this Act can be enforced. Verbal and written contracts are both classed as valid contracts and a buyer is entitled to have either their money back or goods replaced if the contract is broken.

Office of Fair Trading (OFT)
The Office of Fair Trading (OFT) is responsible for the administration of policy competition in the UK. It controls monopolies, mergers and consumer protection, e.g. it investigates consumers' complaints about inaccurate trade descriptions.

Trade Descriptions Act 1968, 1972
This Act makes it a criminal offence to describe goods falsely, and to sell or offer for sale goods which have been so described. It covers many things including advertisements, display cards, oral descriptions and applies to quality, quantity, fitness for purpose and price. The part of the Act passed in 1972 deals with labelling of the country of origin; a product must be clearly labelled so that the consumer can see where it was made.

The Consumer Credit Act 1974
This Act ensures that the actual rate of interest charged for credit facilities must be highlighted to a borrower.

The Prices Act 1974
This ensures that prices should be displayed so as not to give a false impression to potential buyers.

The Resale Prices Act 1964, 1976
This Act prevents manufacturers from enforcing retailers of their products to charge a certain price. However, it does not prevent them from supplying a recommended retail price.

The Consumer Safety Act 1978
This Act identifies the standards for legal safety to reduce the possible risk to consumers from products that may be potentially dangerous or harmful.

The Consumer Protection Act 1987
This Act deals with three main subjects: product liability, general safety requirements and misleading prices. It follows European directives to safeguard the consumer from unsafe products.

Environmental Health and Trading Standards Departments (EHTS)

Trading standards officers are employed by local authorities and their remit is to investigate complaints from consumers against businesses. Having investigated the complaint they have the authority to take the business to court to prevent reoccurrence of the complaint.

The British Standards Institution (kite marks and safety standards)

The British Standard Institution (BSI) is an independent body which sets voluntary standards of reliability and quality. Its objectives are to:

◆ establish quality standards
◆ promote health and safety
◆ protect the environment.

Manufacturers submit their products for testing voluntarily for them to be tested on such things as their safety, quality, strength etc. The kite marks of the institution are displayed by many businesses to provide the consumer with a guarantee that they have recognition from the board, indicating that the product has been tested and approved. Examples of such quality marks include the BSI kite mark, the British Gas Seal of Service and the Investors in People Award (see Fig. 13.6).

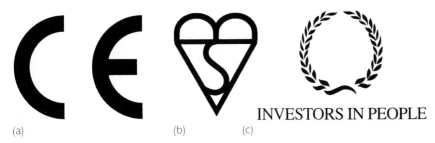

(a)   (b)   (c)

Fig. 13.6 *Quality marks (a) European quality specification; (b) BSI kite mark and (c) Investors in People Award*

Data Protection Act 1984

Practitioners using computers to store personal data on their clients must comply with the Data Protection Act of 1984 which requires them to register with the Data protection Registrar, or they are liable to face prosecution. The Act only applies to computer information stored relating to living persons. It does not cover manually stored records unless these are made under the Consumer Credit Act.

Information and forms are available from Post Offices and there is a fee for a three-year licence, however small business can complete a simplified registration form. The application requires information on what is stored on the computer, its uses, sources and to whom the data may be disclosed.

Anyone who feels that they are affected by lost or incorrect information or disclosure of personally held computer data without their consent may make a claim to the Registrar. They can be told who holds data on them and for a nominal fee are entitled to see these records within 40 days of payment. NB when completing client records careful consideration should be given to the terminology used.

In-salon entertainment

Many hairdressing and beauty salons play background music within their establishments to create the appropriate type of ambience. In beauty and health clinics it is often intended to create a relaxing environment whereas the environment of the hair salon is much more lively. If the owner decides to play recorded music they will need to pay a fee, whereas if they use a television or radio broadcast they will need to buy a licence.

Insurance

Insurance is a way of protecting people and property against unforeseen circumstances. It is possible to insure against almost any risk for a sum of money called a premium. In return for this payment, should the risk which you are insuring against occur, you will receive compensation to indemnify you for the loss (to be put back in the position you were in before the loss).

When operating in a business certain forms of insurance are compulsory by law. They are as follows:

Public liability insurance

This insurance covers claims relating to injury, disease or damage to the property of a third party (the client). It can be extended to cover liability arising out of goods sold or supplied or if the business involves work away from the premises.

Many professional beauty therapy organisations can arrange group cover which is normally included in some form of membership fee which will generally encompass other benefits. It is sensible to look at having a one million pound cover against any injury arising out of the treatments offered.

Employer's liability insurance

Any business employing staff is legally obliged to have this form of insurance. If an employee is injured at work it is normally the employer who is held responsible whether personally at fault or not. The insurance certificate must be prominently displayed. Any injuries that do occur must be recorded in an accident book.

Although not compulsory by law it is sensible to have insurance to cover:

- Theft.
- Damage to premises, stock and equipment by fire, flood, etc.
- Loss of profits through damage to premises.
- Fidelity bonding (insurance cover to protect against the dishonesty of employees).
- Personal accident insurance.
- Life assurance.

ACTIVITY

Draft a plan of a salon layout and decide on the type of establishment and the number of staff to be employed. Pay particular attention to health, safety, hygiene and legislation.

Staff and recruitment

Role of the employer

The employer has overall control of the wellbeing and efficient running of the business whether or not they are directly involved in it.

Role of the manager/manageress

In smaller establishments this role may be performed by the employer. It is not an easy task requiring a great deal of skill and judgement.

The personal qualities that make a good manager are:

- Enthusiasm about the business and the industry in general.
- Willingness to listen and learn.
- Ability to juggle many tasks at the same time; clients, staff, book keeping, wages, etc.
- Patience and tact in dealing with both staff and client problems both on a business and a personal level.
- Knowledge of new trends, e.g. attending exhibitions, reading trade journals, etc.
- Excellent personal and interpersonal skills (tact, diplomacy, punctuality, good communicator, working as a member of a team).
- Immaculate appearance.

The role of the therapist

It goes without saying that the therapist should be well trained and qualified. The therapist needs to be enthusiastic about their work and have a willingness to learn and develop skills. The therapist needs to have a flexible approach and be happy to work as a member of a team, sometimes performing different roles. Again, they should possess excellent personal and interpersonal skills and be of immaculate appearance.

Role of the receptionist

The receptionist is the first point of contact with the salon and therefore an extremely important for the business. The reception area may be staffed by more than one person in larger establishments and by the therapists themselves in smaller concerns. Whoever performs the task needs to be well trained in the workings of the reception area as potential business can be lost through incompetence. (See Chapter 3.)

Support staff

In larger establishments, roles such as cleaning, laundry, handling of stock, preparation of working areas, etc. may be performed by support staff which will obviously add to the overall efficiency of services provided. However it is important that everyone in the establishment can deal with these areas if continuity is to be maintained.

Efficient staff practices

Communication

If the salon is ultimately going to be a successful business it will depend upon efficient levels of communication between all employees thus making the staff more highly motivated and providing a friendly atmosphere for the client.

- Regular staff meetings should be arranged so all employees know what is happening and are allowed to give comments and express their views.
- Staff should be made to feel that they are an important part of the business.
- Staff should be rewarded for anything they do well.
- All employees should be treated equally and fairly.
- Gossip should be discouraged either about clients or fellow employees.
- All employees should be treated with respect.

Staff development

The success of the business lies in expansion and not remaining static. New treatments and ideas should be periodically introduced to increase profit margins, attract new clients and to keep abreast of changes. Staff should be regularly sent on training courses whether they be product knowledge, new skills or further qualifications. This will also help to ensure a highly motivated workforce boosting staff morale.

Appraisal

Appraisal is the term given to a review of an employee's performance over a given period of time, normally annually. The main reason for operating an appraisal system is to help the employee become more effective.

The appraisal is normally categorised into the following areas:

- Review. Looking back over the period concerned, what is the appraisee's job? Has it altered in any way? Is it being performed effectively? Are there any problems?

- Action. What needs to be done? Should there be any training and development? Does the employee need more support/guidance?
- Monitoring. Are the actions being carried out? Are targets being achieved?

Costing of treatments

Many salons do not properly cost out their services so therefore they do not make an adequate profit and wonder why the business is not doing very well even though the appointment book is always full. Costing is very important and should encompass materials, overheads, wages and a profit margin.

The following shows an example of a back massage treatment with an explanation underneath;

Back massage treatment (30 minutes) £15.00

Materials	£1.50
Electricity	£0.80
Laundry	£1.00
Overheads	£1.70
Labour	£6.00
Profit @ 50%	£5.00

- The figures for the materials used are obtained by dividing how much the product would cost at retail by the number of times you can use that product.
- The electricity and overheads costs are calculated by taking the quarterly bills, dividing to find the hourly rate and then dividing again by the number of therapists.
- Laundry is calculated in the same way.
- Labour in this incidence is calculated on the therapist working for £12.00 per hour.
- Profit is calculated on 50% of the total other costs.

Progress Check

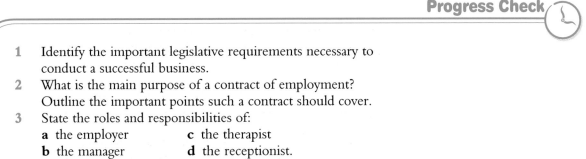

1. Identify the important legislative requirements necessary to conduct a successful business.
2. What is the main purpose of a contract of employment? Outline the important points such a contract should cover.
3. State the roles and responsibilities of:
   a the employer   **c** the therapist
   b the manager   **d** the receptionist.
4. What do you understand by the term 'appraisal'?

Marketing and promotion

Many salon owners may wonder why business is not better when they feel they are offering an excellent service, using top quality products and employing well qualified and highly competent staff. The answer probably lies in the fact that they are not marketing themselves sufficiently.

Marketing is not just about placing an advertisement in the local paper, it is the whole product, the image that the salon wishes to create. In the business of aesthetics this is never more important, attention to detail counts. Marketing your services and appropriate skin care products to the right audience requires foresight, empathy, knowledge, enthusiasm and above all, understanding.

Retailing in the salon

Selling is a very important aspect of salon operations. Profits made on the sales of products and services make the business successful which will ultimately increase the earning potential of all the employees.

The majority of sales in a salon are lost by therapists who think it is not their job to 'sell'. However, a professional therapist realises that a client is not only paying for a service but for the experience and knowledge the therapist has to offer. Many clients are reluctant to ask the therapist which products are right from them but they desperately want to know. It is an essential part of a therapist's job to provide their clients with advice on how to take care of themselves and this includes advice on treatments and products. A therapist must look at each client individually and ensure they link suitable treatments and products not only to the service the client has booked but perhaps also to the client's lifestyle. For example, if a client booked for a back massage informs the therapist she is getting married in nine months, the therapist could link a range of treatments such as facials, waxing, manicures, slimming and toning treatments and make up to help her prepare for her big day. Remember, therapists train for a long time and every year of industrial experience with additional training expands the breadth of knowledge that can be offered to a client.

Cerebral profile of a client

It is paramount that a therapist can identify an individual client's cerebral profile in order to meet their retailing needs. Asking questions and listening to the client's responses can assess this. The therapist must then choose products to match the client's needs and select the appropriate vocabulary (to suit her cerebral profile) to gain a 'yes' response to retailing. A client may actually have several profiles to match her lifestyle, for example one for work and one for her private home life. A therapist must also assess their own profile in order to learn how to identify and strengthen their own weaknesses.

Research has identified four different client profiles:

1. **The rational (intellectual, technical) client**: will analyse every piece of information available, will not want to know about packaging or product texture, but will want pure factual information on ingredients and their effects. The sale of goods to this client will be made more quickly if you give precise information and the correct products and ingredients to gain the appropriate results. This type of client will spend a lot of money if the quality is right.

2. **The insecure client**: needs security, so the therapist must reassure them, be extremely patient and proceed step by step. This client will need a lot of written documentation to peruse (finding security in written rather than spoken information), will want to know how long the product brand has been around, the number of countries where it is available and whether it has been tested, for example in hospitals, etc. This client will have a mental budget before entering the salon and will know what they have available to spend.

   Always reassure this type of client; slowly tell them step by step that they have made a good choice, the right choice and that they will be very pleased with their purchase. This client will need to be given trial sizes with leaflets and brochures. However unwittingly, do not mislead the client. The sale will take a time but once you have established trust and confidence this client will maintain their trust in you.

3. **The 'original' (artist) client**: wants the latest product and wants to be the only one with it! It is important to stimulate this client's imagination; they will not want technical information as they are after the designer 'tag' and like to take risks. As long as you do not mislead you could use phrases like: 'this product is revolutionary', 'extraordinary', 'outstanding' or better still 'it's unique', 'just for you'. The sale to this client does not take so long and they will not have a fixed budget.

4. **The sentimental client**: is extremely talkative, wants to be your friend and to do exactly the same as you. This client is generally very emotional and will talk about their spouse, children, grandparents, animals and so on. It is important to be very attentive, paying close attention to details such as noting their birthday, 'likes' and 'dislikes' etc. If the client talks about their next family holiday, for example, you could direct them to the skin care products they could purchase for use in the sun, discussing the texture, colour and aroma of the product which they will enjoy talking about. The sale with this client may take a long time but they have no mental budget and they will trust your advice.

Objections to sales

In learning to retail, the therapist needs to understand why the various objections to sales are made and whether an objection has occurred because of a misunderstanding. The therapist must put in place a 'discovery step' to establish what is behind the objection and whether it is authentic. To do this the therapist and client need to be face to face, for eye contact, so that the therapist can ascertain the real reason for the objection from the client. That it is a 'real' objection may be evident from the client's non-verbal communication – their body language may be relaxed while they answer questions. A client making a 'fake' objection may be less relaxed and may seek reassurance by frequently touching their face. The therapist should take a positive approach to the challenge of an objection by trying to discover whether there is a misunderstanding, by staying calm and not becoming aggressive, and by respecting the client's wishes and needs.

There are several common objections to making a purchase.

- **Costs**. You could establish why the client thinks the product is expensive by asking them to what they are comparing the product. Perhaps the product seems expensive compared to the brand the client currently uses, so you could compare active ingredients of that brand to the one being recommended or discuss which will give the greater results in a shorter space of time. Never belittle a competitor but state the obvious, for example if the client is using a product with which you are familiar, you may be able to tell her the product is less suitable for her at the moment as her skin is currently dehydrated. Ask the client about her skin and whether she is seeing an improvement in their skin as generally in 'retail' outlets there is no follow-up to check on any improvement once a client has purchased a product. You, however, can provide a professional service and can evaluate and review home care on a monthly basis and recommend the use of high quality professional products with active ingredients prescribed by a professional therapist. Remember, if cost is a problem to a client do not recommend several products to them, prioritise just one.
- **Time**. Establish why the client believes they have no time for skin care by asking what they mean by a long time. Respond that it takes only 5 to 10 minutes a day for basic skin care to maintain the youthful appearance of the skin.
- **Efficiency**. Generally, a client who uses this as an objection with have either a 'rational' or an 'insecure' profile so the therapist needs to respond with the appropriate vocabulary to reassure them. Establish what they mean by 'not efficient' and respond with the appropriate information such as quoting past case studies or data on efficiency tests carried out by the manufacturer.
- **Texture/Aroma**. If the client raises an objection over these points then the therapist is at fault, as they have not listened adequately to the client's preferences, noting the textures and aromas they like, before recommending products.
- **Sensitivity**. If a client states that they are sensitive to products, the therapists must determine what they mean by sensitive. Discuss what ingredients they are sensitive to and respond with information supplied by the manufacturer on dermatological tests they have carried out. Always offer this client a trial size product (it is not a gift to complement a sale but a trial for allergy testing to reassure them) and record this on their record card ensuring a follow-through on its performance at the next visit.

The therapist's body language, volume and speed of voice, appearance and perfume and the salon environment (the temperature, lighting, aroma, etc) will all play an important part in establishing a professional relationship with clients, therefore ultimately affecting the total revenue into the salon from treatments and retail.

To gain information from the client, a therapist must use open questions which allow the client to respond and closed questions to confirm information and gain a 'yes' response to a question. For example, if a client indicates they want to purchase an efficient slimming cream, the therapist should respond by asking what the client means by 'efficient'. The client's response will provide the therapist with a guide to either a further open question or a closed one to take the sale forward. After gaining several 'yes' responses, the therapist must close the sale by asking whether the client would like to buy the product(s) today.

GOOD PRACTICE

- Ensure you offer each client retail and salon treatment advice.
- Listen to each client to identify their profile and select the appropriate vocabulary to gain a 'yes' response.
- Keep up to date with all the commercial and professional products on the market.
- Record all sales and trial sizes on each client's records and evaluate and review the client's progress at their next visit.

It is important to have a thorough understanding of all the products and treatments available in the salon. Many skin care companies offer product knowledge workshops to familiarise the therapist with the products and methods they offer. If this is not available then it will be essential to read all the information available about the products you intend to sell.

Advice for successful selling

1 Find out exactly what the client needs. This means asking questions and listening carefully to the answers. Use 'closed' questions to get short, straightforward answers (usually yes or no); these help to confirm or eliminate information and ideas. Use 'open' questions to invite fuller and more detailed answers. Open questions help to develop the conversation and provide more personal information.

2 Give the client advice. Always relate the benefits of the product specifically to the client.

3 Always smile and talk confidently and positively about the product which you have chosen. Where possible tell the client about your personal experiences with the product.

4 Explain how the product should be used. If possible let the client feel, smell or hold the product. Remember that if the client touches the product and asks the price, then the item is practically sold.

5 Close the sale. Look for signals that tell you the client has decided to take your advice and buy the product; head nodding in agreement, smiles and friendly eye contact are positive buying signals.

6 Where appropriate, explain the benefits of the different sizes available in the product. These will usually be linked to the price. Hesitation or reluctance to mention the price will give the client the impression that you consider the product too expensive.

7 Gain agreement with the client. This is achieved either immediately or after a short period of 'thinking' time. Do not be afraid of silences at this stage. Just keep quiet and wait patiently for the patient to make a decision. Do not talk yourself out of a sale.

8 Use link selling to encourage your client to buy complementary products from the same range, e.g. cleansers and toners, body exfoliants and lotions, etc.

9 Once you have sold the product, wrap it up and process the payment. As you hand over the purchase, check once more that the client understands how to use the product.

10 Enter the details of the purchase on the client's record card and be sure to ask next time how the client is finding the product.

ACTIVITY

Product a treatment plan suitable for a client going on a summer holiday, and design a promotional leaflet for the plan

Sales and selling pointers

- Offer trial sizes to unsure clients to help gain a sale.
- Offer trial sizes when clients purchase a product to introduce them to an additional or complementary product within that range.
- Introduce a client referral scheme into the salon – if a regular client introduces a friend then some kind of incentive such as a discount could be given.
- Introduce a referral scheme with other practitioners – offer incentives to possible sources of client referrals such as hair-dressing salons or health clinics.
- If a therapist goes on maternity leave, send a card informing her regular clients and perhaps offer them a discount for treatments with another therapist until she returns.
- Acknowledge all clients' birthdays – in the month of their birthday send each client an incentive to visit the salon.
- Organise new treatment promotions.
- Have new treatment information printed and hand it out to every client.
- Offer special treatment packages – holidays, Christmas, etc.
- Change display areas very regularly.
- Change salon price lists yearly and date them.
- Change salon décor regularly.
- Set out to promote a product every week knowing all its benefits, effects and ingredients (you will soon know your whole range very thoroughly).
- Organise a salon anniversary promotion yearly inviting local press along.
- Make a feature out of a 'slow' day of the week – give it a name and offer extra incentives when people have an appointment on that day.
- Change your own image regularly.

POINTS TO NOTE

- Use the seasons to your advantage when promoting treatments and highlight the treatments' seasonal benefits to your clients, such as detoxifying treatments for summer exposure.
- Regular newsletters are a way of keeping your clients up to date on your services and staff as well as a way of reminding them of the benefits of existing treatments.
- Enter professional competitions and use these for promoting your business.

Taxation

Tax can be defined as a compulsory financial contribution imposed by the government in order to raise revenue to support the public services that are used and shared by everyone. There are many forms of taxation – on individual earnings, on the profits of a business, Value Added Tax (VAT) and National Insurance (NI). VAT and NI are explained briefly below.

Value Added Tax (VAT)

This is a tax that is levied by the Government on most business transactions known as 'taxable supplies'. If a business has a taxable turnover greater than a certain amount (enquire at your local tax office for the current level) it must register for VAT, filling out the appropriate form from the VAT office. A registration number will then be issued and detailed records will need to be kept of all business transactions. The salon owner will need to charge VAT on services provided and products sold, currently standing at 17.5%, and will be liable to pay VAT on equipment and products purchased from VAT registered companies. These are referred to as outputs and inputs respectively. Every three months (VAT tax period) it will be necessary to fill in a form known as a VAT return. Where output tax exceeds input tax the difference will need to be paid to customs and excise, and the reverse where input tax is greater than the output – then it may be reclaimed from customs and excise.

National Insurance contributions

This is a tax paid by every working person to the inland revenue to support public services, the unemployed and to help towards the payment of a pension in old age. They should be collected by the employer in the case of employees. There are five classes of National Insurance contribution:

- **Class 1**. These are contributions for employed persons.
- **Class 1a**. These are contributions paid when your employer provides you with a car.

- **Class 2**. These are contributions to be paid by the self-employed. They can be paid either by direct debit through a bank or by stamping a card. If earnings fall below the *lower earning limit* it may be possible to apply for exemption, but entitlement to some of the benefits provided may be lost.
- **Class 3**. These are voluntary contributions.
- **Class 4**. These are additional contributions that may be made by the self-employed person and are calculated on the profits of the business.

(More information on NI is available from your local Inland Revenue office.)

Basic business terminology

Insolvency
This is a term used to describe either a business or a person who is unable to pay their debts (bankrupt).

Liquidation
This refers to the winding up of a business to pay off its debts.

Professional standards (ethics)
Every profession has a code of conduct and beauty therapy is no exception. The code stipulates how the therapist should conduct him/herself in order to obtain a high professional standard.

Medical problems

- Do not carry out any medical treatments.
- Do not give injections.
- Do not cut or sever the skin in any way.
- Do not prescribe oral medication.
- Never treat a client under a doctor's care without obtaining written permission.
- Do not criticise any treatment being given by a doctor.
- Always refer to a doctor if you think a client has a medical problem.
- Try to foster good relations with your local medical practitioners.

Salon manners

- Do not enter into discussions on sex, religion, politics or any other potentially controversial subjects with your clients.
- Never discuss one client with another.
- Do not repeat information you have been told in confidence.
- Avoid repeating bad publicity about other therapists or salons.
- Do not act in a manner that may bring the profession into disrepute.

Advertising

- Never make false claims.
- Do not practise undercutting of prices.
- Do not compare yourself in advertisements with other salons.

Banking

Bank statement

A bank statement is a document issued by a bank to all account holders normally on a monthly basis showing all the transactions that have occurred for that period. It will detail how much money is in the account, how much has been put in and taken out.

Cash flow

This can be defined as the flow of money in and out of a business (see p. 372). A cash flow statement is compulsory for all large companies.

Cheque guarantee card

This card will be requested every time you write a cheque as it is a guarantee to the retailer that the bank will honour the cheque to the value shown on the card. If the card limit is for £50.00 then the bank will only honour a cheque drawn to that amount or less.

Credit card

Credit cards offer a method of paying for goods and services without cash. It can be used as a form of credit (in which case interest will be paid) or the amount can be paid off monthly. A statement of account will be sent out detailing exactly how much you have spent each month.

Current account

This is a bank account that traditionally does not pay interest on any money deposited within it but does give the recipient a cheque book and cheque guarantee card to draw off the account.

Deposit account

This is a bank account that pays interest on any monies deposited in it. There may be clauses attached as to how much notice needs to be given for withdrawals without forfeiting interest.

Standing order

A method of paying for regular expenditure such as bills. The bank will ask you to fill in a form detailing the person to whom payment is to be made, their bank details and the amount payable. This amount will then be deducted on a regular basis until the bank is notified otherwise.

Direct debit

This is similar to a standing order only this time it is the person requesting the money who instructs the bank to deduct from your account. You will need to fill out a mandate sanctioning the request. Direct debit is very useful where the sum involved may change monthly.

Overdraft

The account holder and the bank agree a limit to which the account may be overdrawn giving a flexible form of finance. Interest will be paid on amount borrowed.

Loan

A formal arrangement with a bank or financial institution allowing an agreed sum of money to be lent to the account holder for an agreed period of time. This is normally for a longer period than an overdraft.

EXAMPLE OF A CASH FLOW FORECAST										from 20		to 20	
Period (e.g. 4 weeks/Month/Quarter														
	Budget	Actual	Budget	Actual	Budget	Actual	Budget	Actual	Budget	Actual	Budget	Actual
ORDERS												
SALES												
PURCHASES												
RECEIPTS:PURCHASES												
Sales – cash												
– debtors												
Loans/Grants received												
Capital injected												
Asset disposals												
Other income												
TOTAL RECEIPTS (CR)												
PAYMENTS:												
Purchases – cash												
– creditors												
Wages, salaries, PAYE												
Rent, rates												
Light, heat, power												
Insurance												
Transport												
Maintenance												
Advertising												
Telephone												
Postage, packaging												
Professional fees												
VAT (net)												
HP payments/leasing charges												
Bank/finance charges and interest												
Loan repayments												
Tax												
Capital expenditure												
Sundry expenses												
TOTAL PAYMENTS (DR)												
NET CASH FLOW CR												
DR												
OPENING BANK BALANCE/ CR												
BALANCE BROUGHT FORWARD DR												
CLOSING BANK BALANCE CR												
DR												

Fig. 13.7 *Cash flow forecast*

Orders

Advice note

This is a document sent by the supplier to advise when goods will be delivered.

Credit note

This is given by a supplier in exchange for faulty goods and is normally offset against the next invoice.

Delivery note

This document (which is often produced in triplicate) is issued when goods have been ordered and are packed ready for delivery itemising every product. When the driver delivers the goods you are asked to sign the document to confirm that you have received them. One copy is normally given to you, one retained by the supplier and one by the driver.

Pro-forma invoice

This document is issued in particular for a new customer when their credit worthiness is not yet known. It requests payment for goods before they are dispatched.

Book keeping

When setting up in business it will be necessary to keep records of every transaction in a detailed and formal way. The reasons for this are firstly to have documentation of the business's financial position and secondly to allow for an interpretation of the results. It is important to be able to ascertain why things may not be going too well and respond to them.

Whilst it is possible to buy 'off the shelf' book keeping systems, many people who are not expert in the field contract the work out to specialists.

Balance sheet

This is a statement detailing all the assets and liabilities of a business.

Cash book

This book is used to record all payments and receipts carried out on a daily basis together with what has been paid into and taken out of the bank account. It should be periodically checked against bank statements.

Gross profit

This is the term used to describe all profit made before necessary deductions have been taken off.

Net profit

This is a term used to describe the final profit made after all necessary deductions have been made.

PAYE

PAYE stands for 'pay as you earn'. PAYE is applicable to all employees who earn over a specific limit as decided by the government. Earnings related tax and National Insurance contributions are deducted under the scheme by the employer.

Petty cash book

A book to record all minor cash transactions including the date, the amount of cash used and the purpose of the transaction.

Profit and loss account

This document summarises all business transactions for a given period (normally one year).

Purchase day book

This allows you to keep a record of any monies that you owe concerning purchases. It should also detail when goods were supplied and the date by which they must be paid for.

Wages book

This is a record of wage/salary details of every employee and will often include personnel information such as NI number, PAYE number, pension and other deductions.

ACTIVITY

Examine a successful business in your area and try to define the reasons why they have become successful.

Progress Check

1. Explain the importance of marketing and promotion in the salon.
2. What do you understand by the term 'value added tax'?
3. List the key principles involved in setting up a business.

Key Terms

You will need to know what these words and phrases mean. Go back through the chapter to find out.

- Basic business legislation
- Basic business terminology
- Choice and type of premises
- COSHH
- Disability discrimination
- Disciplinary procedures
- Employment legislation
- Fire precautions
- Forms of business arrangement
- Marketing and promotion
- Sex discrimination
- Staff and recruitment
- Taxation
- Termination of employment
- The 'six pack'
- Treatment and consumer legislation
- Unfair dismissal

BIBLIOGRAPHY AND FURTHER READING

Arnould-Taylor, William., *A Textbook of Anatomy and Physiology*, 3rd edition, Stanley Thornes (Publishers) Ltd, 1998.

Brown, Denise, *Aromatherapy*, Headway Lifeguides Series, 1993.

Burns, E. and Blamey, C., 'Soothing Scents in Childbirth' in *International Journal of Aromatherapy*, 1994 vol. 4 no. 1.

Cartwright, Elizabeth, Morris, Gill and Severn, Michelle, *Electro-epilation: A Practical Approach*, 2nd edition, Nelson Thornes, 2001.

Corney, J., *Anthropology for Designers*, Batsford Academic and Educational Ltd, 1980.

Cowmeadow, O., *The Art of Shiatsu*, Element Books Ltd, 1992.

Cullum, Rodney and Mowbray, Leslie, *YMCA Guide to Exercise Music*, YMCA.

Davis, P., *Aromatherapy, an A–Z*, C. W. Daniel Company Ltd, 1990.

Fire, M., 'Providing Massage Therapy in a Psychiatric Hospital' in *International Journal of Alternative and Complementary Medicine*, June 1994.

Franks, B. Don and Howley, Edward T., *Fitness Leader's Handbook*.

Goldberg, Lyn, *Massage and Aromatherapy: A Practical Approach*, 2nd edition, Nelson Thornes, 2001.

Gray FRS, Henry, *Gray's Anatomy*, Senate.

Henry, J. et al, 'Lavender for Night Sedation of People with Dementia' in *International Journal of Aromatherapy*, 1994 vol. 6 no. 2.

International School of Aromatherapy, *A Safety Guide on the Use of Essential Oils*, Nature by Nature Oils Ltd, London, 1993.

Kasner and Tindall, *Ballière's Nurses Dictionary*, Ballière Tindall.

Lavabre, M., *Aromatherapy Worbook*, Healing Arts Press, USA, 1990.

Lawless, Julia, *The Encyclopaedia of Essential Oils*, Element Books Ltd, 1992.

Lewis, Roger and Trevitt, Roger, *Business for Advanced GNVQ*, 2nd edition, Nelson Thornes, 2001.

Mernagh-Ward, Dawn and Cartwright, Jennifer, *Good Practice in Salon Management,* Stanley Thornes (Publishers) Ltd, 1997.

Pitman, V. and MacKenzie, K., *Reflexology: A Practical Approach*, Stanley Thornes (Publishers) Ltd, 1997.

Price, S., *Practical Aromatherapy*, Thorsons Publishing Group, 1987.

Sanderson, H. and Ruddle, J., 'Aromatherapy and Occupational Therapy' in *British Journal of Occupational Therapy*, 1992, 55(8).

Simmons, John V., *The Beauty Salon and its Equipment*, Heinemann.

Simms, Janet, *A Practical Guide to Beauty Therapy*, 2nd edition, Stanley Thornes (Publishers) Ltd, 1998.

Simpkins, J. and Williams, J. J., *Advanced Human Biology*, Collins Educational.

Tisserand, R., 'Aromatherapy Today' in *International Journal of Aromatherapy*, 1993 vol. 5 no. 4.

Winwood, R. S. and Smith, J. L., *Sear's Anatomy and Physiology for Nurses*, Edward Arnold.

Woolfson, A. and Hewitt, D., 'Intensive Aroma Care' in *International Journal of Aromatherapy*, 1992 vol. 4 no. 2.

INDEX

cellulite 58
   treatments 205–6, 220–2
central nervous system 26–8
cerebellum 26, 27
cerebrum 26, 27
chairs
   therapist's 111
   treatment 109–10
chamomile 282
chemical reactivity 151
chemical sterilisation 76, 76
cheque guarantee card 371
chest massage 126–7, 127–8
chloasma 267
cholesterol 46
chromosomes 2
chymotrypsin 40
cinnamon 293
circulatory system 19
   arteries and veins 22–3, 22
   blood 21–2
   heart 19–20, 19
   lymphatic system 23–4, 25
circumduction 12, 13
citric acid 208
clary sage 282
clients
   apprehensive 143
   medical details 98
   personal details 98–9
   profiles 364–5
   see also consultations
clove 293
co-operatives 340
co-ordination 69
cold sores 72
colds 72
collagen 5
colour 271, 272
   skin 272
   in treatment areas 114
compact bone 9, 11
compounds 152
compresses 310
computers 90
concentric musclework 62
conductors (electricity) 153, 154, 156
connective tissue 3, 6, 147
consultations 97–101, 100, 102
   aromatherapy 287–92, 289–91
   artificial nails 319–20
   massage 105, 115–16
   remedial camouflage 265–7, 266
Consumer Credit Act 1974 358
Consumer Protection Act 1987 358
Consumer Safety Act 1978 358
contracts of employment 351
contraindications 98
contrast baths 251–2
Control of Substances Hazardous to
   Health Regulations (COSHH) 1988
   344–7
cool down exercises 64

cosine law 257, 257
cosmetic camouflage see remedial
   camouflage
Cosmolight™ 225–6, 225
costing of treatments 363
couch steps 110
couches 109–10, 110
cranial nerves 28
creams, massage 112
credit cards 371
credit notes 373
cupping 107
current accounts 371
cuticle oil 318
cuticle pusher 318
cypress 293
cytoplasm 2

dappen dishes 318
Data Protection Act 1984 359
DC (direct current) 155, 155
deep stroking 106, 106
deep tissue massage 147
delivery notes 373
dendrites 26
deposit accounts 371
dermal papilla 5
dermis 5–6
diaphragm 35
diastole 20
diet 44, 50–1
   commercial products 53
   eating problems 54
   foods for healthy 45–9
   slimming clubs 53
   types of diet 52–3
diffusion of oils 310–11, 310
digestive system 36–40, 37
direct current (DC) 155, 155
direct debits 371
Disability Discrimination Act 1995 352
disaccharides 44
disciplinary procedures 355–6
disease 72–4
   protection against 74–7
disinfection 76–7
distillation of oils 278, 278
dowager's hump 59
dry floatation tanks 242–4, 243
duodenum 39
dynamic electricity 153

earthing of electrical appliances 155
eating problems 54
eccentric musclework 62
eccrine glands 5, 7
ectomorphs 55, 55
efferent nerves 28
effleurage 105–6, 106
EHTS (Environmental Health and
   Trading Standards) Departments
   359
elastin fibres 5

electric cells 154
electric circuits 153–4, 153
electric current 154, 155, 156–7
electric power 154
electrical equipment 160–1
   brush cleansing treatment 202–3, 202
   care of 161
   electrotherapy treatments 178–201,
      212–16
   mechanical massagers 162–70
   safety precautions 155, 162
   skin sensitivity test 162
   specialised treatments 217–27
   vacuum suction massage 170–7
   vapourisers 201–2, 201
electrical pressure 154
electricity 153–8
Electricity at Work Regulations Act 1990
   343
electrodes
   galvanic treatments 193–4, 194–5
   high frequency electrotherapy 178,
      179, 179–80
   NMES 187–8
electrolytes 156
electromagnetic radiation 157, 254–5,
   254
electromagnets 157
electrons 151
electrotherapy treatments 178
   galvanic 192–201, 194, 197, 199, 200,
      216
   high frequency 178–84, 178, 179–80,
      216
   lifting treatments 218–20, 219
   micro-therapy 212–15, 212, 215, 216
   NMES 185–92, 185, 190
elements 150, 151, 152
emergencies see first aid; health and
   safety
employees 82, 350–7, 361, 361–3
Employment Protection (Consolidation)
   Act 1978 356–7
Employment Rights Act 1996 352–3
EMS (electrical muscle stimulation)
   185–92, 185, 190
Endermologie™ 220–2, 221, 222
endocardium 20
endocrine system 29–33, 30
endomorphs 55, 55
endomysium 14
endoplasmic reticulum 2
endoskeleton 8
enfleurage of oils 279
Environmental Health and Trading
   Standards (EHTS) Departments 359
epidermis 4–5, 5
epiglottis 33
epimysium 14
epinephrine 32
epithelial tissue 3
Equal Pay Act 1970 351
ergosterol 7